U0278796

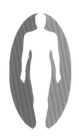

实用人体解剖图谱

Atlas of
Practical Human Anatomy

图谱

头颈分册

Head and Neck Volume

主编
陈金宝

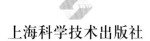

上海科学技术出版社

图书在版编目（CIP）数据

实用人体解剖图谱·头颈分册 / 陈金宝主编 . —上海：
上海科学技术出版社，2015.5
ISBN 978-7-5478-2501-3

Ⅰ. ①实… Ⅱ. ①陈… Ⅲ. ①头部－人体解剖学－图
谱②颈－人体解剖学－图谱 Ⅳ. ① R322-64

中国版本图书馆 CIP 数据核字（2014）第 304197 号

实用人体解剖图谱
头颈分册
主编 陈金宝

上海世纪出版股份有限公司
上 海 科 学 技 术 出 版 社　出版
（上海钦州南路 71 号　邮政编码 200235）

上海世纪出版股份有限公司发行中心发行
200001　上海福建中路 193 号　www.ewen.co
浙江新华印刷技术有限公司印刷
开本 889×1194　1/16　印张 27.75　插页 4
字数 500 千字
2015 年 5 月第 1 版　2015 年 5 月第 1 次印刷
ISBN 978-7-5478-2501-3/R·847
定价：288.00 元

主编简介

发表论文及出版

在国家级杂志发表的论文、编写出版的教材及专著共 140 余篇（部）。其中主编专著《医学摄影》1 部，副主编《断面解剖与 MRI CT ECT 对照图谱》1 部，策划并参加主编的医学彩色图谱《人体解剖学彩色图谱》《组织胚胎学彩色图谱》《寄生虫学彩色图谱》《病理解剖学彩色图谱》《实验诊断学彩色图谱》5 部，策划并参加总主编系列教材 54 种。

承担课题

国家"九五"重点攻关课题"人体解剖学课件""组织胚胎学课件"2 项，国家新世纪网络建设工程课题"人体解剖学网络课程""组织胚胎学网络课程"2 项，教育部重大研究课题子课题 1 项，"药理学"国家级优秀网络课程 1 项，辽宁省科委课题 1 项，辽宁省教育厅课题 1 项。

获得奖励

卫生部奖 6 项，教育部奖 1 项，美国医学电教学会（HESCA）奖 1 项。

辽宁省科技进步一等奖"现代医学教育资源库"1 项，辽宁省优秀教学成果一等奖 1 项，辽宁省优秀教学成果二等奖 2 项，辽宁省优秀教学成果三等奖 1 项，辽宁省优秀课件一等奖 1 项，沈阳市科技进步三等奖 1 项。

曾任职务

中国医科大学教育技术中心主任，网络教育学院常务副院长。卫生部继续医学教育和乡村医生教育的视听教育专家，中华医学会教育技术分会委员、常务委员、副主任委员、主任委员、名誉主任委员，教育部高等医药院校现代教育技术与计算机教学指导委员会委员，中国电化教育协会理事、医学委员会主任委员，辽宁省高等院校电化教育研究会副理事长等职。

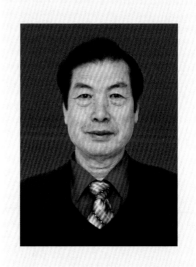

陈金宝

1944 年生，山东单县人，1963 年考入中国医科大学医疗系学习，1969 年毕业。1994 年晋升为教授，2000 年获得国务院特殊津贴。一直在中国医科大学从事医学图像制作和医学图像处理的研究及资源库建设等工作。

编委名单

主 编

陈金宝

副主编

齐亚力　段坤昌　孙桂媛　傅　强
季雪芳　刘　强　周艳芬　段维轶

影像主审

王振宇

编 委

按姓氏笔画排序

于　刚　马　黎　王　顺　王　洋
朱小兵　刘　浩　刘　强　刘自力
齐亚力　孙桂媛　李　亮　杨　雄
陈金宝　邵　博　欧国成　季雪芳
周艳芬　段坤昌　段维轶　傅　强
富长海　黎　宪

标本制作

按姓氏笔画排序

王　顺　王　洋　朱小兵　刘自力
邵　博　段坤昌　富长海　黎　宪

前言

《实用人体解剖图谱》结合临床的实际需要，按照人体的部位进行分册，即头颈分册、躯干内脏分册和四肢分册。为了让读者对人体的结构建立一个立体的概念，我们还设立了概论与断面分册。该图谱主要供普通外科、骨科、心外科、胸外科、泌尿外科、神经外科、血管外科、整形美容外科、乳腺外科、肝脏外科、妇产科、眼科、耳鼻喉科、口腔科、影像科及运动医学等专业的临床医师使用。解剖工作者和医学生也可在教学和科学研究中参考。

该图谱为了充分体现实用性原则，采取了系统解剖、局部解剖、表面解剖、影像解剖和运动解剖相结合，以及正常与变异相结合、大体标本与显微镜切片相结合的方法，充分展示人体的正常结构。此外，在该图谱还包括了有关胚胎学的部分内容。

系统解剖部分重点展示骨骼、肌肉、血管和神经的有关内容。局部解剖部分按照内容的需要，进行逐层解剖，用高分辨率数码相机拍摄，用图像处理技术对拍摄的图像进行加工处理，充分显示浅组织、筋膜、肌肉、骨骼、血管、神经的相互位置关系。断面解剖部分是将人体进行水平、矢状和冠状断层，用高分辨率数码相机拍摄，用图像处理技术对拍摄的图像进行修整，对标本在固定过程中的萎缩部分进行适当处理，使图像更加真实。近年影像技术发展很快，设备的分辨率越来越高，我们应用了超声波、X线、CT、ECT和MRI图像，从不同侧面展示人体的正常结构。表面解剖部分根据内容的要求，采用不同的姿势，充分显示人体的结构，用高分辨率数码相机拍摄后进行加工处理，从而获得高质量的图像。

在本套图谱的编绘过程中，参阅了国内外出版的相关图谱和专著。在此，对出版社和作者表示衷心的感谢。

本套图谱在编绘过程中得到了中国医科大学有关领导，网络教育学院、基础医学院有关教研室，以及临床学院有关科室和专家的大力支持，在此一并表示感谢。

由于作者的水平有限，本套图谱难免存在不当之处或错误，敬请学界专家和读者给予批评指正。

陈金宝

2014 年 10 月

目录

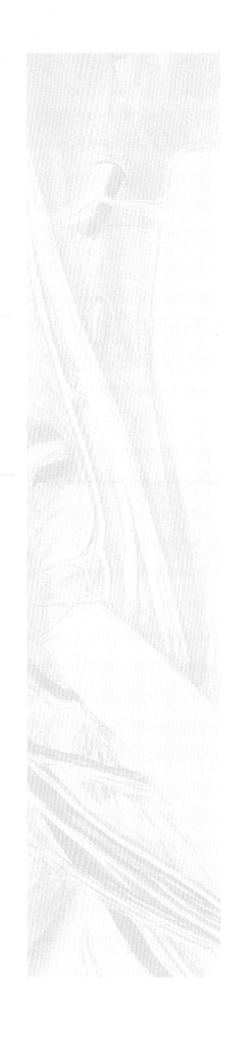

第二章 面部

第三章 颈部

第四章 颈部表面解剖

第五章 脑

第六章 眼

第七章　耳

第八章 鼻

第九章 喉

第十章 甲状腺

第十一章 口部

系统解剖

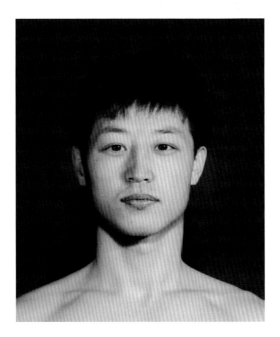

1. 头和颈（前面观）
Head and neck (anterior aspect)

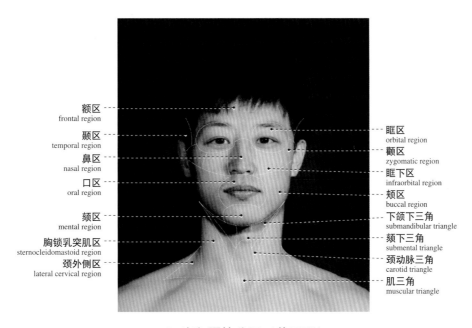

额区
frontal region

颞区
temporal region

鼻区
nasal region

口区
oral region

颏区
mental region

胸锁乳突肌区
sternocleidomastoid region

颈外侧区
lateral cervical region

眶区
orbital region

颧区
zygomatic region

眶下区
infraorbital region

颊区
buccal region

下颌下三角
submandibular triangle

颏下三角
submental triangle

颈动脉三角
carotid triangle

肌三角
muscular triangle

2. 头和颈的分区（前面观）
Regions of the head and neck (anterior aspect)

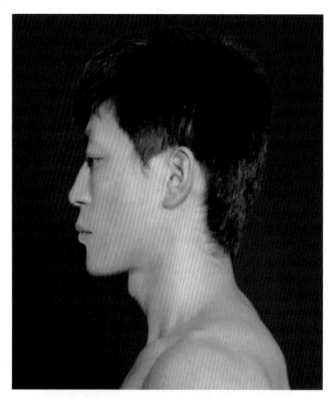

3. 头和颈（侧面观）
Head and neck (lateral aspect)

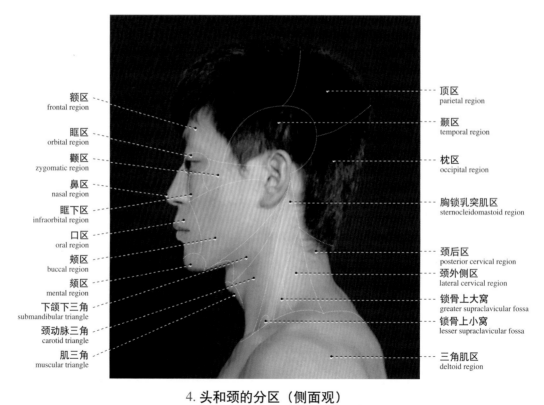

额区
frontal region

眶区
orbital region

颧区
zygomatic region

鼻区
nasal region

眶下区
infraorbital region

口区
oral region

颊区
buccal region

颏区
mental region

下颌下三角
submandibular triangle

颈动脉三角
carotid triangle

肌三角
muscular triangle

顶区
parietal region

颞区
temporal region

枕区
occipital region

胸锁乳突肌区
sternocleidomastoid region

颈后区
posterior cervical region

颈外侧区
lateral cervical region

锁骨上大窝
greater supraclavicular fossa

锁骨上小窝
lesser supraclavicular fossa

三角肌区
deltoid region

4. 头和颈的分区（侧面观）
Regions of the head and neck (lateral aspect)

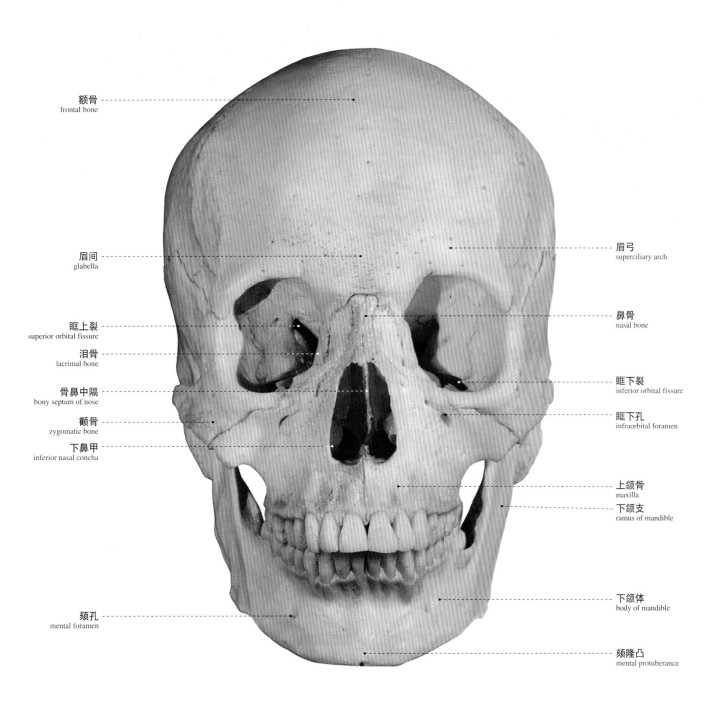

额骨
frontal bone

眉弓
superciliary arch

眉间
glabella

鼻骨
nasal bone

眶上裂
superior orbital fissure

泪骨
lacrimal bone

眶下裂
inferior orbital fissure

骨鼻中隔
bony septum of nose

眶下孔
infraorbital foramen

颧骨
zygomatic bone

下鼻甲
inferior nasal concha

上颌骨
maxilla

下颌支
ramus of mandible

下颌体
body of mandible

颏孔
mental foramen

颏隆凸
mental protuberance

5. 颅（前面观 1）
Skull (anterior aspect 1)

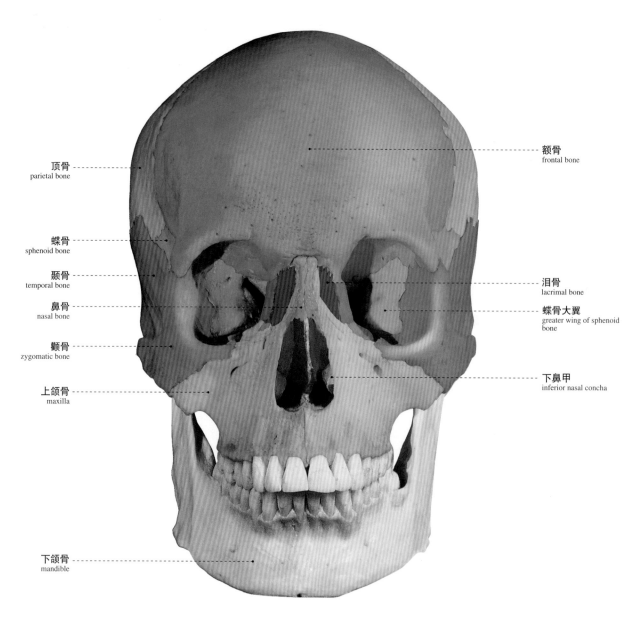

顶骨
parietal bone

蝶骨
sphenoid bone

颞骨
temporal bone

鼻骨
nasal bone

颧骨
zygomatic bone

上颌骨
maxilla

下颌骨
mandible

额骨
frontal bone

泪骨
lacrimal bone

蝶骨大翼
greater wing of sphenoid bone

下鼻甲
inferior nasal concha

6. 颅（前面观 2）
Skull (anterior aspect 2)

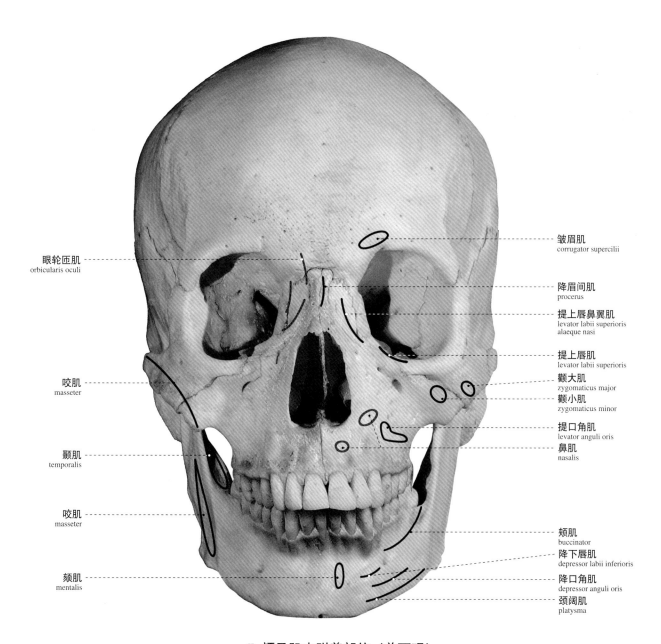

眼轮匝肌
orbicularis oculi

咬肌
masseter

颞肌
temporalis

咬肌
masseter

颏肌
mentalis

皱眉肌
corrugator supercilii

降眉间肌
procerus

提上唇鼻翼肌
levator labii superioris
alaeque nasi

提上唇肌
levator labii superioris

颧大肌
zygomaticus major

颧小肌
zygomaticus minor

提口角肌
levator anguli oris

鼻肌
nasalis

颊肌
buccinator

降下唇肌
depressor labii inferioris

降口角肌
depressor anguli oris

颈阔肌
platysma

7. 颅骨肌肉附着部位（前面观）
Muscle attachment sites of the skull (anterior aspect)

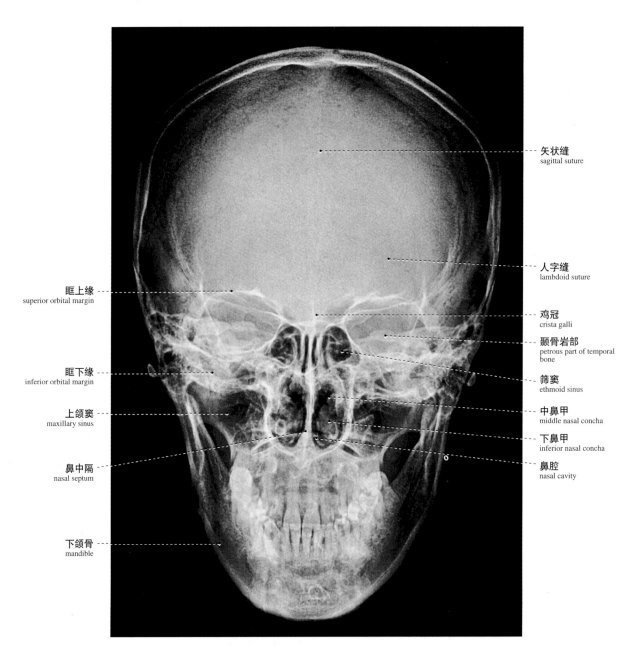

眶上缘
superior orbital margin

眶下缘
inferior orbital margin

上颌窦
maxillary sinus

鼻中隔
nasal septum

下颌骨
mandible

矢状缝
sagittal suture

人字缝
lambdoid suture

鸡冠
crista galli

颞骨岩部
petrous part of temporal bone

筛窦
ethmoid sinus

中鼻甲
middle nasal concha

下鼻甲
inferior nasal concha

鼻腔
nasal cavity

8. 颅 X 线像（前后位）
Radiograph of the skull (anteroposterior view)

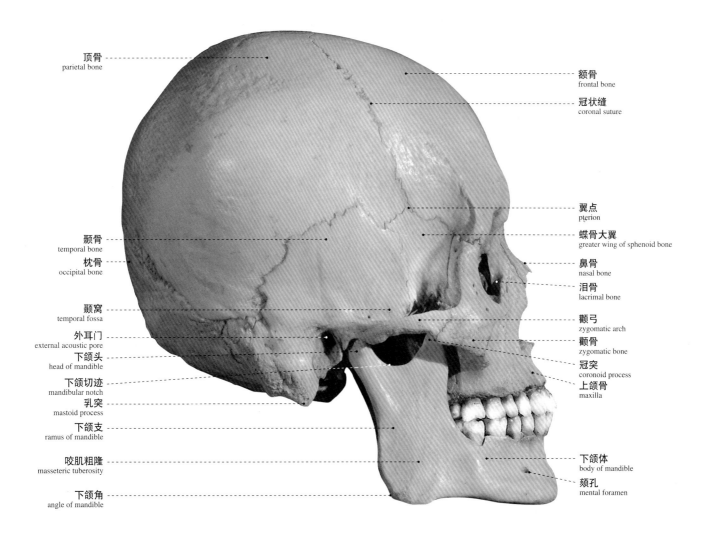

顶骨
parietal bone

额骨
frontal bone

冠状缝
coronal suture

翼点
pterion

颞骨
temporal bone

枕骨
occipital bone

蝶骨大翼
greater wing of sphenoid bone

鼻骨
nasal bone

泪骨
lacrimal bone

颞窝
temporal fossa

外耳门
external acoustic pore

下颌头
head of mandible

颧弓
zygomatic arch

颧骨
zygomatic bone

冠突
coronoid process

下颌切迹
mandibular notch

乳突
mastoid process

上颌骨
maxilla

下颌支
ramus of mandible

咬肌粗隆
masseteric tuberosity

下颌体
body of mandible

颏孔
mental foramen

下颌角
angle of mandible

9. 颅（侧面观）

Skull (lateral aspect)

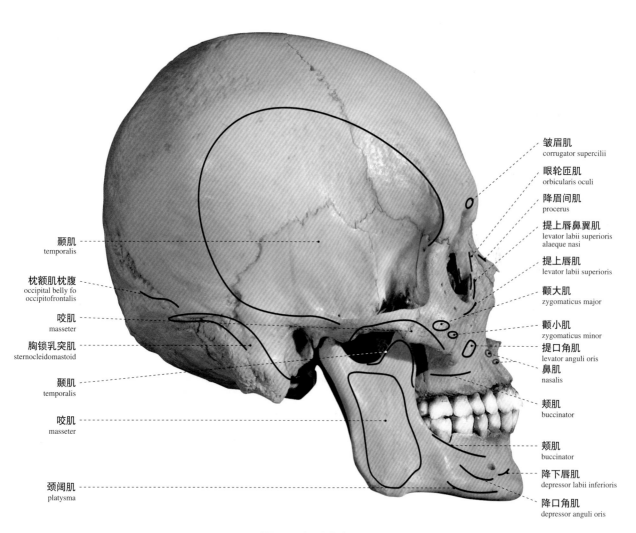

颞肌
temporalis

枕额肌枕腹
occipital belly fo
occipitofrontalis

咬肌
masseter

胸锁乳突肌
sternocleidomastoid

颞肌
temporalis

咬肌
masseter

颈阔肌
platysma

皱眉肌
corrugator supercilii

眼轮匝肌
orbicularis oculi

降眉间肌
procerus

提上唇鼻翼肌
levator labii superioris
alaeque nasi

提上唇肌
levator labii superioris

颧大肌
zygomaticus major

颧小肌
zygomaticus minor

提口角肌
levator anguli oris

鼻肌
nasalis

颊肌
buccinator

颊肌
buccinator

降下唇肌
depressor labii inferioris

降口角肌
depressor anguli oris

10. 颅骨肌肉附着部位（侧面观）
Muscle attachment sites of the skull (lateral aspect)

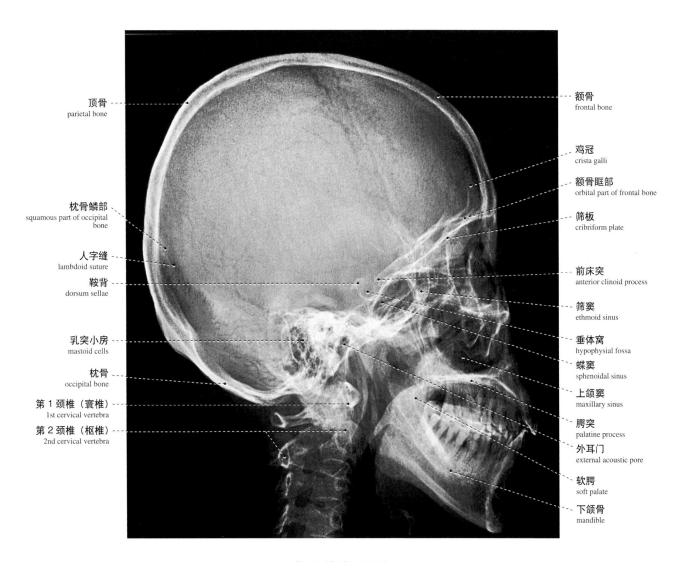

顶骨
parietal bone

枕骨鳞部
squamous part of occipital bone

人字缝
lambdoid suture

鞍背
dorsum sellae

乳突小房
mastoid cells

枕骨
occipital bone

第 1 颈椎（寰椎）
1st cervical vertebra

第 2 颈椎（枢椎）
2nd cervical vertebra

额骨
frontal bone

鸡冠
crista galli

额骨眶部
orbital part of frontal bone

筛板
cribriform plate

前床突
anterior clinoid process

筛窦
ethmoid sinus

垂体窝
hypophysial fossa

蝶窦
sphenoidal sinus

上颌窦
maxillary sinus

腭突
palatine process

外耳门
external acoustic pore

软腭
soft palate

下颌骨
mandible

11. 颅 X 线像（侧位）

Radiograph of the skull (lateral view)

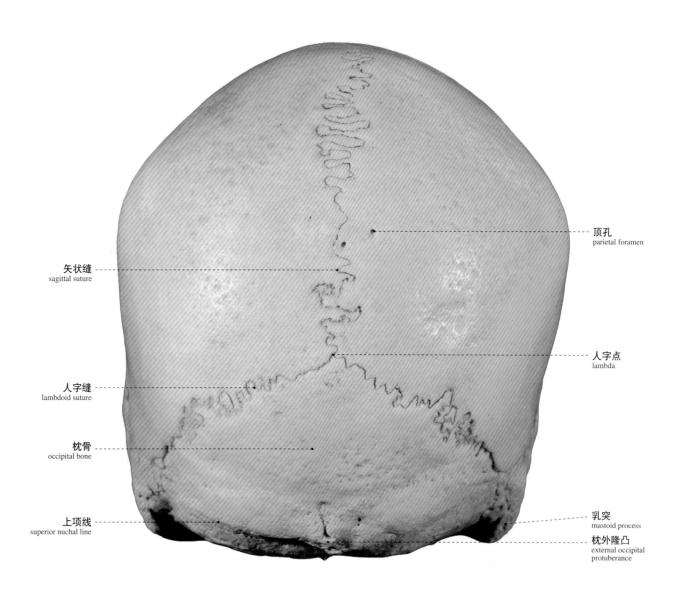

顶孔
parietal foramen

矢状缝
sagittal suture

人字点
lambda

人字缝
lambdoid suture

枕骨
occipital bone

上项线
superior nuchal line

乳突
mastoid process

枕外隆凸
external occipital protuberance

12. 颅（后面观）
Skull (posterior aspect)

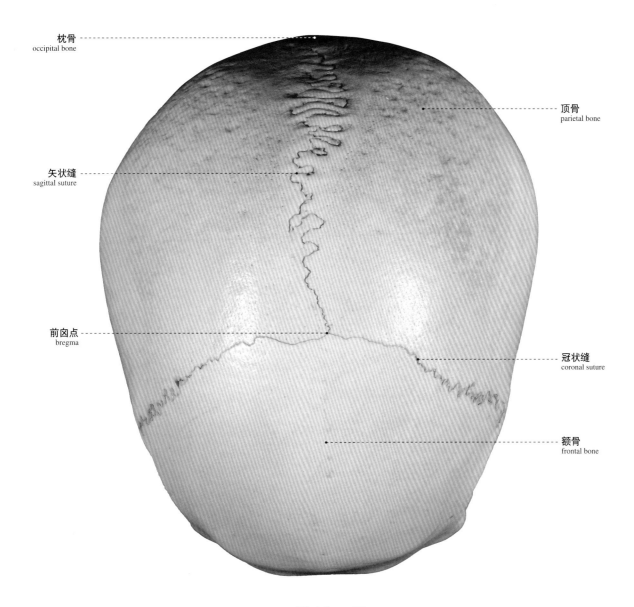

枕骨
occipital bone

顶骨
parietal bone

矢状缝
sagittal suture

前囟点
bregma

冠状缝
coronal suture

额骨
frontal bone

13. 颅（上面观）
Skull (superior aspect)

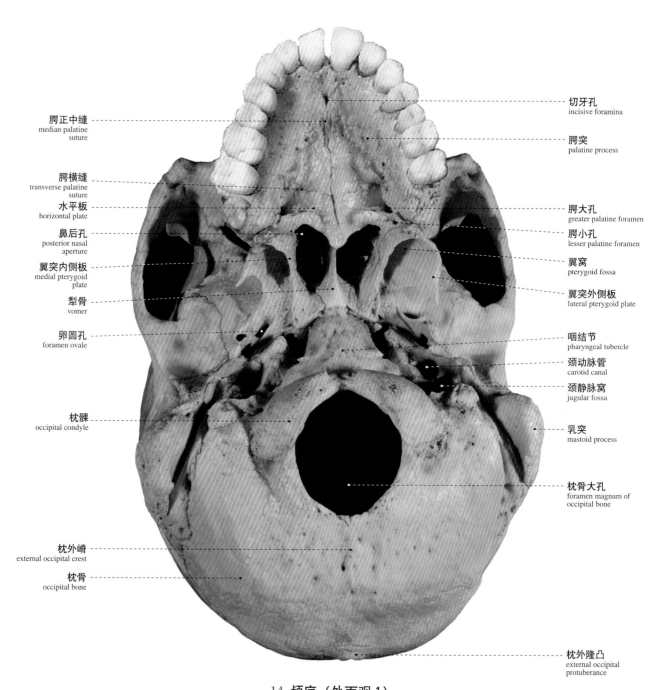

腭正中缝
median palatine
suture

腭横缝
transverse palatine
suture

水平板
horizontal plate

鼻后孔
posterior nasal
aperture

翼突内侧板
medial pterygoid
plate

犁骨
vomer

卵圆孔
foramen ovale

枕髁
occipital condyle

枕外嵴
external occipital crest

枕骨
occipital bone

切牙孔
incisive foramina

腭突
palatine process

腭大孔
greater palatine foramen

腭小孔
lesser palatine foramen

翼窝
pterygoid fossa

翼突外侧板
lateral pterygoid plate

咽结节
pharyngeal tubercle

颈动脉管
carotid canal

颈静脉窝
jugular fossa

乳突
mastoid process

枕骨大孔
foramen magnum of
occipital bone

枕外隆凸
external occipital
protuberance

14. 颅底（外面观 1）
Base of the skull (external aspect 1)

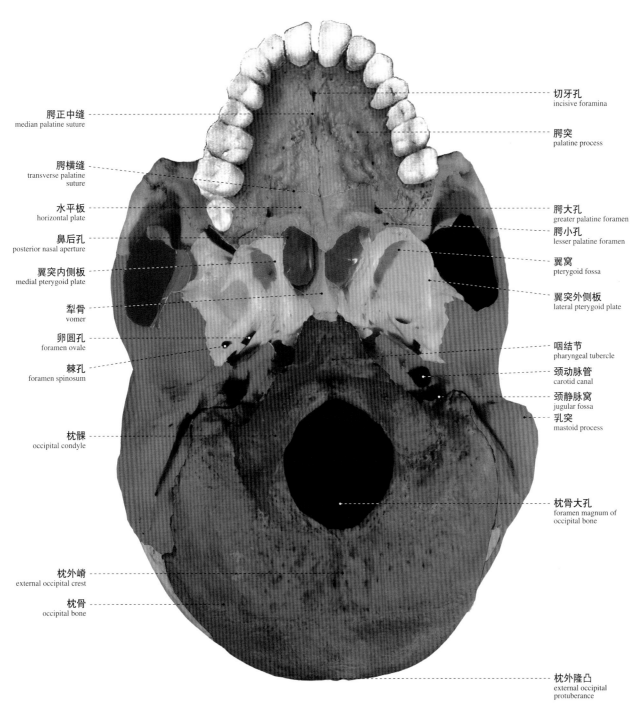

腭正中缝
median palatine suture

腭横缝
transverse palatine suture

水平板
horizontal plate

鼻后孔
posterior nasal aperture

翼突内侧板
medial pterygoid plate

犁骨
vomer

卵圆孔
foramen ovale

棘孔
foramen spinosum

枕髁
occipital condyle

枕外嵴
external occipital crest

枕骨
occipital bone

切牙孔
incisive foramina

腭突
palatine process

腭大孔
greater palatine foramen

腭小孔
lesser palatine foramen

翼窝
pterygoid fossa

翼突外侧板
lateral pterygoid plate

咽结节
pharyngeal tubercle

颈动脉管
carotid canal

颈静脉窝
jugular fossa

乳突
mastoid process

枕骨大孔
foramen magnum of occipital bone

枕外隆凸
external occipital protuberance

15. 颅底（外面观 2）
Base of the skull (external aspect 2)

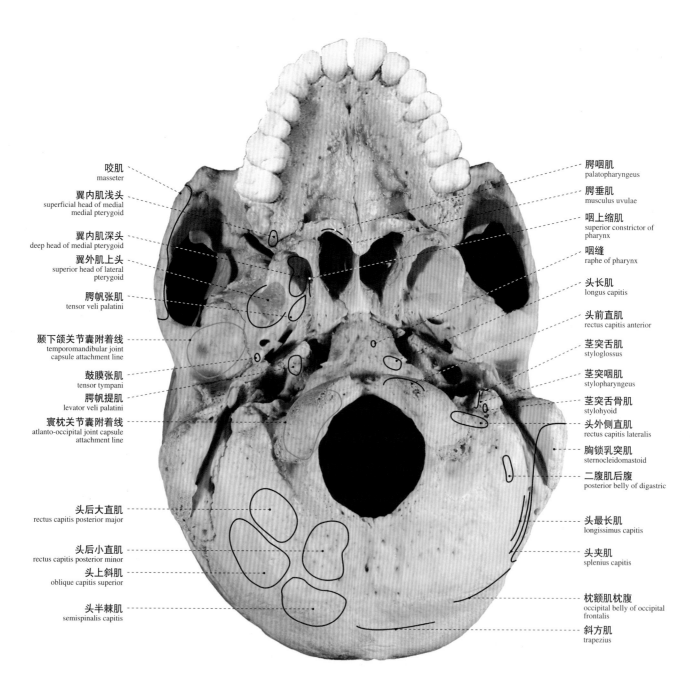

咬肌
masseter

翼内肌浅头
superficial head of medial
medial pterygoid

翼内肌深头
deep head of medial pterygoid

翼外肌上头
superior head of lateral
pterygoid

腭帆张肌
tensor veli palatini

颞下颌关节囊附着线
temporomandibular joint
capsule attachment line

鼓膜张肌
tensor tympani

腭帆提肌
levator veli palatini

寰枕关节囊附着线
atlanto-occipital joint capsule
attachment line

头后大直肌
rectus capitis posterior major

头后小直肌
rectus capitis posterior minor

头上斜肌
oblique capitis superior

头半棘肌
semispinalis capitis

腭咽肌
palatopharyngeus

腭垂肌
musculus uvulae

咽上缩肌
superior constrictor of
pharynx

咽缝
raphe of pharynx

头长肌
longus capitis

头前直肌
rectus capitis anterior

茎突舌肌
styloglossus

茎突咽肌
stylopharyngeus

茎突舌骨肌
stylohyoid

头外侧直肌
rectus capitis lateralis

胸锁乳突肌
sternocleidomastoid

二腹肌后腹
posterior belly of digastric

头最长肌
longissimus capitis

头夹肌
splenius capitis

枕额肌枕腹
occipital belly of occipital
frontalis

斜方肌
trapezius

16. 颅底肌肉附着部位（外面观）
Muscle attachment sites of the base of the skull (external aspect)

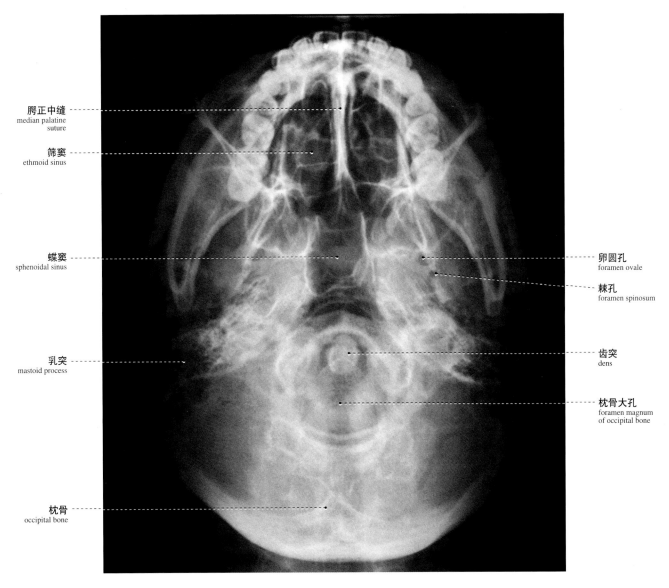

腭正中缝
median palatine
suture

筛窦
ethmoid sinus

蝶窦
sphenoidal sinus

乳突
mastoid process

枕骨
occipital bone

卵圆孔
foramen ovale

棘孔
foramen spinosum

齿突
dens

枕骨大孔
foramen magnum
of occipital bone

17. 颅 X 线像（颌顶位）
Radiograph of the base of the skull (SMV)

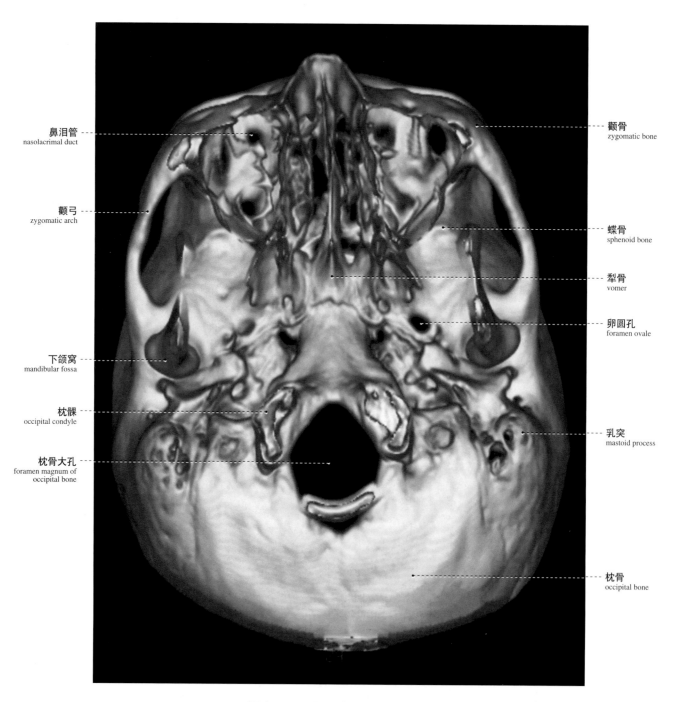

鼻泪管
nasolacrimal duct

颧弓
zygomatic arch

下颌窝
mandibular fossa

枕髁
occipital condyle

枕骨大孔
foramen magnum of
occipital bone

颧骨
zygomatic bone

蝶骨
sphenoid bone

犁骨
vomer

卵圆孔
foramen ovale

乳突
mastoid process

枕骨
occipital bone

18. 颅底 CT 三维重建图像（颌顶位）

CT 3D reconstruction image of the base of the skull (SMV)

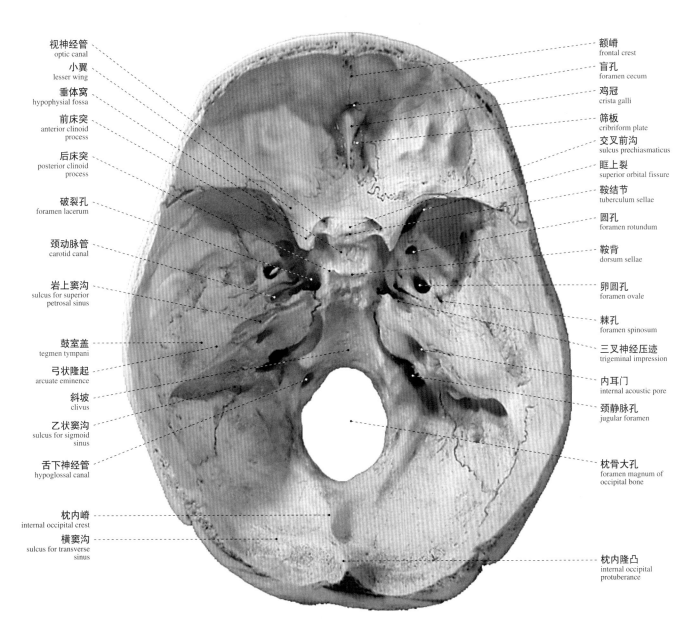

视神经管
optic canal

小翼
lesser wing

垂体窝
hypophysial fossa

前床突
anterior clinoid process

后床突
posterior clinoid process

破裂孔
foramen lacerum

颈动脉管
carotid canal

岩上窦沟
sulcus for superior petrosal sinus

鼓室盖
tegmen tympani

弓状隆起
arcuate eminence

斜坡
clivus

乙状窦沟
sulcus for sigmoid sinus

舌下神经管
hypoglossal canal

枕内嵴
internal occipital crest

横窦沟
sulcus for transverse sinus

额嵴
frontal crest

盲孔
foramen cecum

鸡冠
crista galli

筛板
cribriform plate

交叉前沟
sulcus prechiasmaticus

眶上裂
superior orbital fissure

鞍结节
tuberculum sellae

圆孔
foramen rotundum

鞍背
dorsum sellae

卵圆孔
foramen ovale

棘孔
foramen spinosum

三叉神经压迹
trigeminal impression

内耳门
internal acoustic pore

颈静脉孔
jugular foramen

枕骨大孔
foramen magnum of occipital bone

枕内隆凸
internal occipital protuberance

19. 颅底（内面观 1）

Base of the skull (internal aspect 1)

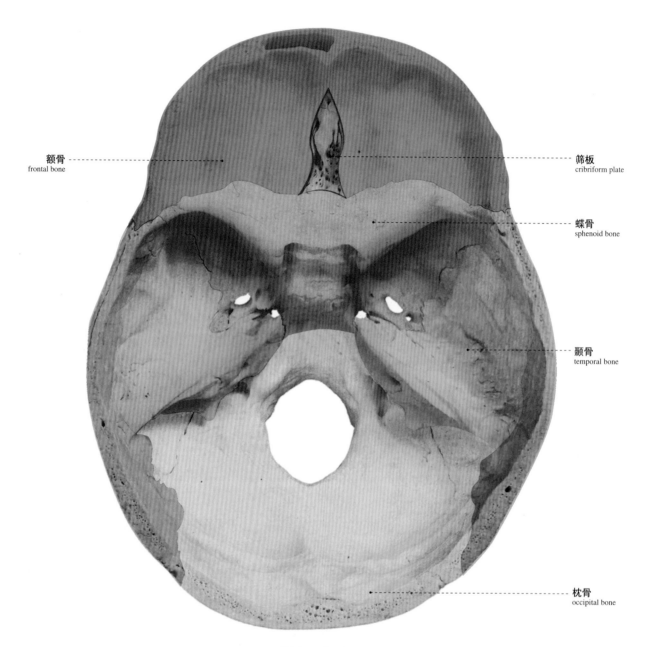

额骨
frontal bone

筛板
cribriform plate

蝶骨
sphenoid bone

颞骨
temporal bone

枕骨
occipital bone

20. 颅底（内面观 2）
Base of the skull (internal aspect 2)

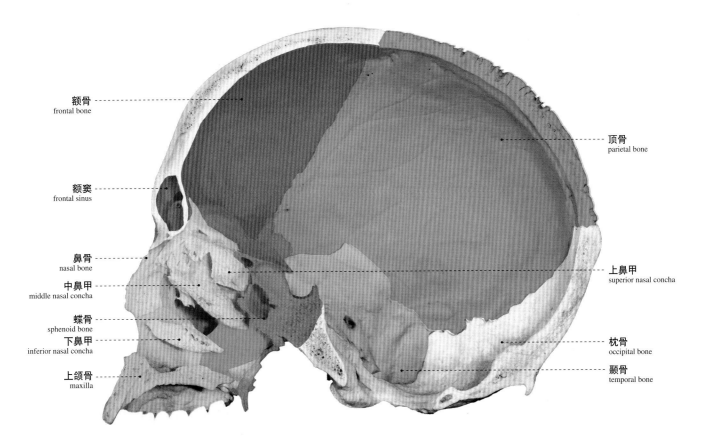

额骨
frontal bone

额窦
frontal sinus

鼻骨
nasal bone

中鼻甲
middle nasal concha

蝶骨
sphenoid bone

下鼻甲
inferior nasal concha

上颌骨
maxilla

顶骨
parietal bone

上鼻甲
superior nasal concha

枕骨
occipital bone

颞骨
temporal bone

21. 右半侧颅（内面观）
Right half of the skull (internal aspect)

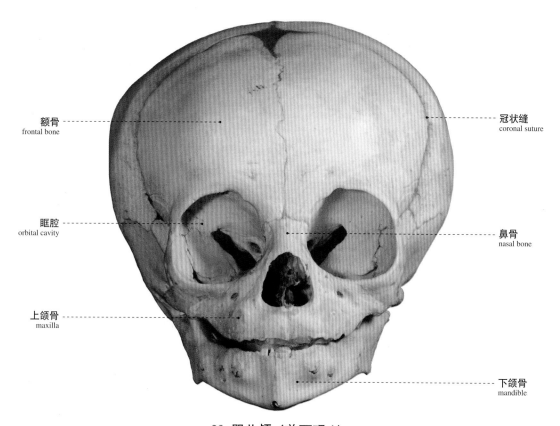

额骨
frontal bone

冠状缝
coronal suture

眶腔
orbital cavity

鼻骨
nasal bone

上颌骨
maxilla

下颌骨
mandible

22. 婴儿颅（前面观 1）

Skull of an infant (anterior aspect 1)

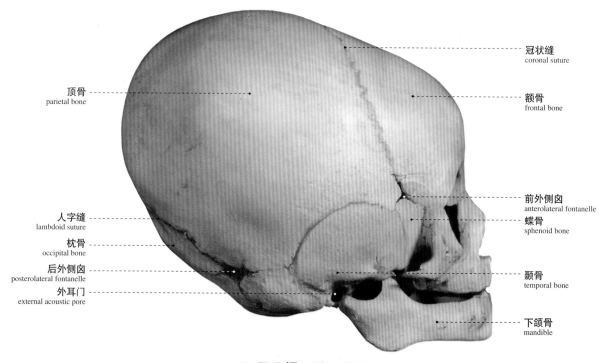

顶骨
parietal bone

冠状缝
coronal suture

额骨
frontal bone

人字缝
lambdoid suture

枕骨
occipital bone

后外侧囟
posterolateral fontanelle

外耳门
external acoustic pore

前外侧囟
anterolateral fontanelle

蝶骨
sphenoid bone

颞骨
temporal bone

下颌骨
mandible

23. 婴儿颅（侧面观 1）

Skull of an infant (lateral aspect 1)

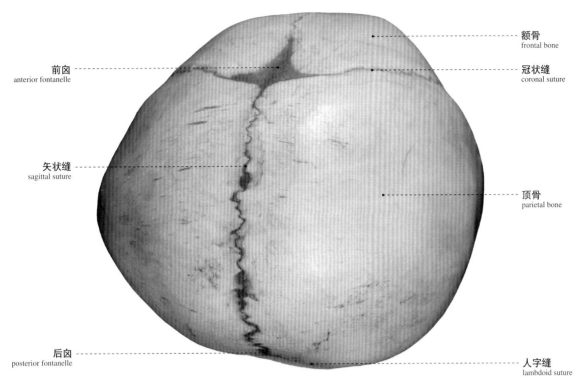

前囟
anterior fontanelle

矢状缝
sagittal suture

后囟
posterior fontanelle

额骨
frontal bone

冠状缝
coronal suture

顶骨
parietal bone

人字缝
lambdoid suture

24. 婴儿颅（上面观）
Skull of an infant (superior aspect)

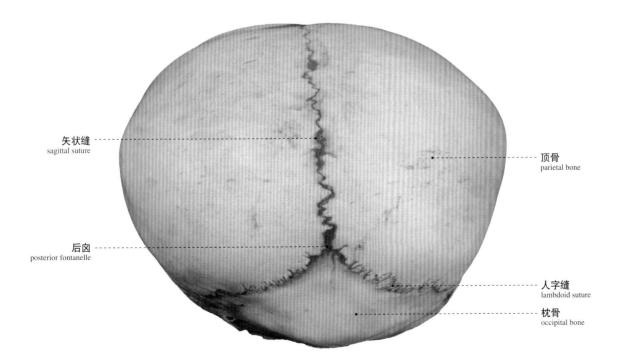

矢状缝
sagittal suture

后囟
posterior fontanelle

顶骨
parietal bone

人字缝
lambdoid suture

枕骨
occipital bone

25. 婴儿颅（后面观）
Skull of an infant (posterior aspect)

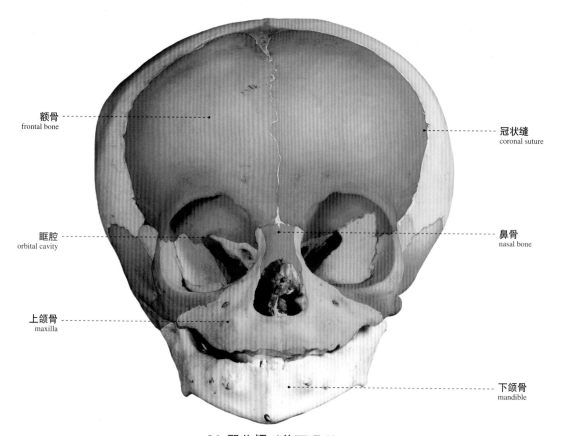

额骨
frontal bone

冠状缝
coronal suture

眶腔
orbital cavity

鼻骨
nasal bone

上颌骨
maxilla

下颌骨
mandible

26. 婴儿颅（前面观 2）

Skull of an infant (anterior aspect 2)

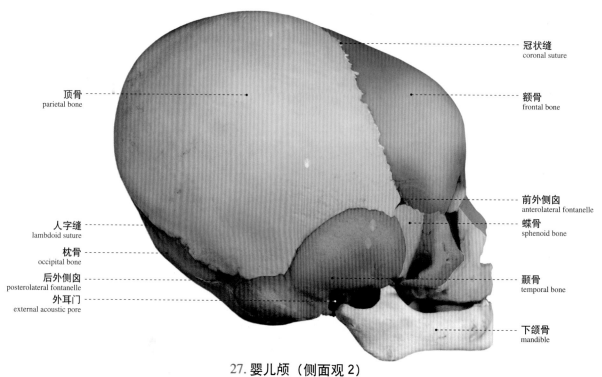

顶骨
parietal bone

冠状缝
coronal suture

额骨
frontal bone

前外侧囟
anterolateral fontanelle

蝶骨
sphenoid bone

人字缝
lambdoid suture

枕骨
occipital bone

后外侧囟
posterolateral fontanelle

外耳门
external acoustic pore

颞骨
temporal bone

下颌骨
mandible

27. 婴儿颅（侧面观 2）

Skull of an infant (lateral aspect 2)

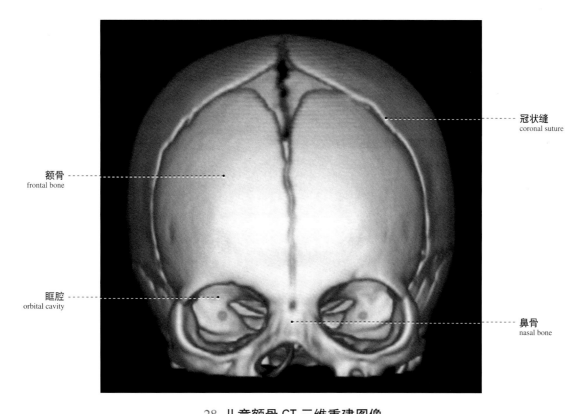

冠状缝
coronal suture

额骨
frontal bone

眶腔
orbital cavity

鼻骨
nasal bone

28. 儿童额骨 CT 三维重建图像

CT 3D reconstruction image of the child frontal bone

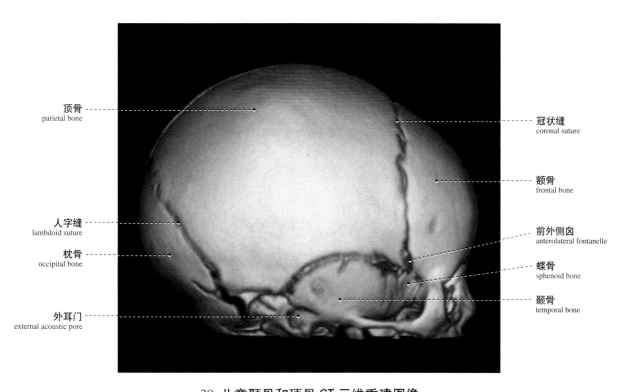

顶骨
parietal bone

冠状缝
coronal suture

额骨
frontal bone

人字缝
lambdoid suture

前外侧囟
anterolateral fontanelle

枕骨
occipital bone

蝶骨
sphenoid bone

颞骨
temporal bone

外耳门
external acoustic pore

29. 儿童颞骨和顶骨 CT 三维重建图像

CT 3D reconstruction image of the child temporal bone and parietal bone

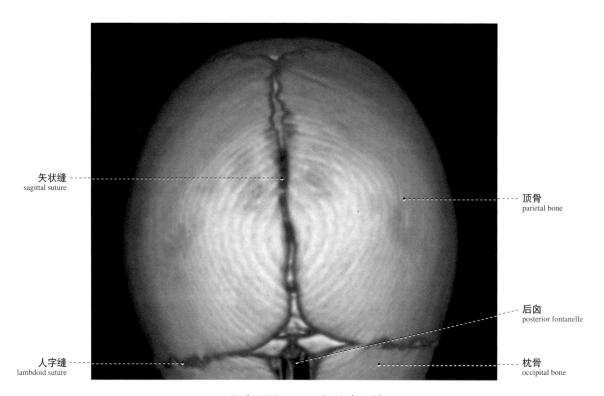

矢状缝
sagittal suture

顶骨
parietal bone

后囟
posterior fontanelle

人字缝
lambdoid suture

枕骨
occipital bone

30. 儿童顶骨 CT 三维重建图像
CT 3D reconstruction image of the child parietal bone

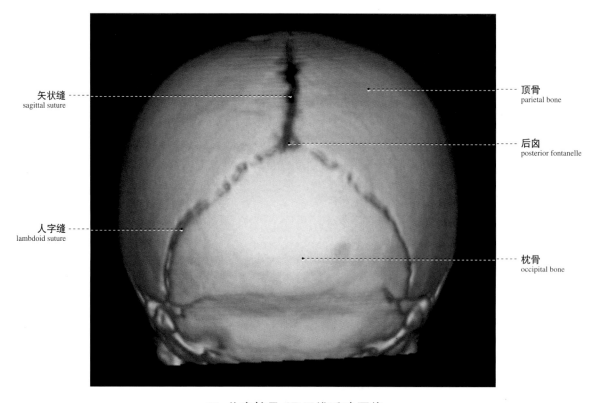

矢状缝
sagittal suture

顶骨
parietal bone

后囟
posterior fontanelle

人字缝
lambdoid suture

枕骨
occipital bone

31. 儿童枕骨 CT 三维重建图像
CT 3D reconstruction image of the child occipital bone

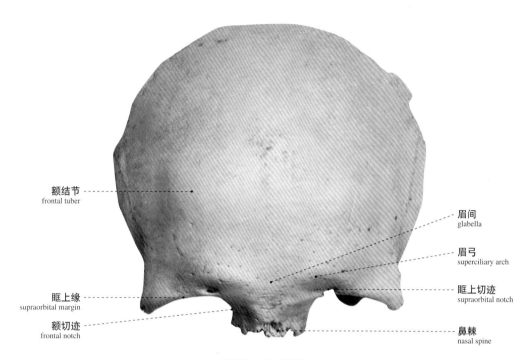

额结节
frontal tuber

眉间
glabella

眉弓
superciliary arch

眶上缘
supraorbital margin

眶上切迹
supraorbital notch

额切迹
frontal notch

鼻棘
nasal spine

32. 额骨（前面观）
Frontal bone (anterior aspect)

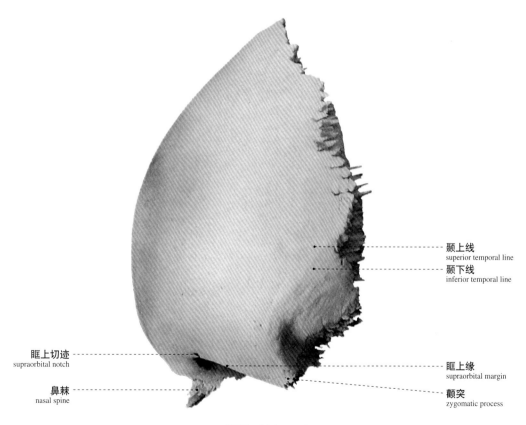

颞上线
superior temporal line

颞下线
inferior temporal line

眶上切迹
supraorbital notch

鼻棘
nasal spine

眶上缘
supraorbital margin

颧突
zygomatic process

33. 额骨（侧面观）
Frontal bone (lateral aspect)

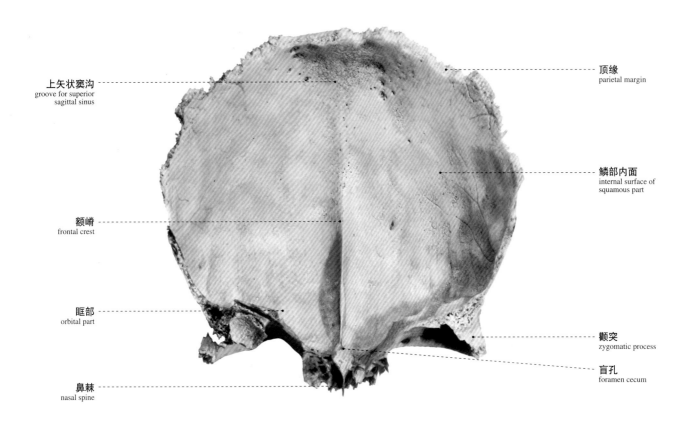

顶缘
parietal margin

上矢状窦沟
groove for superior
sagittal sinus

鳞部内面
internal surface of
squamous part

额嵴
frontal crest

眶部
orbital part

颧突
zygomatic process

盲孔
foramen cecum

鼻棘
nasal spine

34. 额骨（内面观）
Frontal bone (internal aspect)

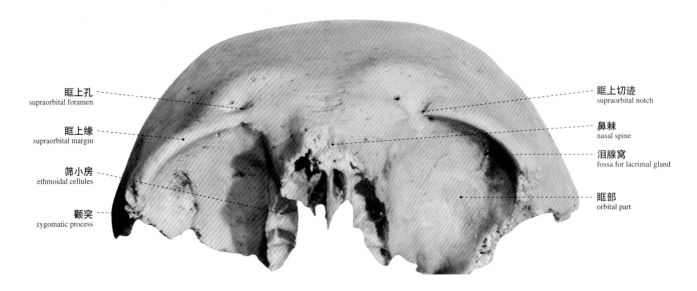

眶上孔
supraorbital foramen

眶上缘
supraorbital margin

筛小房
ethmoidal cellules

颧突
zygomatic process

眶上切迹
supraorbital notch

鼻棘
nasal spine

泪腺窝
fossa for lacrimal gland

眶部
orbital part

35. 额骨（下面观）
Frontal bone (inferior aspect)

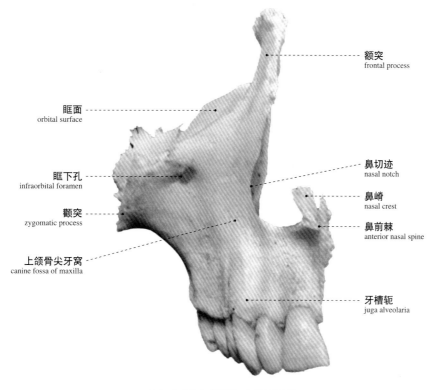

额突
frontal process

眶面
orbital surface

眶下孔
infraorbital foramen

颧突
zygomatic process

上颌骨尖牙窝
canine fossa of maxilla

鼻切迹
nasal notch

鼻嵴
nasal crest

鼻前棘
anterior nasal spine

牙槽轭
juga alveolaria

36. 右侧上颌骨（前面观）
Right maxillary (anterior aspect)

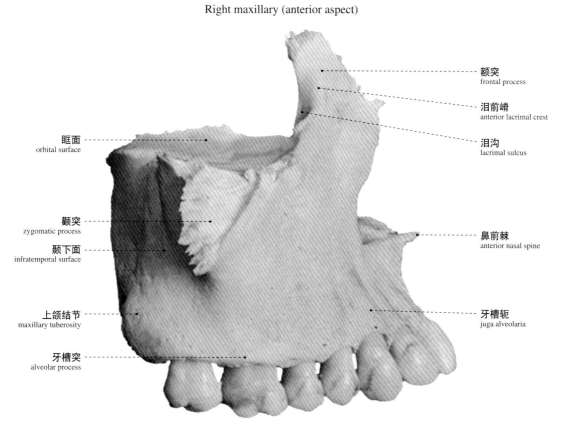

额突
frontal process

泪前嵴
anterior lacrimal crest

泪沟
lacrimal sulcus

眶面
orbital surface

颧突
zygomatic process

颞下面
infratemporal surface

上颌结节
maxillary tuberosity

牙槽突
alveolar process

鼻前棘
anterior nasal spine

牙槽轭
juga alveolaria

37. 右侧上颌骨（外侧面观）
Right maxillary (lateral aspect)

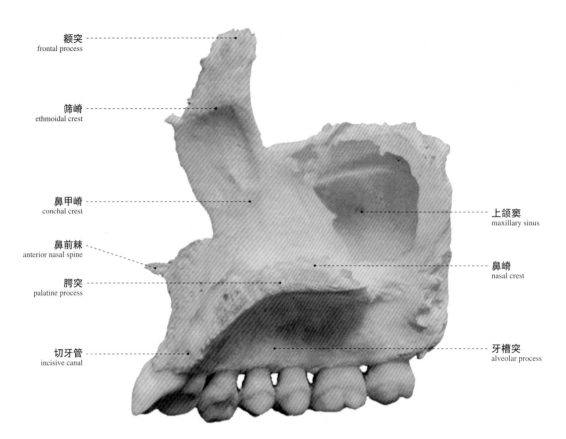

额突
frontal process

筛嵴
ethmoidal crest

鼻甲嵴
conchal crest

鼻前棘
anterior nasal spine

腭突
palatine process

切牙管
incisive canal

上颌窦
maxillary sinus

鼻嵴
nasal crest

牙槽突
alveolar process

38. 右侧上颌骨（内侧面观）
Right maxillary (medial aspect)

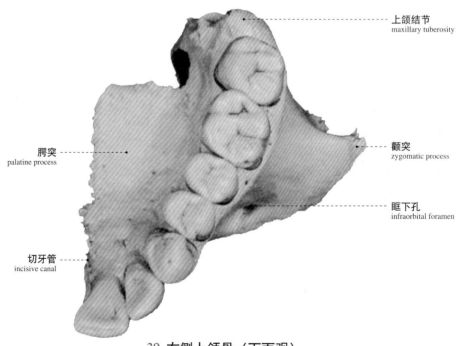

上颌结节
maxillary tuberosity

腭突
palatine process

颧突
zygomatic process

眶下孔
infraorbital foramen

切牙管
incisive canal

39. 右侧上颌骨（下面观）
Right maxillary (inferior aspect)

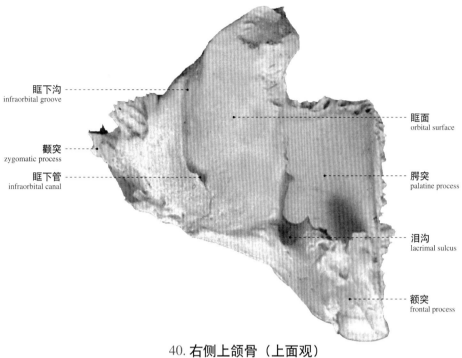

眶下沟
infraorbital groove

颧突
zygomatic process

眶下管
infraorbital canal

眶面
orbital surface

腭突
palatine process

泪沟
lacrimal sulcus

额突
frontal process

40. 右侧上颌骨（上面观）
Right maxillary (superior aspect)

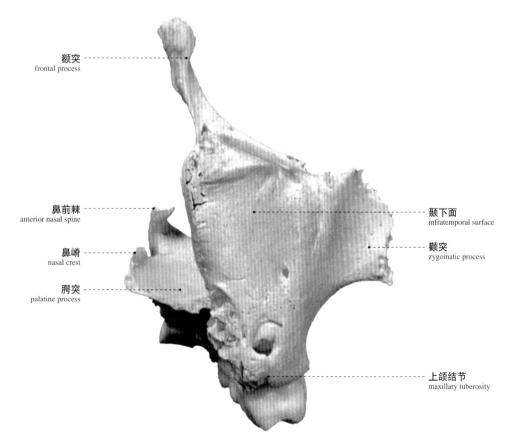

额突
frontal process

鼻前棘
anterior nasal spine

鼻嵴
nasal crest

腭突
palatine process

颞下面
infratemporal surface

颧突
zygomatic process

上颌结节
maxillary tuberosity

41. 右侧上颌骨（后面观）
Right maxillary (posterior aspect)

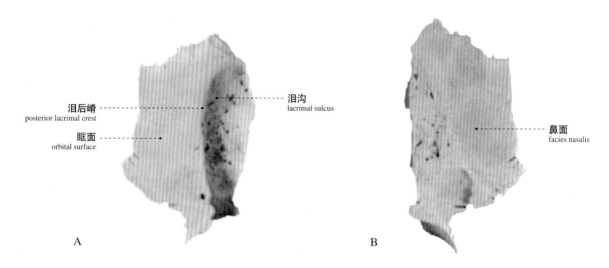

泪后嵴
posterior lacrimal crest

眶面
orbital surface

泪沟
lacrimal sulcus

鼻面
facies nasalis

A

B

42. 右侧泪骨
Right lacrimal bone

A. 外侧面观；B. 内侧面观

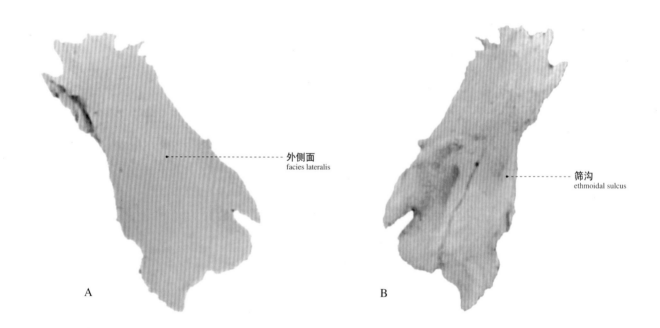

外侧面
facies lateralis

筛沟
ethmoidal sulcus

A

B

43. 右侧鼻骨
Right nasal bone

A. 外侧面观；B. 内侧面观

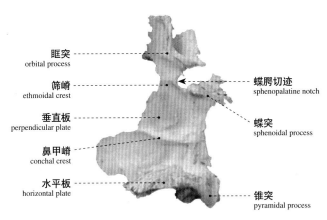

眶突
orbital process

筛嵴
ethmoidal crest

垂直板
perpendicular plate

鼻甲嵴
conchal crest

水平板
horizontal plate

蝶腭切迹
sphenopalatine notch

蝶突
sphenoidal process

锥突
pyramidal process

44. 右侧腭骨（内侧面观）
Right palatine bone (medial aspect)

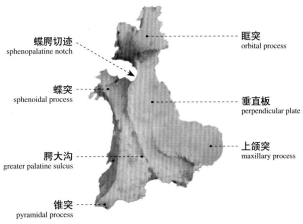

蝶腭切迹
sphenopalatine notch

蝶突
sphenoidal process

腭大沟
greater palatine sulcus

锥突
pyramidal process

眶突
orbital process

垂直板
perpendicular plate

上颌突
maxillary process

45. 右侧腭骨（外侧面观）
Right palatine bone (lateral aspect)

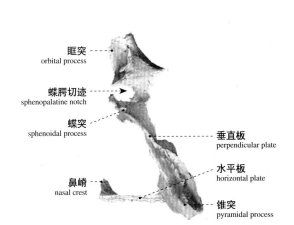

眶突
orbital process

蝶腭切迹
sphenopalatine notch

蝶突
sphenoidal process

鼻嵴
nasal crest

垂直板
perpendicular plate

水平板
horizontal plate

锥突
pyramidal process

46. 右侧腭骨（后面观）
Right palatine bone (posterior aspect)

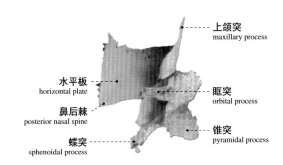

上颌突
maxillary process

水平板
horizontal plate

鼻后棘
posterior nasal spine

蝶突
sphenoidal process

眶突
orbital process

锥突
pyramidal process

47. 右侧腭骨（上面观）
Right palatine bone (superior aspect)

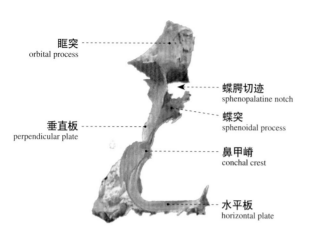

眶突
orbital process

蝶腭切迹
sphenopalatine notch

蝶突
sphenoidal process

垂直板
perpendicular plate

鼻甲嵴
conchal crest

水平板
horizontal plate

48. 右侧腭骨（前面观）
Right palatine bone (anterior aspect)

上颌突
maxillary process

腭大沟
greater palatine sulcus

水平板
horizontal plate

腭小孔
lesser palatine foramina

锥突
pyramidal process

蝶突
sphenoidal process

49. 右侧腭骨（下面观）
Right palatine bone (inferior aspect)

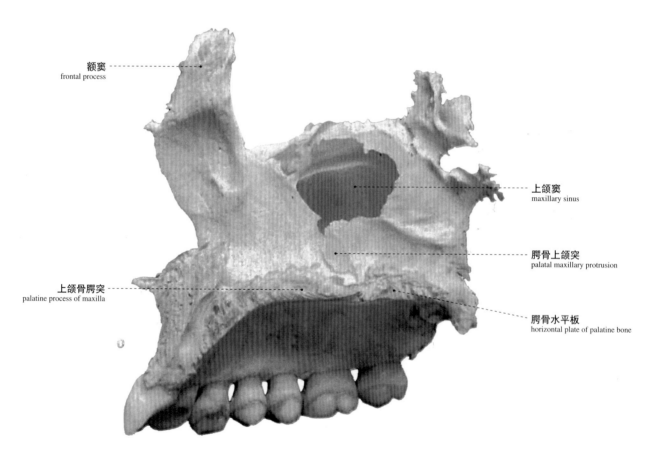

额窦
frontal process

上颌窦
maxillary sinus

腭骨上颌突
palatal maxillary protrusion

上颌骨腭突
palatine process of maxilla

腭骨水平板
horizontal plate of palatine bone

50. 上颌骨和腭骨（内侧面观）
Maxillary bone and palatine bone (medial aspect)

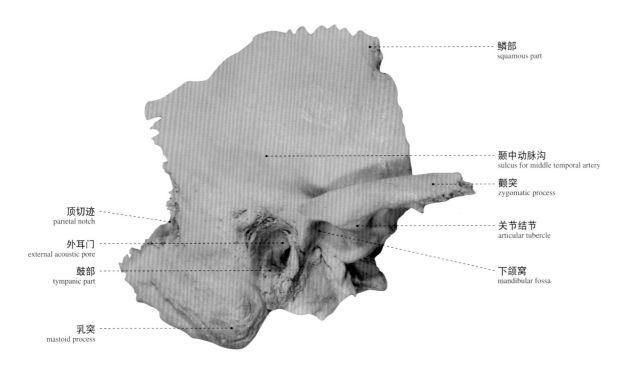

鳞部
squamous part

颞中动脉沟
sulcus for middle temporal artery

颧突
zygomatic process

关节结节
articular tubercle

下颌窝
mandibular fossa

顶切迹
parietal notch

外耳门
external acoustic pore

鼓部
tympanic part

乳突
mastoid process

51. 颞骨（外侧面观）
Temporal bone (lateral aspect)

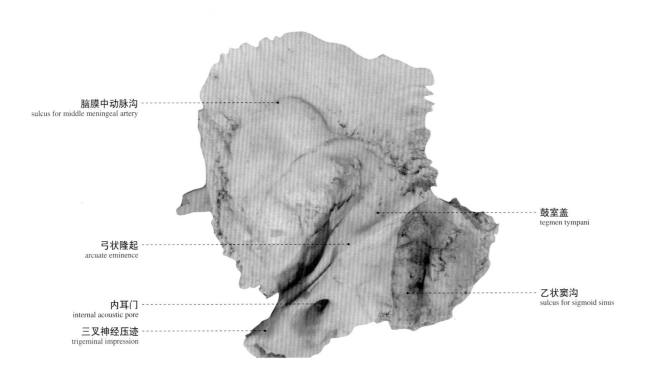

脑膜中动脉沟
sulcus for middle meningeal artery

鼓室盖
tegmen tympani

弓状隆起
arcuate eminence

乙状窦沟
sulcus for sigmoid sinus

内耳门
internal acoustic pore

三叉神经压迹
trigeminal impression

52. 颞骨（内侧面观）
Temporal bone (medial aspect)

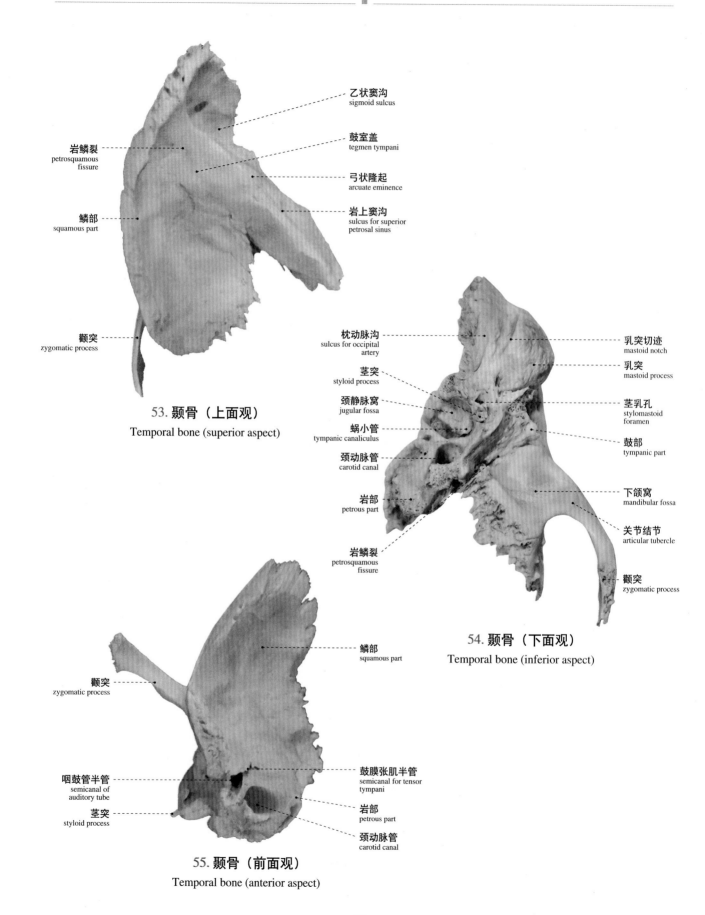

乙状窦沟
sigmoid sulcus

鼓室盖
tegmen tympani

弓状隆起
arcuate eminence

岩上窦沟
sulcus for superior
petrosal sinus

岩鳞裂
petrosquamous
fissure

鳞部
squamous part

颧突
zygomatic process

53. 颞骨（上面观）
Temporal bone (superior aspect)

枕动脉沟
sulcus for occipital
artery

茎突
styloid process

颈静脉窝
jugular fossa

蜗小管
tympanic canaliculus

颈动脉管
carotid canal

岩部
petrous part

岩鳞裂
petrosquamous
fissure

乳突切迹
mastoid notch

乳突
mastoid process

茎乳孔
stylomastoid
foramen

鼓部
tympanic part

下颌窝
mandibular fossa

关节结节
articular tubercle

颧突
zygomatic process

54. 颞骨（下面观）
Temporal bone (inferior aspect)

鳞部
squamous part

颧突
zygomatic process

咽鼓管半管
semicanal of
auditory tube

茎突
styloid process

鼓膜张肌半管
semicanal for tensor
tympani

岩部
petrous part

颈动脉管
carotid canal

55. 颞骨（前面观）
Temporal bone (anterior aspect)

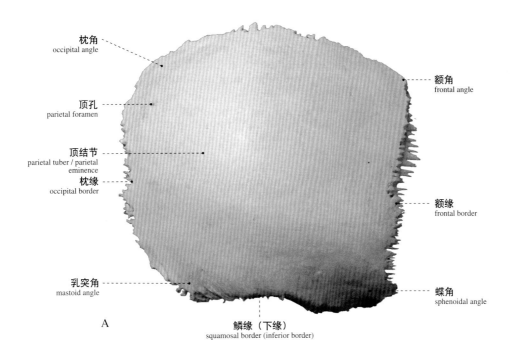

枕角
occipital angle

顶孔
parietal foramen

顶结节
parietal tuber / parietal eminence

枕缘
occipital border

乳突角
mastoid angle

额角
frontal angle

额缘
frontal border

蝶角
sphenoidal angle

鳞缘（下缘）
squamosal border (inferior border)

A

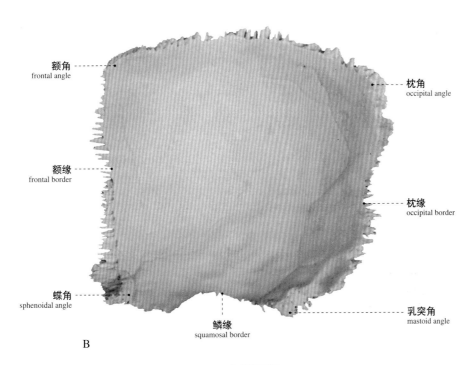

额角
frontal angle

额缘
frontal border

蝶角
sphenoidal angle

鳞缘
squamosal border

枕角
occipital angle

枕缘
occipital border

乳突角
mastoid angle

B

56. 右侧顶骨
Right parietal bone
A. 外侧面观；B. 内侧面观

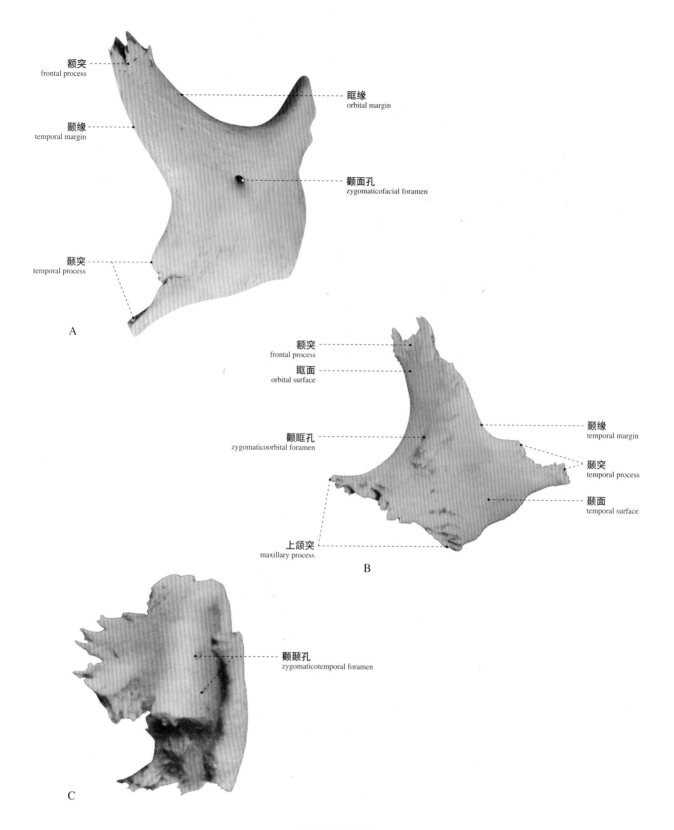

额突
frontal process

眶缘
orbital margin

颞缘
temporal margin

颧面孔
zygomaticofacial foramen

颞突
temporal process

A

额突
frontal process

眶面
orbital surface

颧眶孔
zygomaticoorbital foramen

颞缘
temporal margin

颞突
temporal process

颞面
temporal surface

上颌突
maxillary process

B

颧颞孔
zygomaticotemporal foramen

C

57.右侧颧骨
Right zygomatic bone

A.外侧面观；B.内侧面观；C.后面观

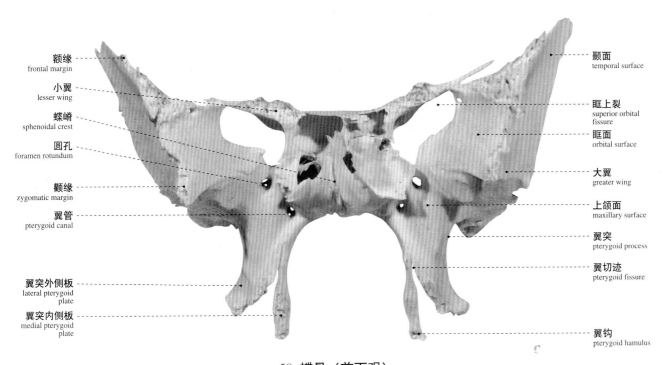

额缘 frontal margin
小翼 lesser wing
蝶嵴 sphenoidal crest
圆孔 foramen rotundum
颧缘 zygomatic margin
翼管 pterygoid canal
翼突外侧板 lateral pterygoid plate
翼突内侧板 medial pterygoid plate

颞面 temporal surface
眶上裂 superior orbital fissure
眶面 orbital surface
大翼 greater wing
上颌面 maxillary surface
翼突 pterygoid process
翼切迹 pterygoid fissure
翼钩 pterygoid hamulus

58. 蝶骨（前面观）
Sphenoid bone (anterior aspect)

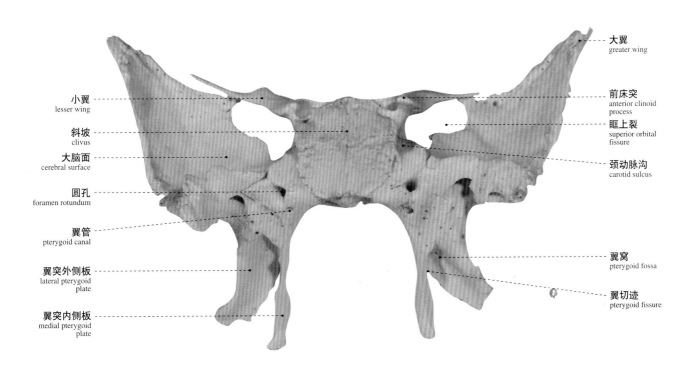

小翼 lesser wing
斜坡 clivus
大脑面 cerebral surface
圆孔 foramen rotundum
翼管 pterygoid canal
翼突外侧板 lateral pterygoid plate
翼突内侧板 medial pterygoid plate

大翼 greater wing
前床突 anterior clinoid process
眶上裂 superior orbital fissure
颈动脉沟 carotid sulcus
翼窝 pterygoid fossa
翼切迹 pterygoid fissure

59. 蝶骨（后面观）
Sphenoid bone (posterior aspect)

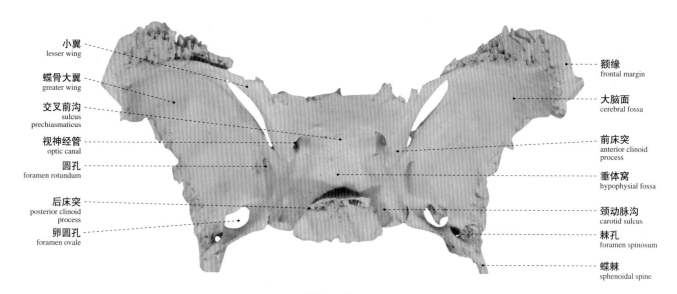

小翼
lesser wing

蝶骨大翼
greater wing

交叉前沟
sulcus prechiasmaticus

视神经管
optic canal

圆孔
foramen rotundum

后床突
posterior clinoid process

卵圆孔
foramen ovale

额缘
frontal margin

大脑面
cerebral fossa

前床突
anterior clinoid process

垂体窝
hypophysial fossa

颈动脉沟
carotid sulcus

棘孔
foramen spinosum

蝶棘
sphenoidal spine

60. 蝶骨（上面观）
Sphenoid bone (superior aspect)

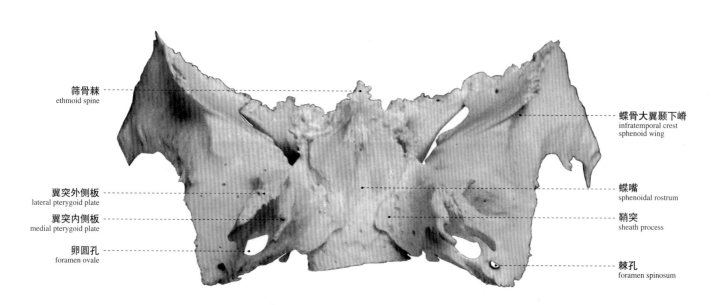

筛骨棘
ethmoid spine

翼突外侧板
lateral pterygoid plate

翼突内侧板
medial pterygoid plate

卵圆孔
foramen ovale

蝶骨大翼颞下嵴
infratemporal crest sphenoid wing

蝶嘴
sphenoidal rostrum

鞘突
sheath process

棘孔
foramen spinosum

61. 蝶骨（下面观）
Sphenoid (inferior aspect)

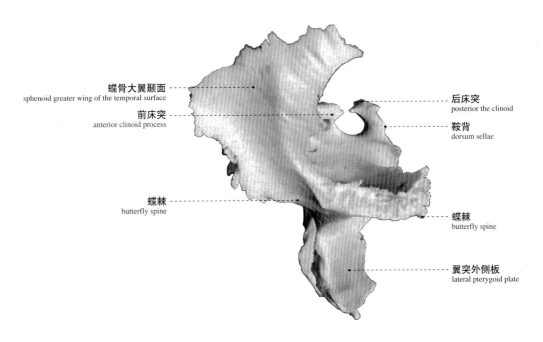

蝶骨大翼颞面
sphenoid greater wing of the temporal surface

前床突
anterior clinoid process

蝶棘
butterfly spine

后床突
posterior the clinoid

鞍背
dorsum sellae

蝶棘
butterfly spine

翼突外侧板
lateral pterygoid plate

62. 蝶骨（左侧面观）
Sphenoid bone (left lateral aspect)

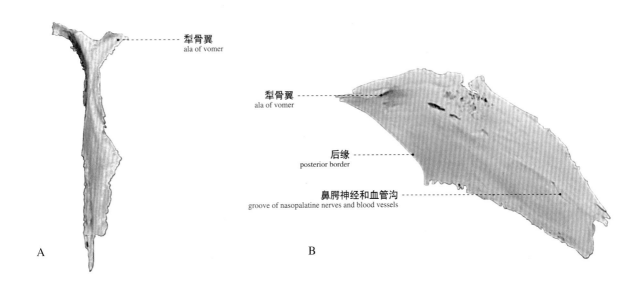

犁骨翼
ala of vomer

犁骨翼
ala of vomer

后缘
posterior border

鼻腭神经和血管沟
groove of nasopalatine nerves and blood vessels

A

B

63. 犁骨
Vomer

A. 后面观；B. 右侧面观

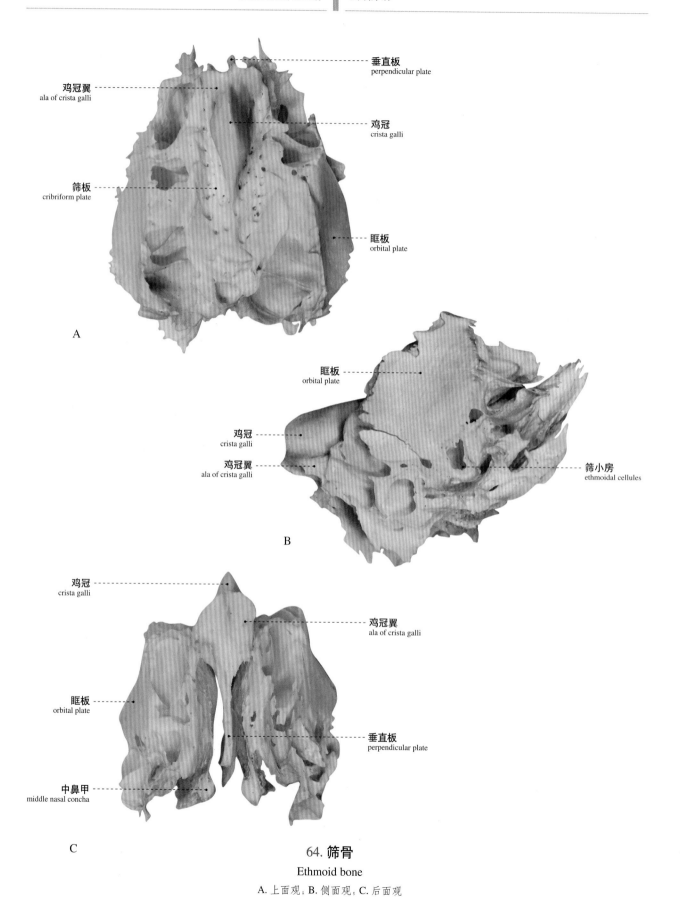

垂直板
perpendicular plate

鸡冠翼
ala of crista galli

鸡冠
crista galli

筛板
cribriform plate

眶板
orbital plate

A

眶板
orbital plate

鸡冠
crista galli

鸡冠翼
ala of crista galli

筛小房
ethmoidal cellules

B

鸡冠
crista galli

鸡冠翼
ala of crista galli

眶板
orbital plate

垂直板
perpendicular plate

中鼻甲
middle nasal concha

C

64. 筛骨
Ethmoid bone
A. 上面观；B. 侧面观；C. 后面观

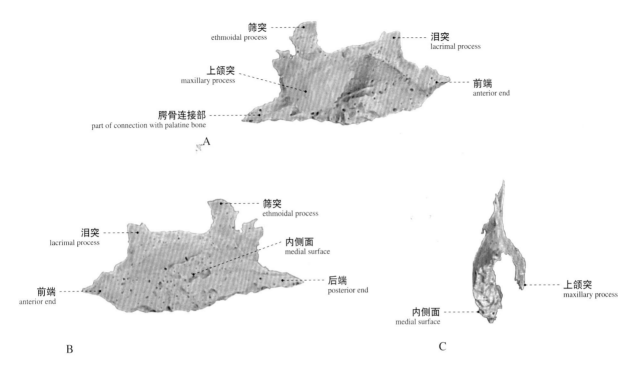

65. 右侧下鼻甲

Right inferior nasal concha

A. 外侧面观；B. 内侧面观；C. 后面观

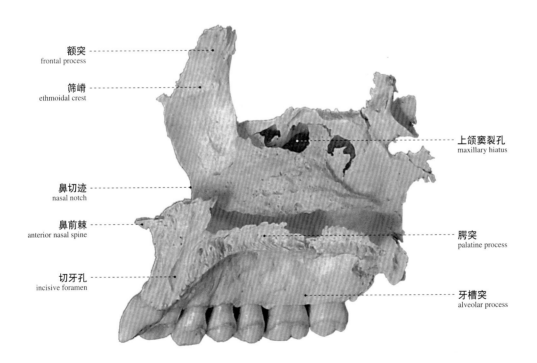

66. 右侧上颌骨、腭骨和下鼻甲（内侧面观）

Right maxilla, palatine bone and inferior nasal concha (medial aspect)

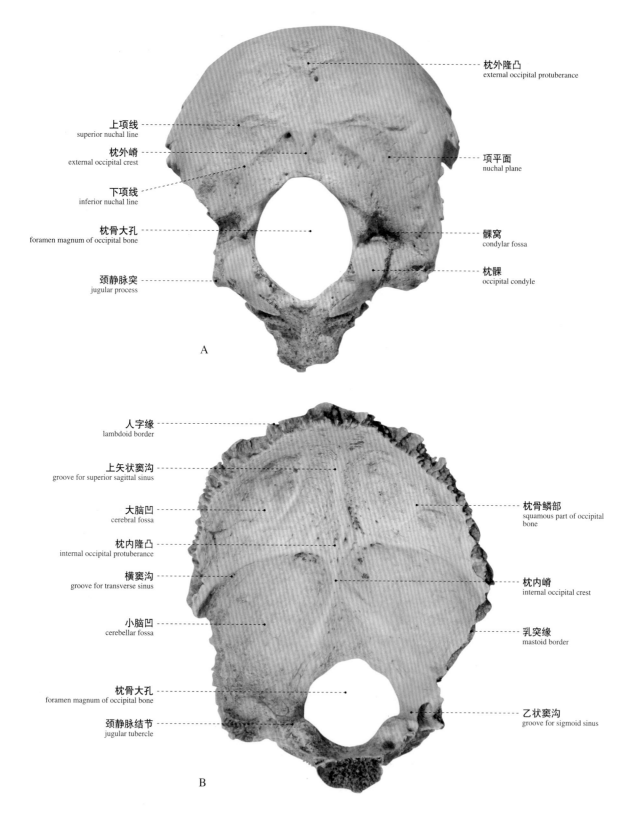

枕外隆凸
external occipital protuberance

上项线
superior nuchal line

枕外嵴
external occipital crest

下项线
inferior nuchal line

枕骨大孔
foramen magnum of occipital bone

颈静脉突
jugular process

项平面
nuchal plane

髁窝
condylar fossa

枕髁
occipital condyle

A

人字缘
lambdoid border

上矢状窦沟
groove for superior sagittal sinus

大脑凹
cerebral fossa

枕内隆凸
internal occipital protuberance

横窦沟
groove for transverse sinus

小脑凹
cerebellar fossa

枕骨大孔
foramen magnum of occipital bone

颈静脉结节
jugular tubercle

枕骨鳞部
squamous part of occipital bone

枕内嵴
internal occipital crest

乳突缘
mastoid border

乙状窦沟
groove for sigmoid sinus

B

67. 枕骨

Occipital bone

A. 外面观；B. 内面观

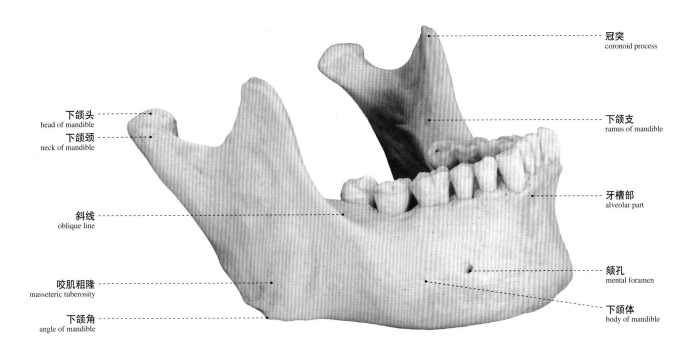

冠突
coronoid process

下颌头
head of mandible

下颌颈
neck of mandible

下颌支
ramus of mandible

斜线
oblique line

牙槽部
alveolar part

咬肌粗隆
masseteric tuberosity

颏孔
mental foramen

下颌角
angle of mandible

下颌体
body of mandible

68. 下颌骨（外侧面观）
Mandible (lateral aspect)

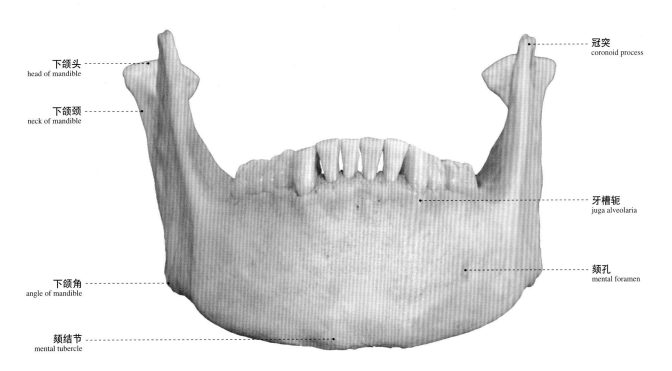

冠突
coronoid process

下颌头
head of mandible

下颌颈
neck of mandible

牙槽轭
juga alveolaria

下颌角
angle of mandible

颏孔
mental foramen

颏结节
mental tubercle

69. 下颌骨（前面观）
Mandible (anterior aspect)

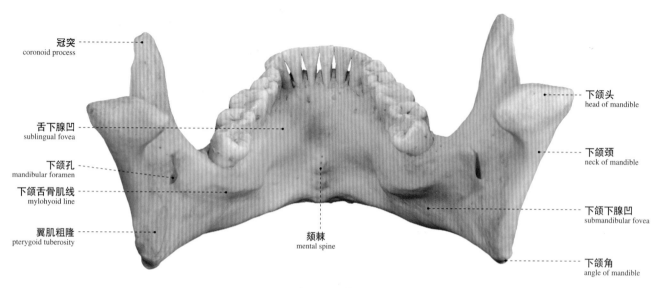

冠突
coronoid process

舌下腺凹
sublingual fovea

下颌孔
mandibular foramen

下颌舌骨肌线
mylohyoid line

翼肌粗隆
pterygoid tuberosity

下颌头
head of mandible

下颌颈
neck of mandible

下颌下腺凹
submandibular fovea

下颌角
angle of mandible

颏棘
mental spine

70. 下颌骨（后面观）
Mandible (posterior aspect)

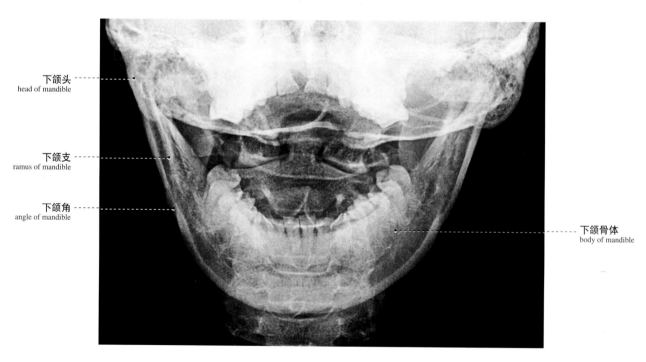

下颌头
head of mandible

下颌支
ramus of mandible

下颌角
angle of mandible

下颌骨体
body of mandible

71. 下颌骨 X 线像（前后位）
Radiograph of the mandible (anteroposterior view)

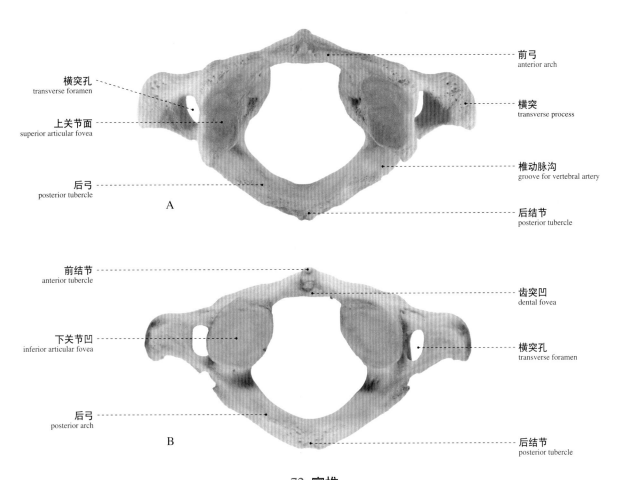

横突孔
transverse foramen

上关节面
superior articular fovea

后弓
posterior tubercle

A

前弓
anterior arch

横突
transverse process

椎动脉沟
groove for vertebral artery

后结节
posterior tubercle

前结节
anterior tubercle

下关节凹
inferior articular fovea

后弓
posterior arch

B

齿突凹
dental fovea

横突孔
transverse foramen

后结节
posterior tubercle

72. 寰椎
Atlas

A. 上面观；B. 下面观

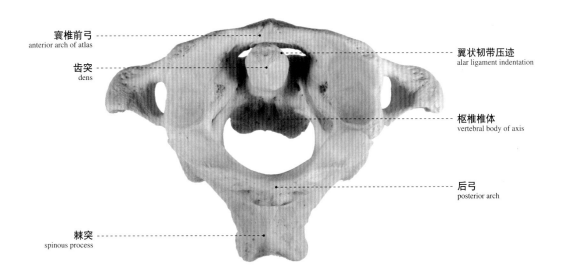

寰椎前弓
anterior arch of atlas

齿突
dens

棘突
spinous process

翼状韧带压迹
alar ligament indentation

枢椎椎体
vertebral body of axis

后弓
posterior arch

73. 寰枢关节（上面观）
Atlantoaxial joint (superior aspect)

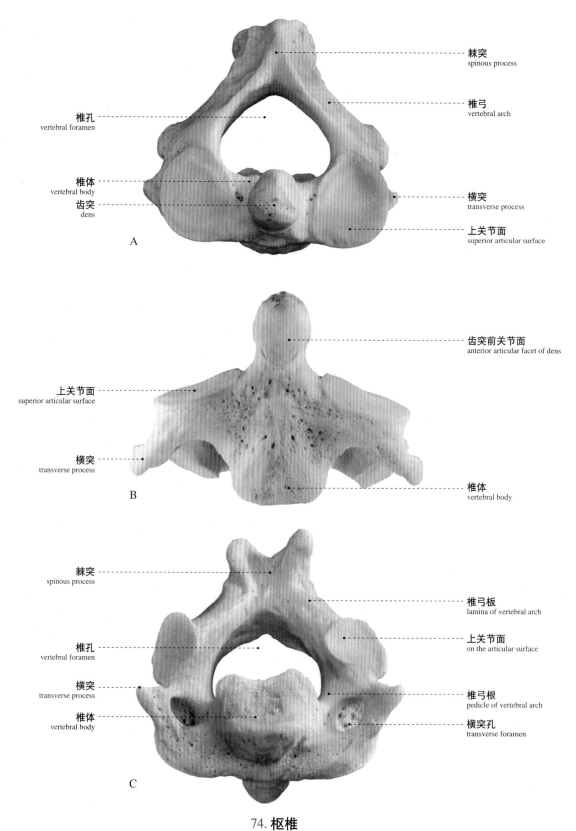

棘突
spinous process

椎弓
vertebral arch

椎孔
vertebral foramen

椎体
vertebral body

齿突
dens

横突
transverse process

上关节面
superior articular surface

A

齿突前关节面
anterior articular facet of dens

上关节面
superior articular surface

横突
transverse process

椎体
vertebral body

B

棘突
spinous process

椎弓板
lamina of vertebral arch

椎孔
vertebral foramen

上关节面
on the articular surface

横突
transverse process

椎体
vertebral body

椎弓根
pedicle of vertebral arch

横突孔
transverse foramen

C

74. 枢椎

Axis

A.上面观；B.前面观；C.下面观

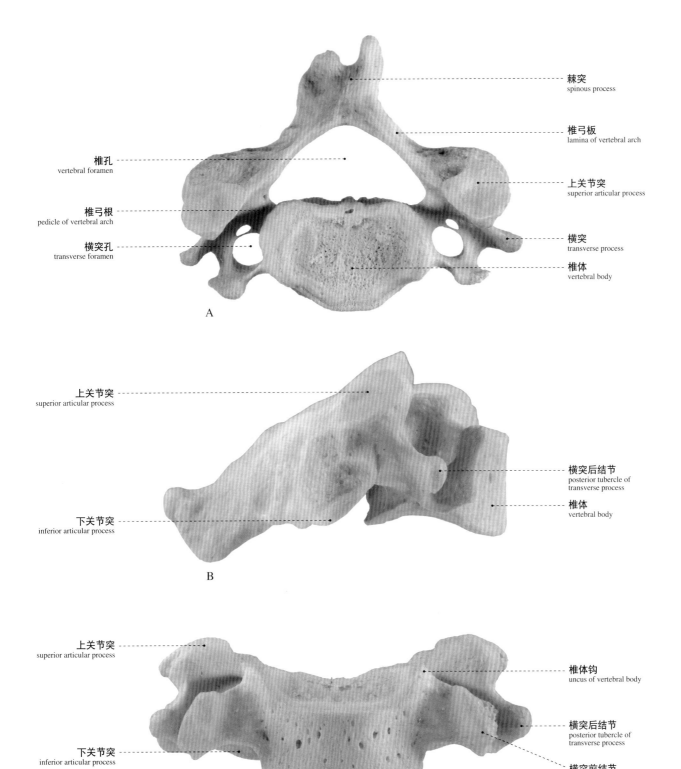

棘突
spinous process

椎弓板
lamina of vertebral arch

椎孔
vertebral foramen

上关节突
superior articular process

椎弓根
pedicle of vertebral arch

横突
transverse process

横突孔
transverse foramen

椎体
vertebral body

A

上关节突
superior articular process

横突后结节
posterior tubercle of transverse process

椎体
vertebral body

下关节突
inferior articular process

B

上关节突
superior articular process

椎体钩
uncus of vertebral body

横突后结节
posterior tubercle of transverse process

下关节突
inferior articular process

横突前结节
anterior tubercle of transverse process

椎体
vertebral body

C

75. 颈椎
Cervical vertebra
A. 上面观；B. 侧面观；C. 前面观

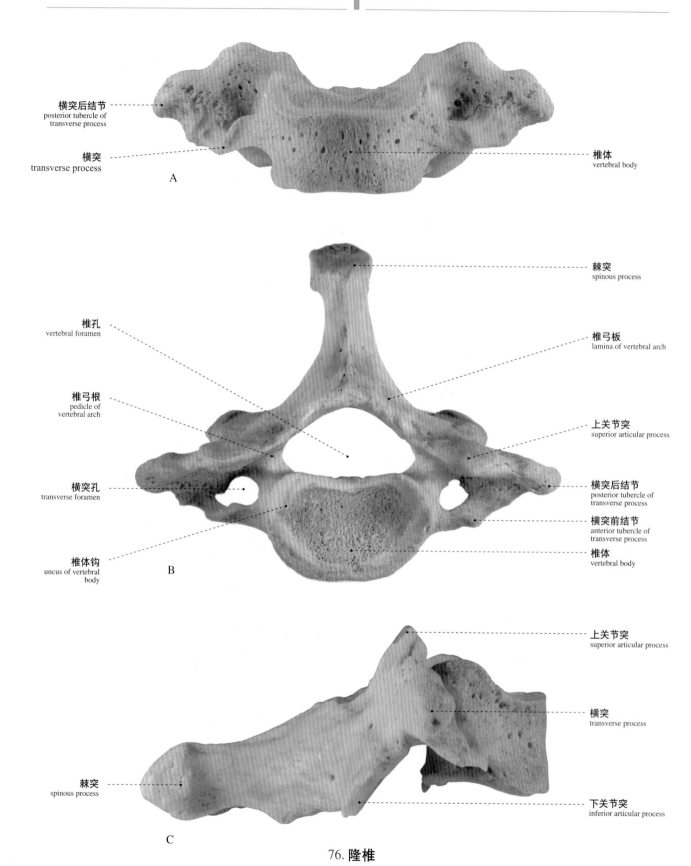

横突后结节
posterior tubercle of
transverse process

横突
transverse process

A

椎体
vertebral body

椎孔
vertebral foramen

椎弓根
pedicle of
vertebral arch

横突孔
transverse foramen

椎体钩
uncus of vertebral
body

B

棘突
spinous process

椎弓板
lamina of vertebral arch

上关节突
superior articular process

横突后结节
posterior tubercle of
transverse process

横突前结节
anterior tubercle of
transverse process

椎体
vertebral body

棘突
spinous process

C

上关节突
superior articular process

横突
transverse process

下关节突
inferior articular process

76. 隆椎

Vertebra prominens

A. 前面观；B. 上面观；C. 侧面观

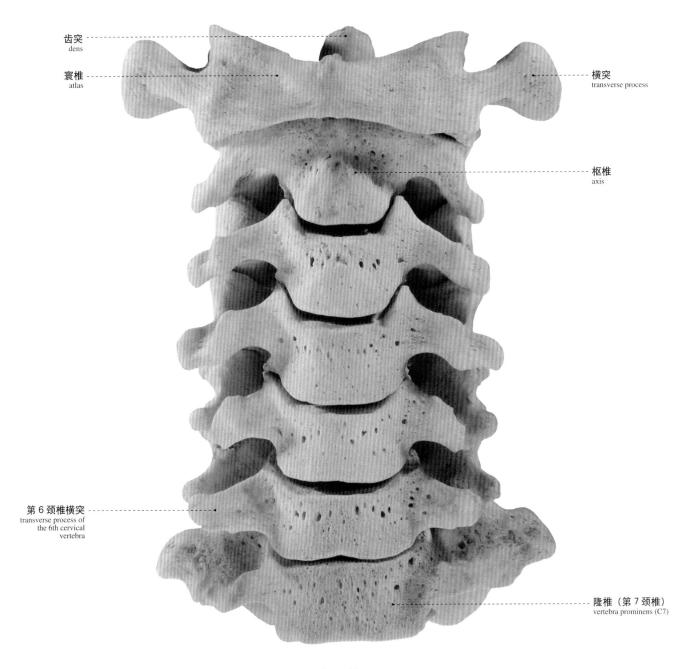

齿突
dens

寰椎
atlas

横突
transverse process

枢椎
axis

第 6 颈椎横突
transverse process of
the 6th cervical
vertebra

隆椎（第 7 颈椎）
vertebra prominens (C7)

77. 颈椎（前面观）
Cervical vertebra (anterior aspect)

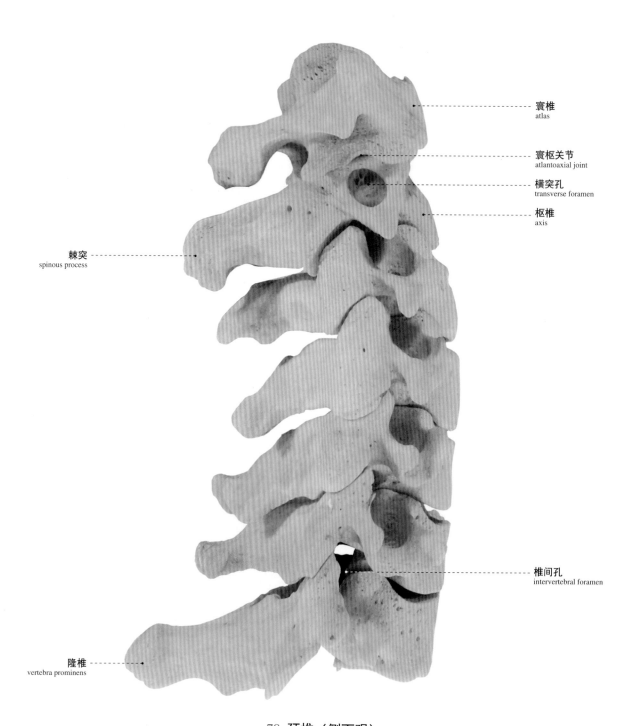

寰椎
atlas

寰枢关节
atlantoaxial joint

横突孔
transverse foramen

枢椎
axis

棘突
spinous process

椎间孔
intervertebral foramen

隆椎
vertebra prominens

78. 颈椎（侧面观）
Cervical vertebra (lateral aspect)

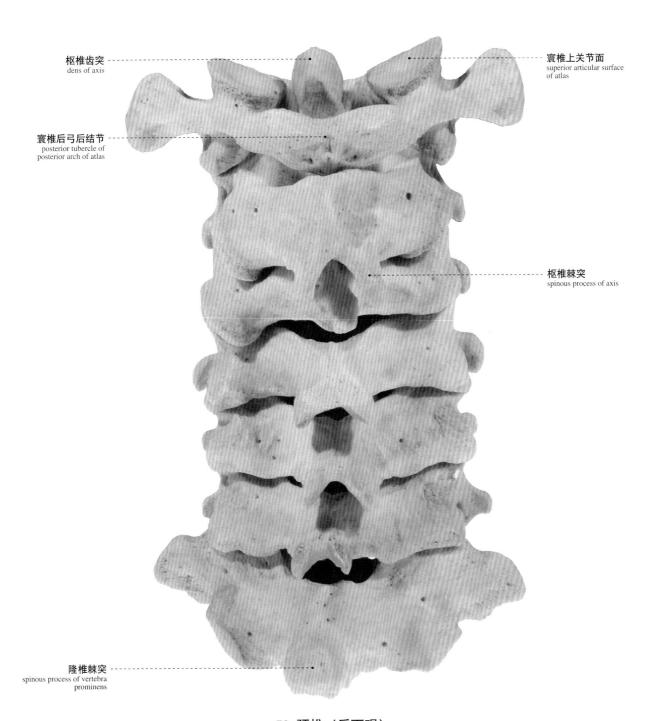

枢椎齿突
dens of axis

寰椎上关节面
superior articular surface
of atlas

寰椎后弓后结节
posterior tubercle of
posterior arch of atlas

枢椎棘突
spinous process of axis

隆椎棘突
spinous process of vertebra
prominens

79. 颈椎（后面观）
Cervical vertebra (posterior aspect)

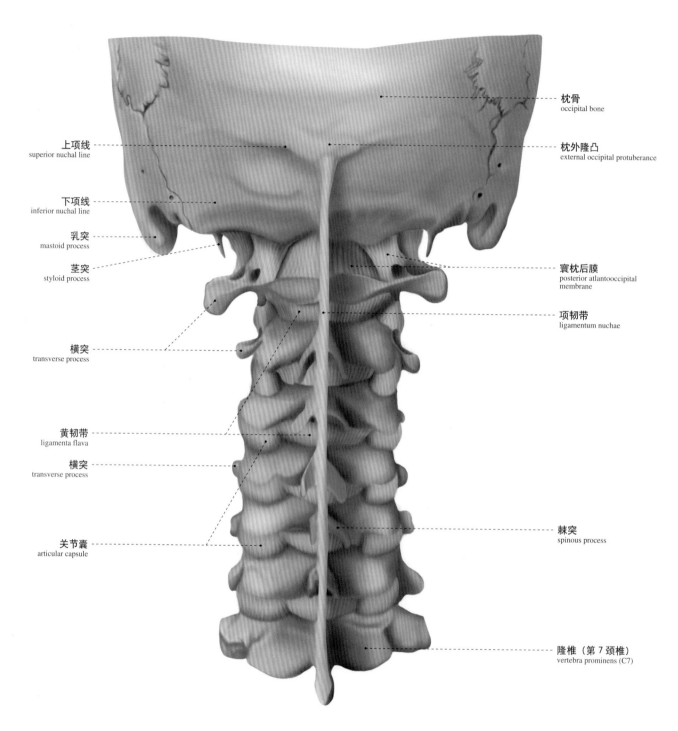

枕骨
occipital bone

上项线
superior nuchal line

枕外隆凸
external occipital protuberance

下项线
inferior nuchal line

乳突
mastoid process

茎突
styloid process

寰枕后膜
posterior atlantooccipital membrane

项韧带
ligamentum nuchae

横突
transverse process

黄韧带
ligamenta flava

横突
transverse process

棘突
spinous process

关节囊
articular capsule

隆椎（第7颈椎）
vertebra prominens (C7)

80. 颈椎的韧带（后面观）
Ligaments of the cervical vertebrae (posterior aspect)

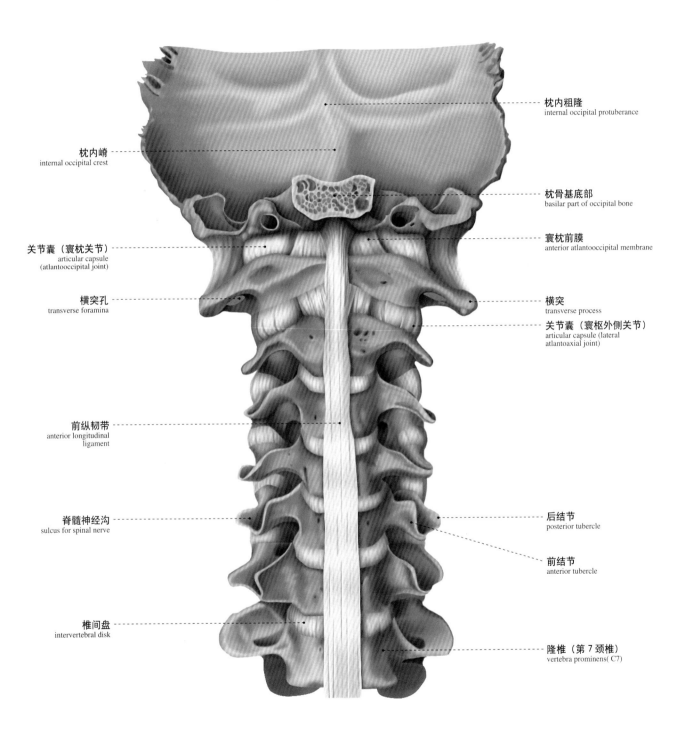

枕内粗隆
internal occipital protuberance

枕内嵴
internal occipital crest

枕骨基底部
basilar part of occipital bone

关节囊（寰枕关节）
articular capsule
(atlantooccipital joint)

寰枕前膜
anterior atlantooccipital membrane

横突孔
transverse foramina

横突
transverse process

关节囊（寰枢外侧关节）
articular capsule (lateral
atlantoaxial joint)

前纵韧带
anterior longitudinal
ligament

脊髓神经沟
sulcus for spinal nerve

后结节
posterior tubercle

前结节
anterior tubercle

椎间盘
intervertebral disk

隆椎（第7颈椎）
vertebra prominens(C7)

81. 颈椎的韧带（前面观）
Ligaments of the cervical vertebrae (anterior aspect)

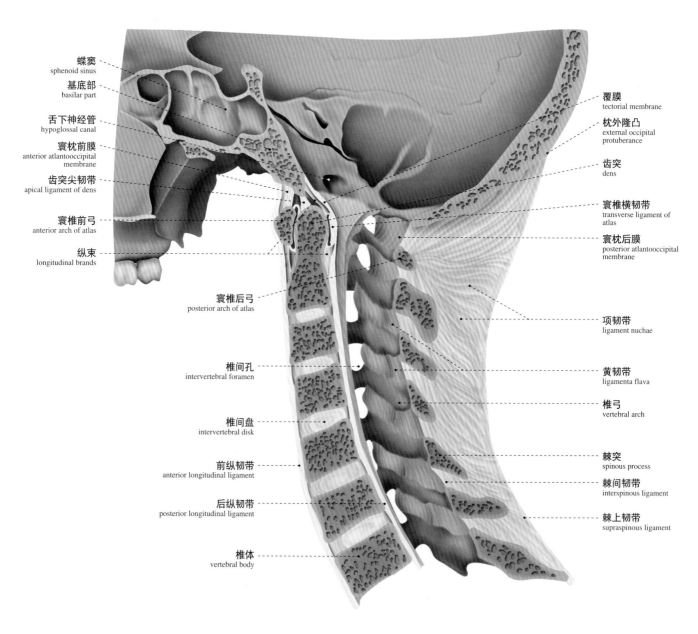

蝶窦
sphenoid sinus

基底部
basilar part

舌下神经管
hypoglossal canal

寰枕前膜
anterior atlantooccipital
membrane

齿突尖韧带
apical ligament of dens

寰椎前弓
anterior arch of atlas

纵束
longitudinal brands

寰椎后弓
posterior arch of atlas

椎间孔
intervertebral foramen

椎间盘
intervertebral disk

前纵韧带
anterior longitudinal ligament

后纵韧带
posterior longitudinal ligament

椎体
vertebral body

覆膜
tectorial membrane

枕外隆凸
external occipital
protuberance

齿突
dens

寰椎横韧带
transverse ligament of
atlas

寰枕后膜
posterior atlantooccipital
membrane

项韧带
ligament nuchae

黄韧带
ligamenta flava

椎弓
vertebral arch

棘突
spinous process

棘间韧带
interspinous ligament

棘上韧带
supraspinous ligament

82. 颈椎的韧带（侧面观）
Ligaments of the cervical vertebrae (lateral aspect)

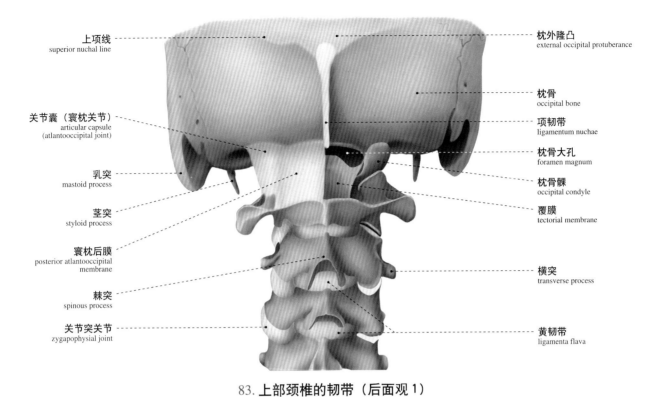

上项线
superior nuchal line

枕外隆凸
external occipital protuberance

枕骨
occipital bone

关节囊（寰枕关节）
articular capsule
(atlantooccipital joint)

项韧带
ligamentum nuchae

枕骨大孔
foramen magnum

乳突
mastoid process

枕骨髁
occipital condyle

茎突
styloid process

覆膜
tectorial membrane

寰枕后膜
posterior atlantooccipital
membrane

棘突
spinous process

横突
transverse process

关节突关节
zygapophysial joint

黄韧带
ligamenta flava

83. 上部颈椎的韧带（后面观 1）

Ligaments of the upper cervical spine (posterior aspect 1)

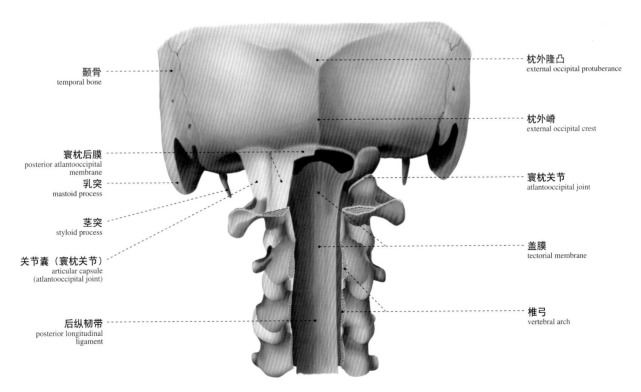

颞骨
temporal bone

枕外隆凸
external occipital protuberance

枕外嵴
external occipital crest

寰枕后膜
posterior atlantooccipital
membrane

乳突
mastoid process

寰枕关节
atlantooccipital joint

茎突
styloid process

关节囊（寰枕关节）
articular capsule
(atlantooccipital joint)

盖膜
tectorial membrane

后纵韧带
posterior longitudinal
ligament

椎弓
vertebral arch

84. 上部颈椎的韧带（后面观 2）

Ligaments of the upper cervical spine (posterior aspect 2)

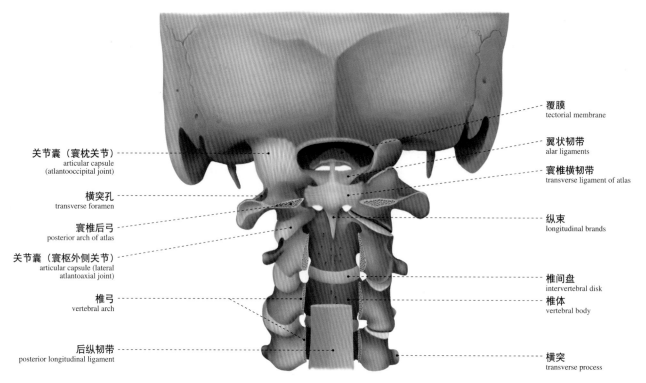

关节囊（寰枕关节）
articular capsule
(atlantooccipital joint)

横突孔
transverse foramen

寰椎后弓
posterior arch of atlas

关节囊（寰枢外侧关节）
articular capsule (lateral
atlantoaxial joint)

椎弓
vertebral arch

后纵韧带
posterior longitudinal ligament

覆膜
tectorial membrane

翼状韧带
alar ligaments

寰椎横韧带
transverse ligament of atlas

纵束
longitudinal brands

椎间盘
intervertebral disk

椎体
vertebral body

横突
transverse process

85. 上部颈椎的韧带（后面观 3）
Ligaments of the upper cervical spine (posterior aspect 3)

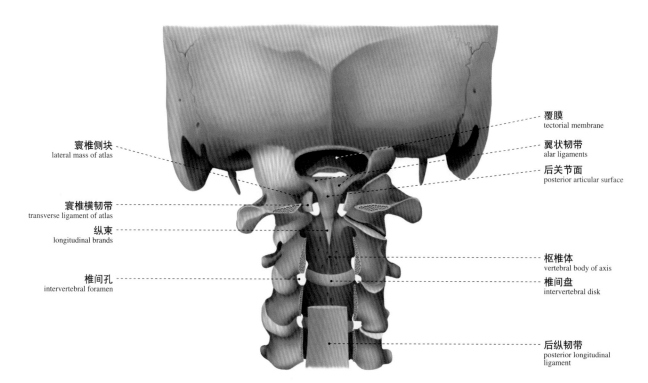

寰椎侧块
lateral mass of atlas

寰椎横韧带
transverse ligament of atlas

纵束
longitudinal brands

椎间孔
intervertebral foramen

覆膜
tectorial membrane

翼状韧带
alar ligaments

后关节面
posterior articular surface

枢椎体
vertebral body of axis

椎间盘
intervertebral disk

后纵韧带
posterior longitudinal
ligament

86. 上部颈椎的韧带（后面观 4）
Ligaments of the upper cervical spine (posterior aspect 4)

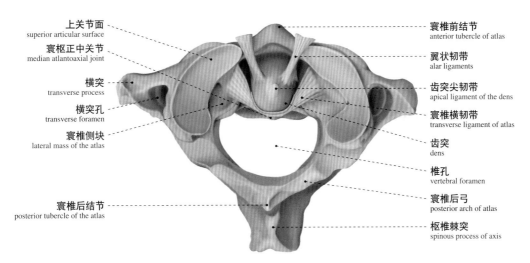

上关节面
superior articular surface

寰枢正中关节
median atlantoaxial joint

横突
transverse process

横突孔
transverse foramen

寰椎侧块
lateral mass of the atlas

寰椎后结节
posterior tubercle of the atlas

寰椎前结节
anterior tubercle of atlas

翼状韧带
alar ligaments

齿突尖韧带
apical ligament of the dens

寰椎横韧带
transverse ligament of atlas

齿突
dens

椎孔
vertebral foramen

寰椎后弓
posterior arch of atlas

枢椎棘突
spinous process of axis

87. 寰枢正中关节韧带
Ligaments of the median atlanto-axial joint

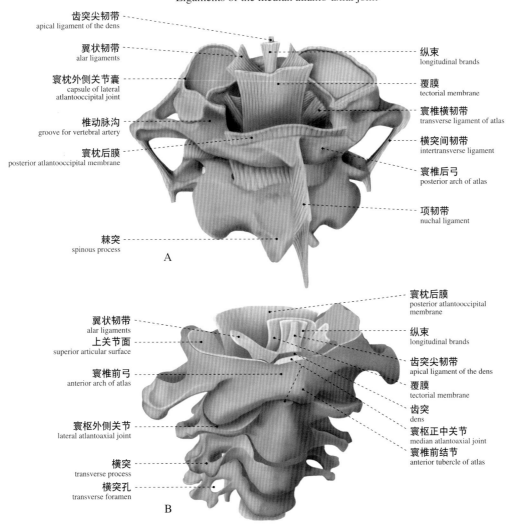

齿突尖韧带
apical ligament of the dens

翼状韧带
alar ligaments

寰枕外侧关节囊
capsule of lateral
atlantooccipital joint

椎动脉沟
groove for vertebral artery

寰枕后膜
posterior atlantooccipital membrane

棘突
spinous process

纵束
longitudinal brands

覆膜
tectorial membrane

寰椎横韧带
transverse ligament of atlas

横突间韧带
intertransverse ligament

寰椎后弓
posterior arch of atlas

项韧带
nuchal ligament

A

寰枕后膜
posterior atlantooccipital
membrane

纵束
longitudinal brands

齿突尖韧带
apical ligament of the dens

覆膜
tectorial membrane

齿突
dens

寰枢正中关节
median atlantoaxial joint

寰椎前结节
anterior tubercle of atlas

翼状韧带
alar ligaments

上关节面
superior articular surface

寰椎前弓
anterior arch of atlas

寰枢外侧关节
lateral atlantoaxial joint

横突
transverse process

横突孔
transverse foramen

B

88. 颅颈关节韧带
Ligaments of the craniovertebral joints

A. 后上面观；B. 前上面观

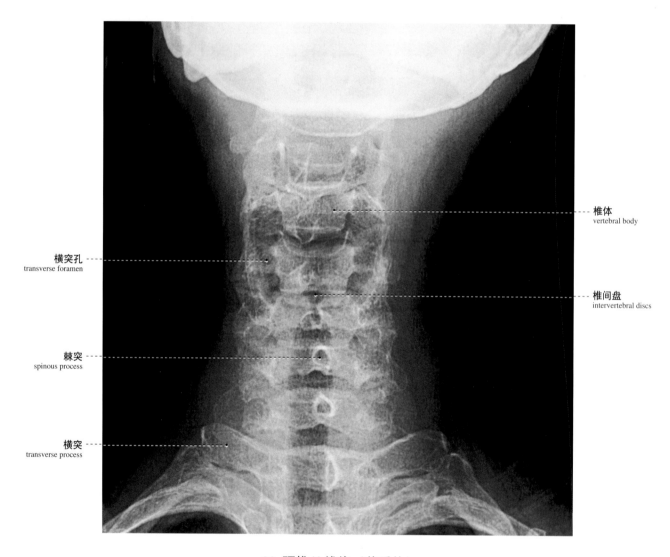

横突孔
transverse foramen

棘突
spinous process

横突
transverse process

椎体
vertebral body

椎间盘
intervertebral discs

89. 颈椎 X 线像（前后位）
Radiograph of the cervical vertebra (anteroposterior view)

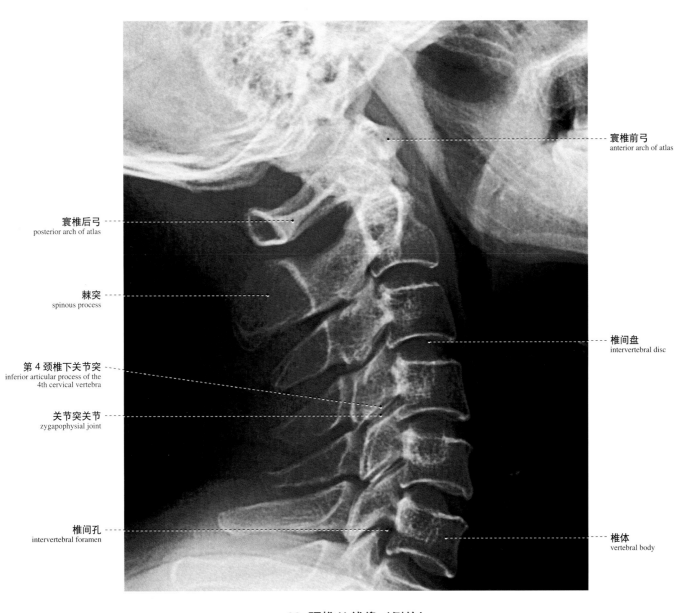

寰椎前弓
anterior arch of atlas

寰椎后弓
posterior arch of atlas

棘突
spinous process

第 4 颈椎下关节突
inferior articular process of the
4th cervical vertebra

关节突关节
zygapophysial joint

椎间盘
intervertebral disc

椎间孔
intervertebral foramen

椎体
vertebral body

90. 颈椎 X 线像（侧位）
Radiograph of the cervical vertebra (lateral view)

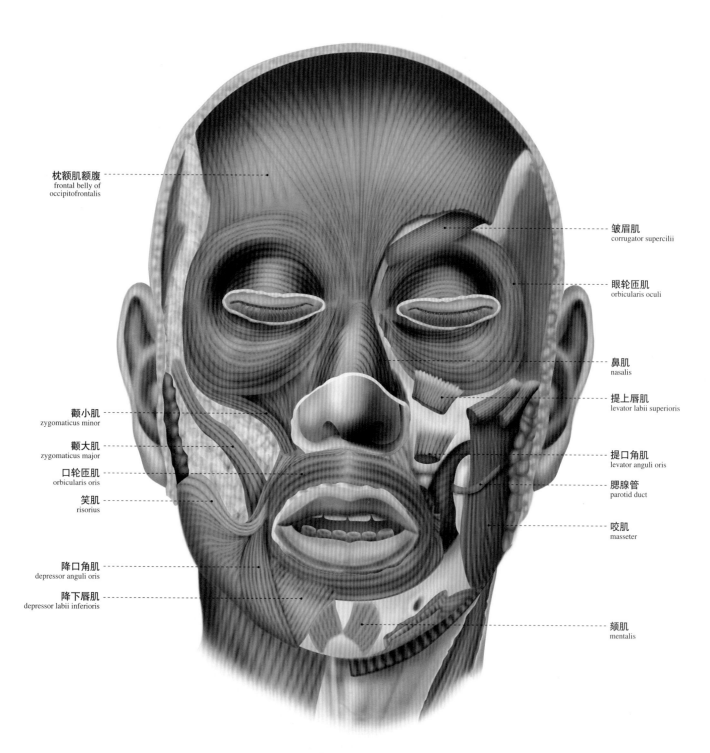

枕额肌额腹
frontal belly of
occipitofrontalis

皱眉肌
corrugator supercilii

眼轮匝肌
orbicularis oculi

鼻肌
nasalis

提上唇肌
levator labii superioris

颧小肌
zygomaticus minor

颧大肌
zygomaticus major

口轮匝肌
orbicularis oris

笑肌
risorius

提口角肌
levator anguli oris

腮腺管
parotid duct

咬肌
masseter

降口角肌
depressor anguli oris

降下唇肌
depressor labii inferioris

颏肌
mentalis

91. 头颈肌（前面观）
Muscles of the head and neck (anterior aspect)

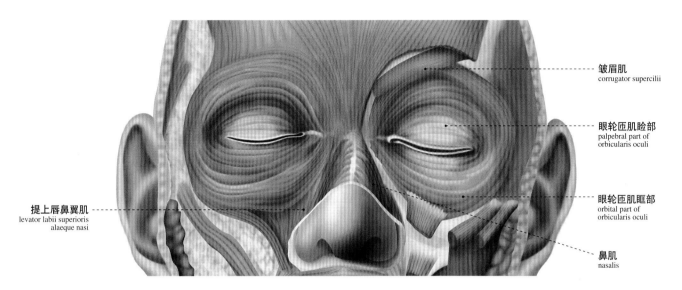

皱眉肌
corrugator supercilii

眼轮匝肌睑部
palpebral part of
orbicularis oculi

眼轮匝肌眶部
orbital part of
orbicularis oculi

鼻肌
nasalis

提上唇鼻翼肌
levator labii superioris
alaeque nasi

92. 眼部肌肉
Ocular muscles

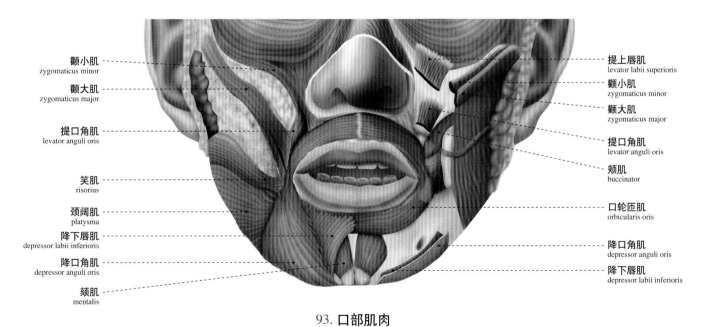

颧小肌
zygomaticus minor

颧大肌
zygomaticus major

提口角肌
levator anguli oris

笑肌
risorius

颈阔肌
platysma

降下唇肌
depressor labii inferioris

降口角肌
depressor anguli oris

颏肌
mentalis

提上唇肌
levator labii superioris

颧小肌
zygomaticus minor

颧大肌
zygomaticus major

提口角肌
levator anguli oris

颊肌
buccinator

口轮匝肌
orbicularis oris

降口角肌
depressor anguli oris

降下唇肌
depressor labii inferioris

93. 口部肌肉
Mouth muscles

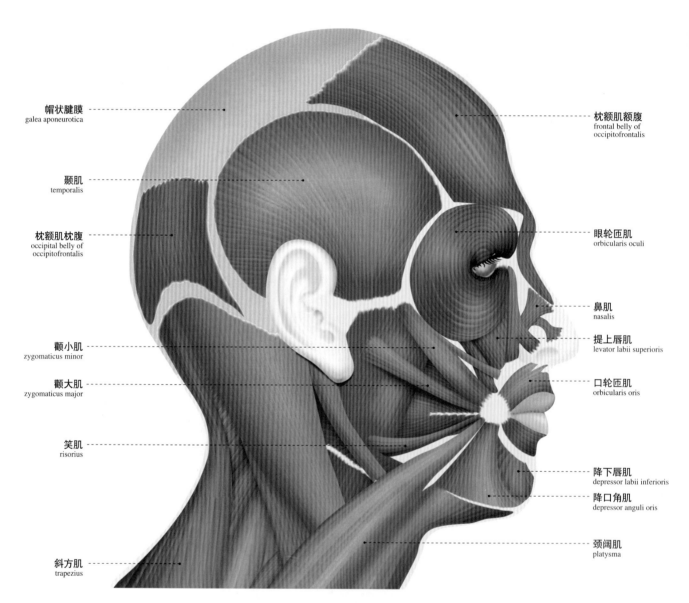

帽状腱膜
galea aponeurotica

颞肌
temporalis

枕额肌枕腹
occipital belly of
occipitofrontalis

颧小肌
zygomaticus minor

颧大肌
zygomaticus major

笑肌
risorius

斜方肌
trapezius

枕额肌额腹
frontal belly of
occipitofrontalis

眼轮匝肌
orbicularis oculi

鼻肌
nasalis

提上唇肌
levator labii superioris

口轮匝肌
orbicularis oris

降下唇肌
depressor labii inferioris

降口角肌
depressor anguli oris

颈阔肌
platysma

94. 头颈肌（侧面观）

Muscles of the head and neck (lateral aspect)

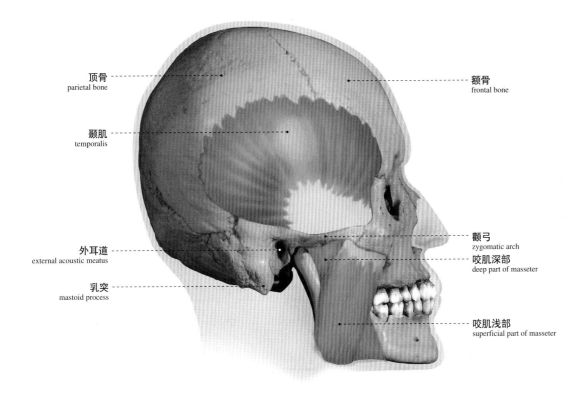

95. 咀嚼肌浅层（侧面观）
Superficial layer of the masticatory muscles (lateral aspect)

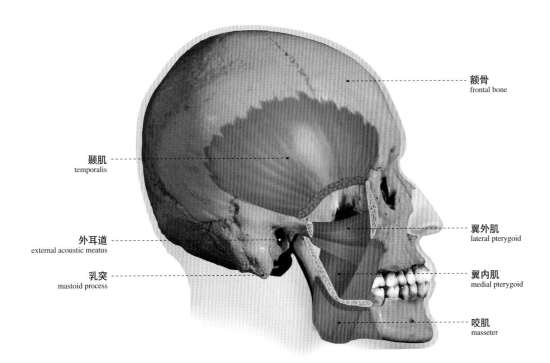

96. 咀嚼肌深层（侧面观）
Deep layer of the masticatory muscles (lateral aspect)

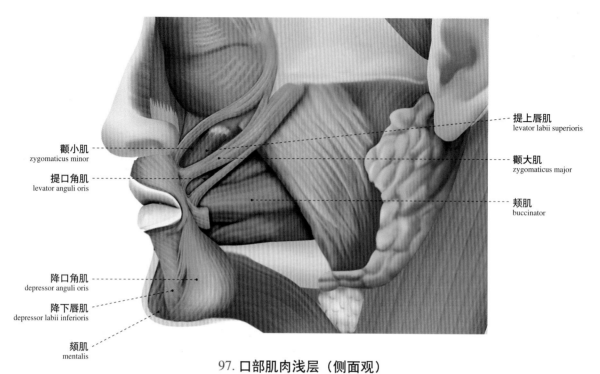

颧小肌
zygomaticus minor

提口角肌
levator anguli oris

降口角肌
depressor anguli oris

降下唇肌
depressor labii inferioris

颏肌
mentalis

提上唇肌
levator labii superioris

颧大肌
zygomaticus major

颊肌
buccinator

97. 口部肌肉浅层（侧面观）
Superficial layer of the mouth muscles (lateral aspect)

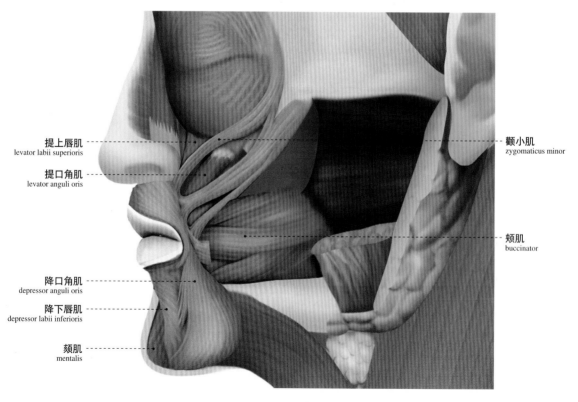

提上唇肌
levator labii superioris

提口角肌
levator anguli oris

降口角肌
depressor anguli oris

降下唇肌
depressor labii inferioris

颏肌
mentalis

颧小肌
zygomaticus minor

颊肌
buccinator

98. 口部肌肉深层（侧面观）
Deep layer of the mouth muscles (lateral aspect)

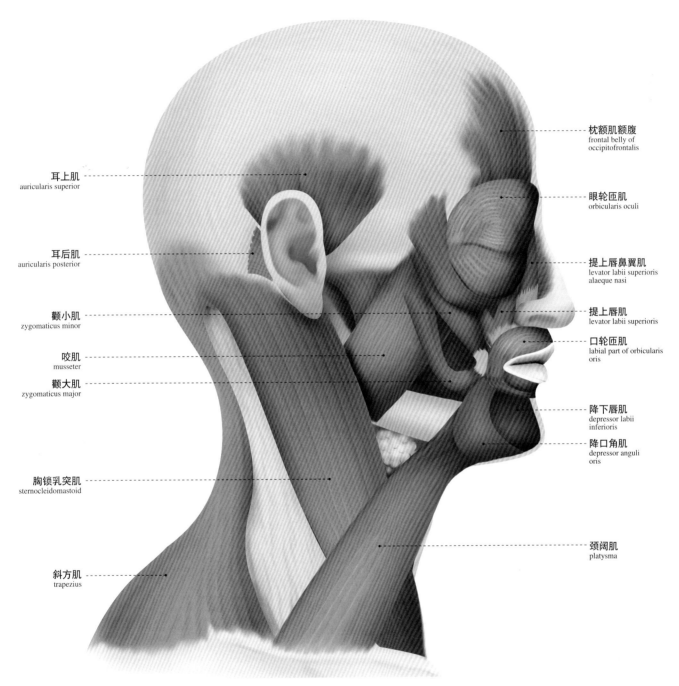

耳上肌
auricularis superior

耳后肌
auricularis posterior

颧小肌
zygomaticus minor

咬肌
musseter

颧大肌
zygomaticus major

胸锁乳突肌
sternocleidomastoid

斜方肌
trapezius

枕额肌额腹
frontal belly of
occipitofrontalis

眼轮匝肌
orbicularis oculi

提上唇鼻翼肌
levator labii superioris
alaeque nasi

提上唇肌
levator labii superioris

口轮匝肌
labial part of orbicularis
oris

降下唇肌
depressor labii
inferioris

降口角肌
depressor anguli
oris

颈阔肌
platysma

99. 面部表情肌（侧面观）
Muscles of facial expression (lateral aspect)

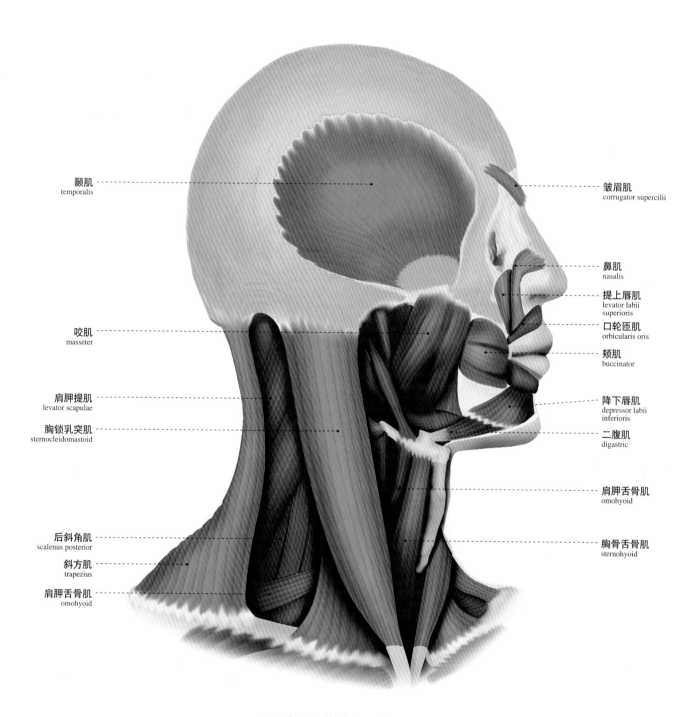

颞肌
temporalis

皱眉肌
corrugator supercilii

鼻肌
nasalis

提上唇肌
levator labii superioris

咬肌
masseter

口轮匝肌
orbicularis oris

颊肌
buccinator

肩胛提肌
levator scapulae

胸锁乳突肌
sternocleidomastoid

降下唇肌
depressor labii inferioris

二腹肌
digastric

肩胛舌骨肌
omohyoid

后斜角肌
scalenus posterior

斜方肌
trapezius

胸骨舌骨肌
sternohyoid

肩胛舌骨肌
omohyoid

100. 头颈肌的浅层（外侧面观）
Superficial layer of the muscles of the head and neck (lateral aspect)

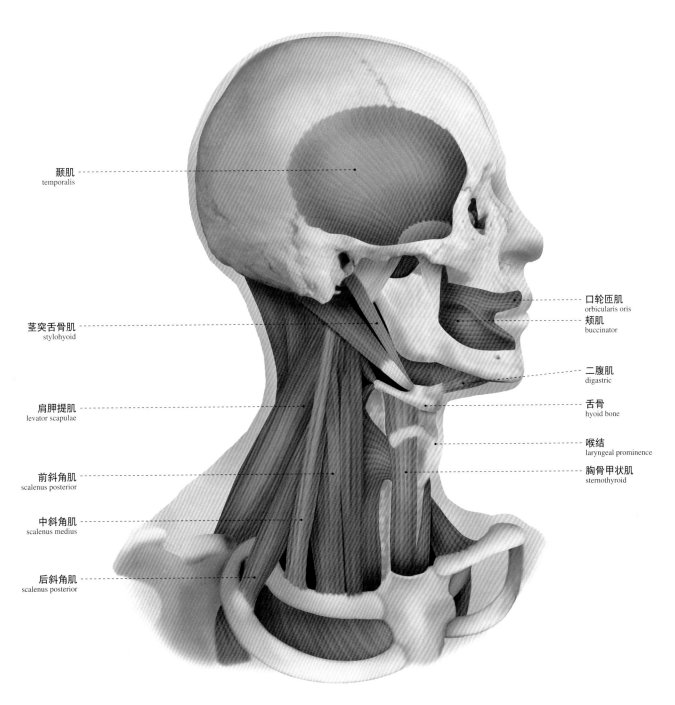

颞肌
temporalis

茎突舌骨肌
stylohyoid

肩胛提肌
levator scapulae

前斜角肌
scalenus posterior

中斜角肌
scalenus medius

后斜角肌
scalenus posterior

口轮匝肌
orbicularis oris

颊肌
buccinator

二腹肌
digastric

舌骨
hyoid bone

喉结
laryngeal prominence

胸骨甲状肌
sternothyroid

101. 头颈肌的深层（外侧面观）
Deep layer of the muscles of the head and neck (lateral aspect)

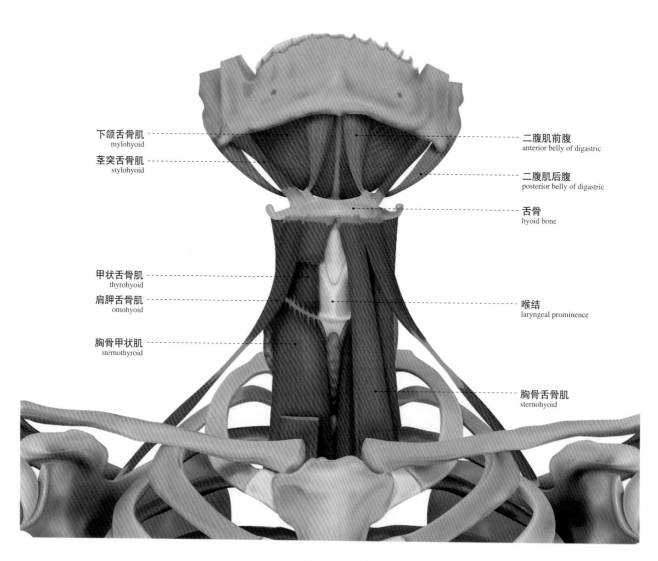

下颌舌骨肌
mylohyoid

茎突舌骨肌
stylohyoid

甲状舌骨肌
thyrohyoid

肩胛舌骨肌
omohyoid

胸骨甲状肌
sternothyroid

二腹肌前腹
anterior belly of digastric

二腹肌后腹
posterior belly of digastric

舌骨
hyoid bone

喉结
laryngeal prominence

胸骨舌骨肌
sternohyoid

102. 舌骨上下肌群（前面观）
Hyoid upper and lower muscles (anterior aspect)

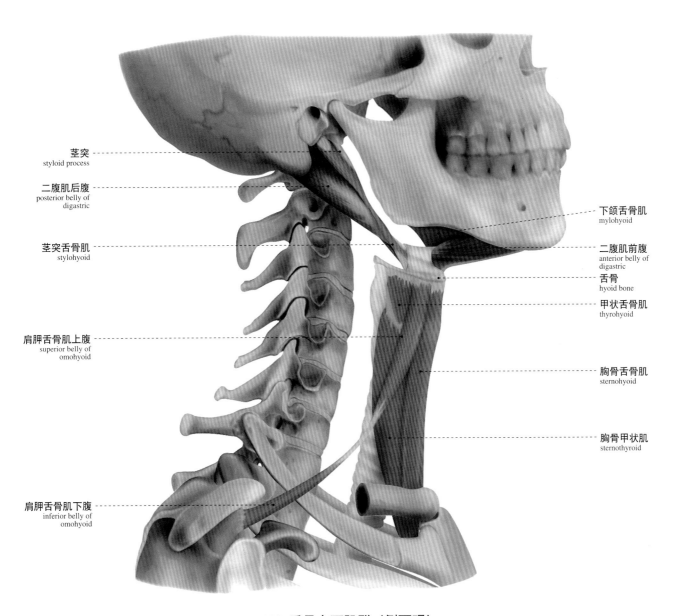

茎突
styloid process

二腹肌后腹
posterior belly of
digastric

茎突舌骨肌
stylohyoid

肩胛舌骨肌上腹
superior belly of
omohyoid

肩胛舌骨肌下腹
inferior belly of
omohyoid

下颌舌骨肌
mylohyoid

二腹肌前腹
anterior belly of
digastric

舌骨
hyoid bone

甲状舌骨肌
thyrohyoid

胸骨舌骨肌
sternohyoid

胸骨甲状肌
sternothyroid

103. 舌骨上下肌群（侧面观）
Hyoid upper and lower muscles (lateral aspect)

表1　头部肌肉

肌　名		起　点	止　点	主要作用	神经支配
面肌	枕额肌额腹	帽状腱膜	眉部皮肤	提眉，下牵皮肤	面神经
	枕额肌枕腹	上项线	帽状腱膜	后牵头皮	
	眼轮匝肌	围绕睑裂周围		闭合睑裂	
	口轮匝肌	围绕口裂周围		闭合口裂	
	提上唇肌	上唇上方的骨面	口角或唇的皮肤等	提口角与上唇	
	提口角肌				
	颧肌				
	降口角肌	下唇下方 下颌骨前面		提口角与上唇	
	降下唇肌				
	颊肌	面颊深层		使唇颊贴紧牙齿，帮助咀嚼和吸吮，牵口角向外侧	
咀嚼肌	咬肌	颧弓	下颌骨的咬肌粗隆	上提下颌（闭口）	三叉神经
	颞肌	颞窝	下颌骨冠突		
	翼内肌	翼窝	下颌骨内面的翼肌粗隆		
	翼外肌	翼突外侧面	下颌颈、颞下颌关节的关节盘等处	两侧收缩拉下颌向前（张口），单侧收缩拉下颌骨向对侧	

表2　颈部肌肉

肌　名			起　点	止　点	主要作用	神经支配
颈浅肌	颈外侧肌	颈阔肌	三角肌、胸大肌筋膜	口角	紧张颈部皮肤	面神经
		胸锁乳突肌	胸骨柄、锁骨的胸骨端	颞骨乳突	一侧收缩使头向同侧屈，两侧收缩使头向后仰	副神经
颈前肌	舌骨上肌群	二腹肌	后腹：乳突；前腹：下颌体	以中间腱附于舌骨体	降下颌骨，上提舌骨	前腹：三叉神经 后腹：面神经
		下颌舌骨肌	下颌体面	舌骨体	上提舌骨	三叉神经
		茎突舌骨肌	茎突	舌骨	上提舌骨	面神经
		颏舌骨肌	颏棘	舌骨	上提舌骨	第1颈神经前支
	舌骨下肌群	肩胛舌骨肌	与名称一致		下降舌骨	颈襻
		胸骨舌骨肌				
		胸骨甲状肌				
		甲状舌骨肌				
颈深肌	外侧群	前斜角肌	颈椎横突	第1肋上面	上提第1～2肋助吸气	颈神经前支
		中斜角肌				
		后斜角肌		第2肋上面		

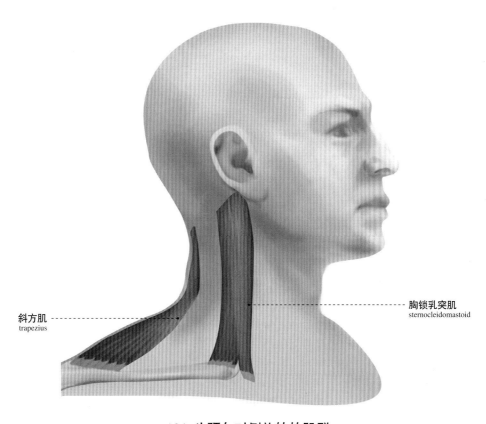

斜方肌
trapezius

胸锁乳突肌
sternocleidomastoid

104. 头颈向对侧旋转的肌群
Muscles of the contralateral rotation of the head and neck

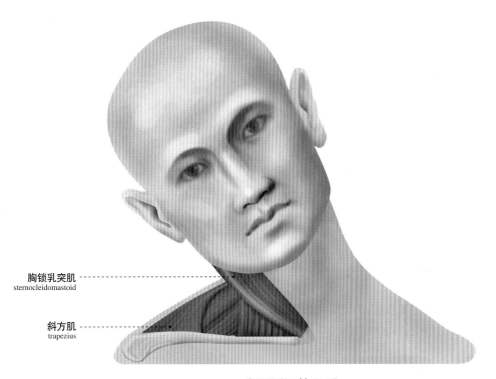

胸锁乳突肌
sternocleidomastoid

斜方肌
trapezius

105. 头颈侧屈的肌群
Muscles of the lateral flexion of the head and neck

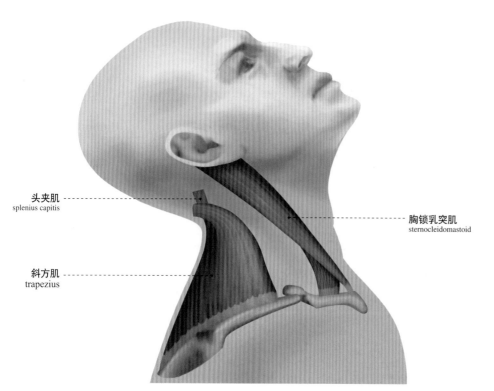

头夹肌
splenius capitis

斜方肌
trapezius

胸锁乳突肌
sternocleidomastoid

106. 头颈部的伸肌群
Stretch muscles of the head and neck

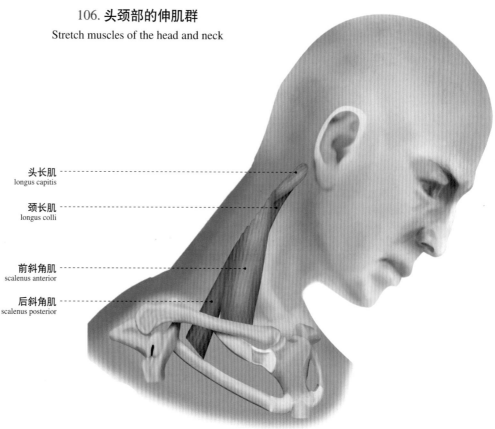

头长肌
longus capitis

颈长肌
longus colli

前斜角肌
scalenus anterior

后斜角肌
scalenus posterior

107. 头颈部的屈肌群
Flexor muscles of the head and neck

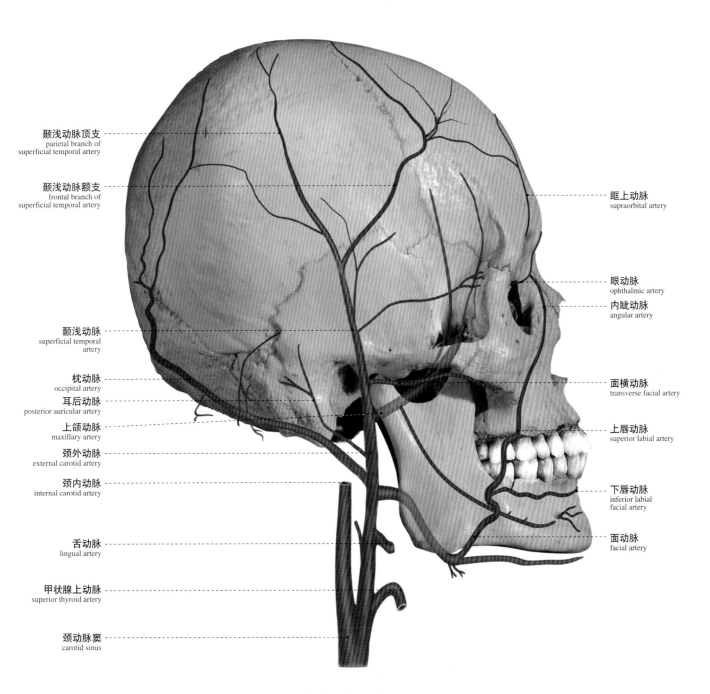

颞浅动脉顶支
parietal branch of
superficial temporal artery

颞浅动脉额支
frontal branch of
superficial temporal artery

颞浅动脉
superficial temporal
artery

枕动脉
occipital artery

耳后动脉
posterior auricular artery

上颌动脉
maxillary artery

颈外动脉
external carotid artery

颈内动脉
internal carotid artery

舌动脉
lingual artery

甲状腺上动脉
superior thyroid artery

颈动脉窦
carotid sinus

眶上动脉
supraorbital artery

眼动脉
ophthalmic artery

内眦动脉
angular artery

面横动脉
transverse facial artery

上唇动脉
superior labial artery

下唇动脉
inferior labial
facial artery

面动脉
facial artery

108. 颅的动脉（外侧面观）
Arteries of the skull (lateral aspect)

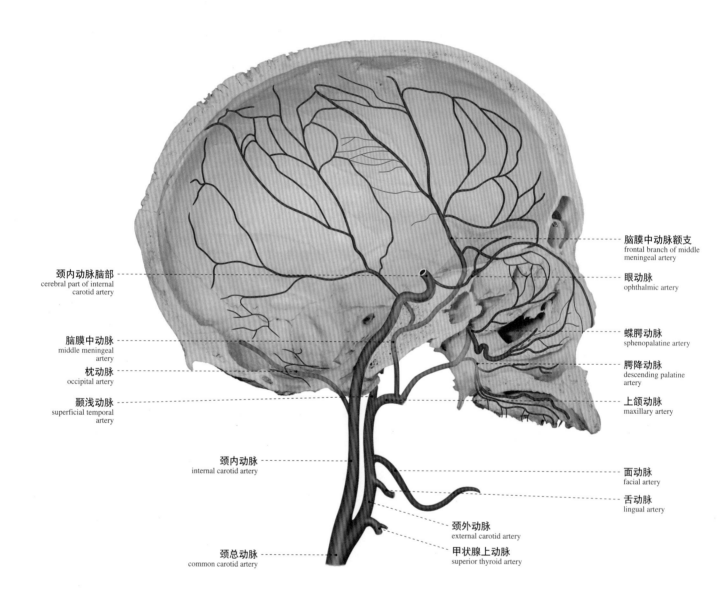

颈内动脉脑部
cerebral part of internal
carotid artery

脑膜中动脉
middle meningeal
artery

枕动脉
occipital artery

颞浅动脉
superficial temporal
artery

颈内动脉
internal carotid artery

颈总动脉
common carotid artery

脑膜中动脉额支
frontal branch of middle
meningeal artery

眼动脉
ophthalmic artery

蝶腭动脉
sphenopalatine artery

腭降动脉
descending palatine
artery

上颌动脉
maxillary artery

面动脉
facial artery

舌动脉
lingual artery

颈外动脉
external carotid artery

甲状腺上动脉
superior thyroid artery

109. 颅的动脉（内侧面观）
Arteries of the skull (medial aspect)

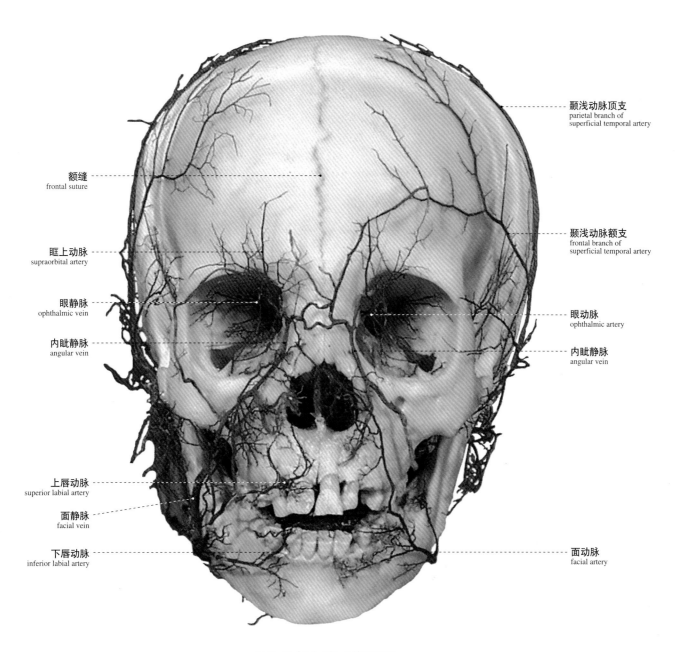

颞浅动脉顶支
parietal branch of
superficial temporal artery

额缝
frontal suture

颞浅动脉额支
frontal branch of
superficial temporal artery

眶上动脉
supraorbital artery

眼动脉
ophthalmic artery

眼静脉
ophthalmic vein

内眦静脉
angular vein

内眦静脉
angular vein

上唇动脉
superior labial artery

面静脉
facial vein

下唇动脉
inferior labial artery

面动脉
facial artery

110. 头部血管（前面观）
Blood vessels of the head (anterior aspect)

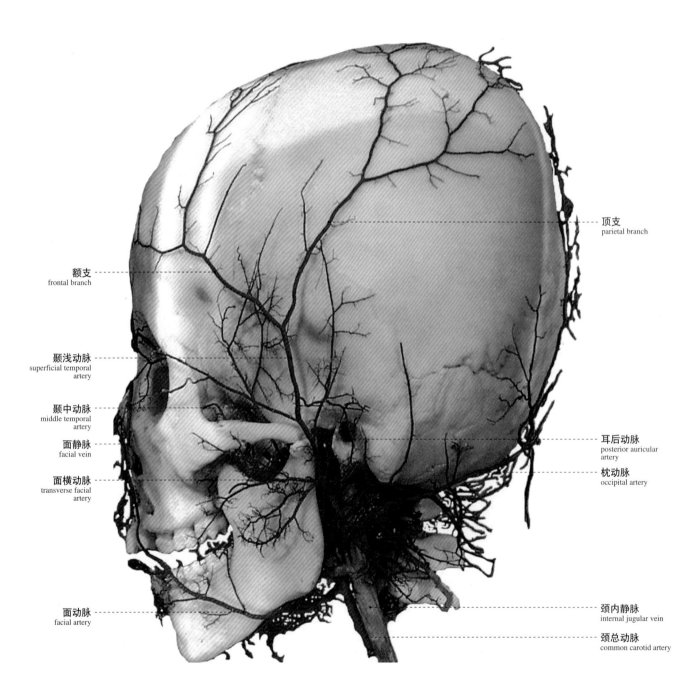

顶支
parietal branch

额支
frontal branch

颞浅动脉
superficial temporal
artery

颞中动脉
middle temporal
artery

面静脉
facial vein

面横动脉
transverse facial
artery

耳后动脉
posterior auricular
artery

枕动脉
occipital artery

面动脉
facial artery

颈内静脉
internal jugular vein

颈总动脉
common carotid artery

111. 头部血管（侧面观）
Blood vessels of the head (lateral aspect)

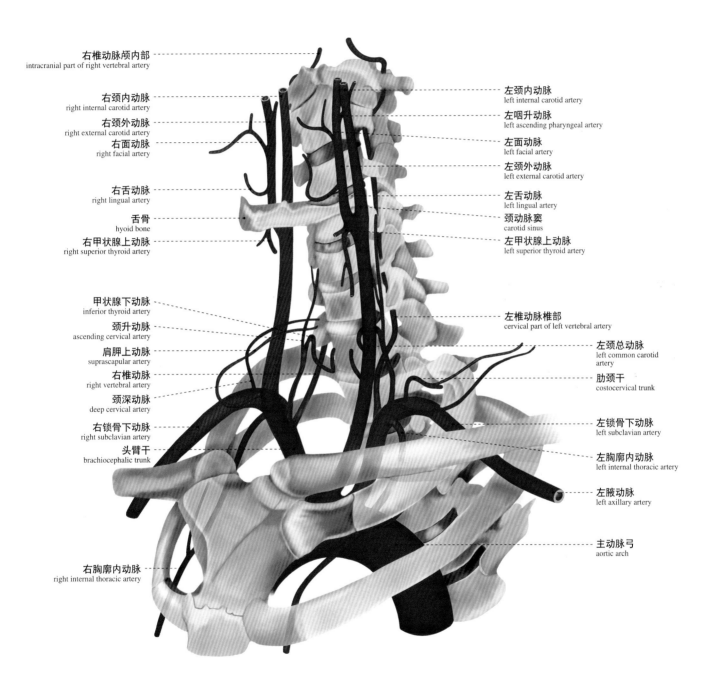

右椎动脉颅内部
intracranial part of right vertebral artery

右颈内动脉
right internal carotid artery

右颈外动脉
right external carotid artery

右面动脉
right facial artery

右舌动脉
right lingual artery

舌骨
hyoid bone

右甲状腺上动脉
right superior thyroid artery

甲状腺下动脉
inferior thyroid artery

颈升动脉
ascending cervical artery

肩胛上动脉
suprascapular artery

右椎动脉
right vertebral artery

颈深动脉
deep cervical artery

右锁骨下动脉
right subclavian artery

头臂干
brachiocephalic trunk

右胸廓内动脉
right internal thoracic artery

左颈内动脉
left internal carotid artery

左咽升动脉
left ascending pharyngeal artery

左面动脉
left facial artery

左颈外动脉
left external carotid artery

左舌动脉
left lingual artery

颈动脉窦
carotid sinus

左甲状腺上动脉
left superior thyroid artery

左椎动脉椎部
cervical part of left vertebral artery

左颈总动脉
left common carotid artery

肋颈干
costocervical trunk

左锁骨下动脉
left subclavian artery

左胸廓内动脉
left internal thoracic artery

左腋动脉
left axillary artery

主动脉弓
aortic arch

112. 颈部动脉（左前斜位观）
Arteries of the neck (left anterior oblique aspect)

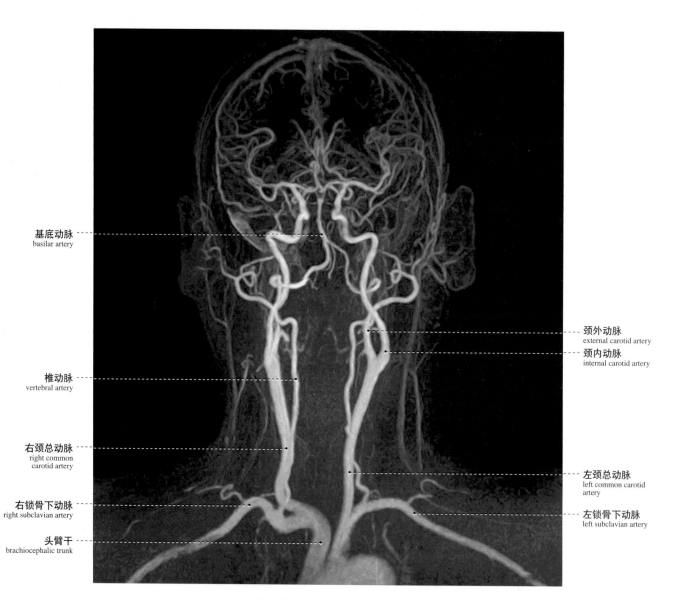

基底动脉
basilar artery

椎动脉
vertebral artery

右颈总动脉
right common
carotid artery

右锁骨下动脉
right subclavian artery

头臂干
brachiocephalic trunk

颈外动脉
external carotid artery

颈内动脉
internal carotid artery

左颈总动脉
left common carotid
artery

左锁骨下动脉
left subclavian artery

113. 头颈部数字减影血管造影（前后位）
DSA of the head and neck (anteroposterior view)

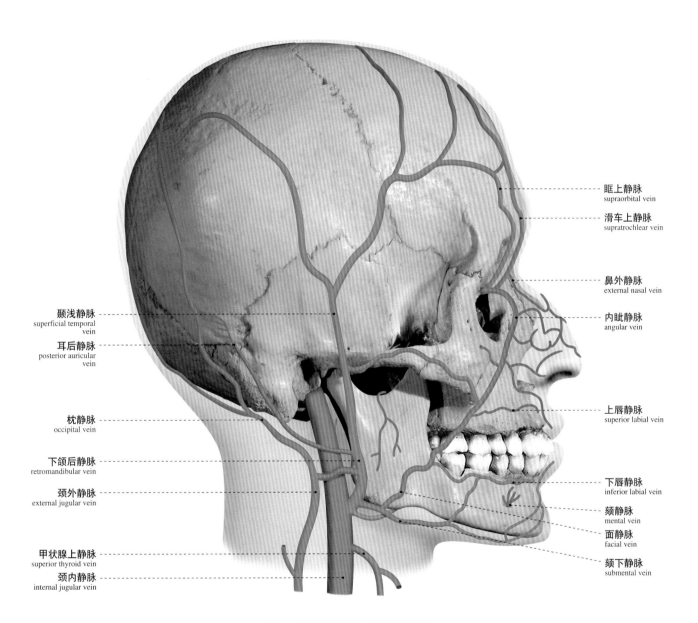

颞浅静脉
superficial temporal
vein

耳后静脉
posterior auricular
vein

枕静脉
occipital vein

下颌后静脉
retromandibular vein

颈外静脉
external jugular vein

甲状腺上静脉
superior thyroid vein

颈内静脉
internal jugular vein

眶上静脉
supraorbital vein

滑车上静脉
supratrochlear vein

鼻外静脉
external nasal vein

内眦静脉
angular vein

上唇静脉
superior labial vein

下唇静脉
inferior labial vein

颏静脉
mental vein

面静脉
facial vein

颏下静脉
submental vein

114. 头部浅静脉（侧面观 1）
Superficial veins of the head (lateral aspect 1)

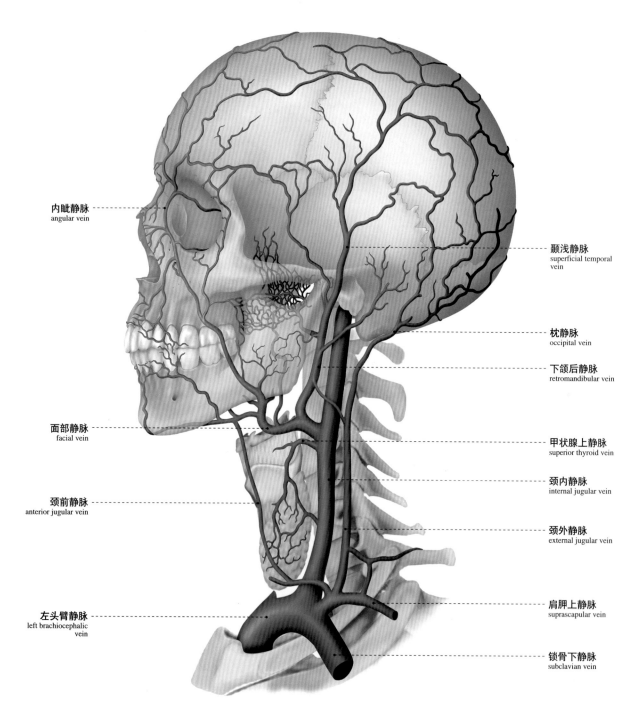

内眦静脉
angular vein

面部静脉
facial vein

颈前静脉
anterior jugular vein

左头臂静脉
left brachiocephalic
vein

颞浅静脉
superficial temporal
vein

枕静脉
occipital vein

下颌后静脉
retromandibular vein

甲状腺上静脉
superior thyroid vein

颈内静脉
internal jugular vein

颈外静脉
external jugular vein

肩胛上静脉
suprascapular vein

锁骨下静脉
subclavian vein

115. 头部浅静脉（侧面观 2）
Superficial veins of the head (lateral aspect 2)

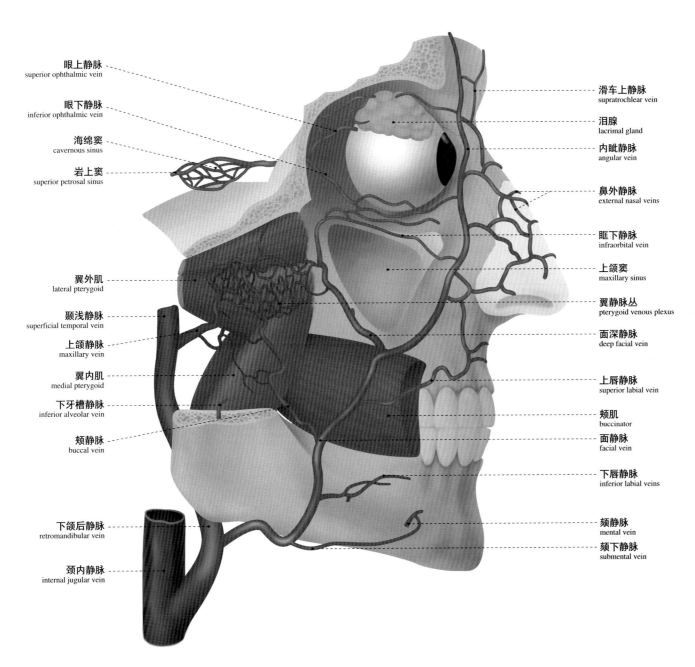

眼上静脉
superior ophthalmic vein

眼下静脉
inferior ophthalmic vein

海绵窦
cavernous sinus

岩上窦
superior petrosal sinus

翼外肌
lateral pterygoid

颞浅静脉
superficial temporal vein

上颌静脉
maxillary vein

翼内肌
medial pterygoid

下牙槽静脉
inferior alveolar vein

颊静脉
buccal vein

下颌后静脉
retromandibular vein

颈内静脉
internal jugular vein

滑车上静脉
supratrochlear vein

泪腺
lacrimal gland

内眦静脉
angular vein

鼻外静脉
external nasal veins

眶下静脉
infraorbital vein

上颌窦
maxillary sinus

翼静脉丛
pterygoid venous plexus

面深静脉
deep facial vein

上唇静脉
superior labial vein

颊肌
buccinator

面静脉
facial vein

下唇静脉
inferior labial veins

颏静脉
mental vein

颏下静脉
submental vein

116. 头部深静脉（侧面观）
Deep veins of the head (lateral aspect)

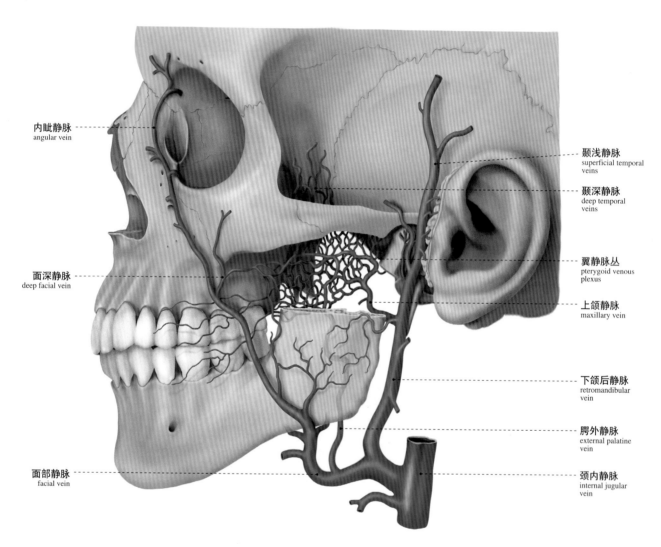

内眦静脉
angular vein

面深静脉
deep facial vein

面部静脉
facial vein

颞浅静脉
superficial temporal veins

颞深静脉
deep temporal veins

翼静脉丛
pterygoid venous plexus

上颌静脉
maxillary vein

下颌后静脉
retromandibular vein

腭外静脉
external palatine vein

颈内静脉
internal jugular vein

117. 头部深静脉（左侧面观）
Deep veins of the head (left lateral aspect)

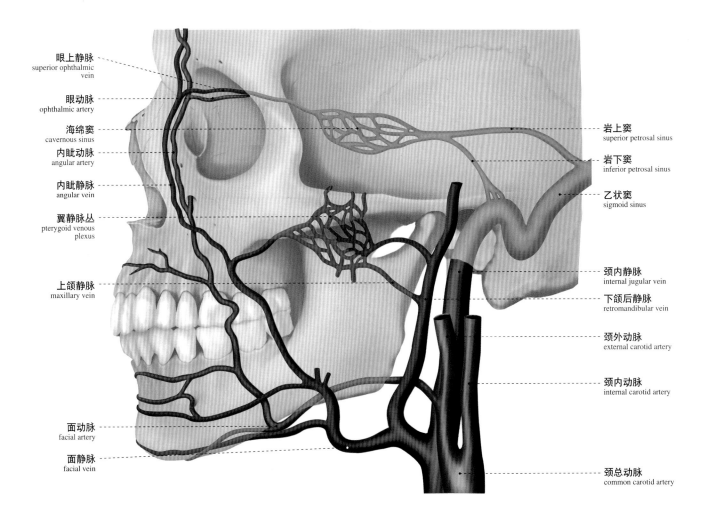

眼上静脉
superior ophthalmic vein

眼动脉
ophthalmic artery

海绵窦
cavernous sinus

内眦动脉
angular artery

内眦静脉
angular vein

翼静脉丛
pterygoid venous plexus

上颌静脉
maxillary vein

面动脉
facial artery

面静脉
facial vein

岩上窦
superior petrosal sinus

岩下窦
inferior petrosal sinus

乙状窦
sigmoid sinus

颈内静脉
internal jugular vein

下颌后静脉
retromandibular vein

颈外动脉
external carotid artery

颈内动脉
internal carotid artery

颈总动脉
common carotid artery

118. 面部血管（侧面观）
Facial blood vessels (lateral aspect)

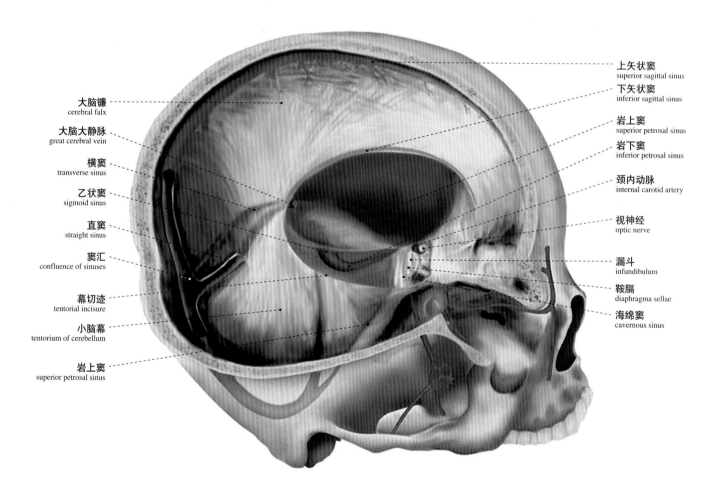

大脑镰
cerebral falx

大脑大静脉
great cerebral vein

横窦
transverse sinus

乙状窦
sigmoid sinus

直窦
straight sinus

窦汇
confluence of sinuses

幕切迹
tentorial incisure

小脑幕
tentorium of cerebellum

岩上窦
superior petrosal sinus

上矢状窦
superior sagittal sinus

下矢状窦
inferior sagittal sinus

岩上窦
superior petrosal sinus

岩下窦
inferior petrosal sinus

颈内动脉
internal carotid artery

视神经
optic nerve

漏斗
infundibulum

鞍膈
diaphragma sellae

海绵窦
cavernous sinus

119. 硬脑膜及硬脑膜静脉窦
Cerebral dura mater and the venous sinuses of the dura mater

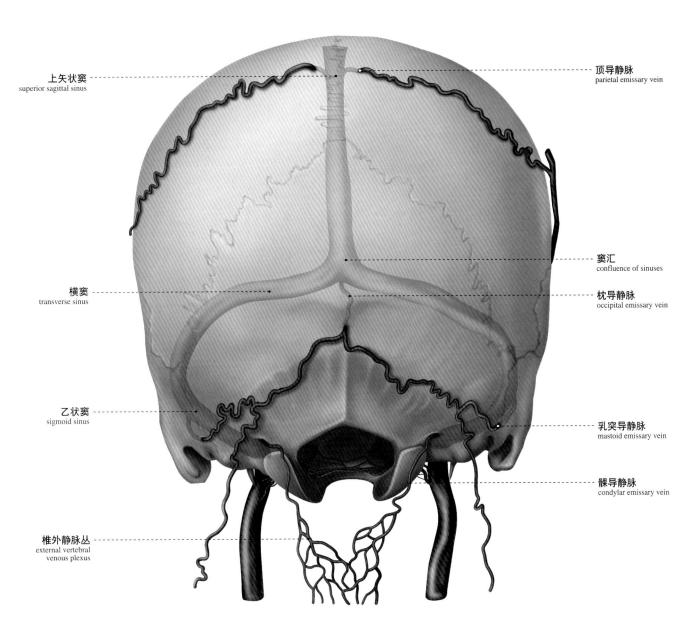

上矢状窦
superior sagittal sinus

顶导静脉
parietal emissary vein

窦汇
confluence of sinuses

横窦
transverse sinus

枕导静脉
occipital emissary vein

乙状窦
sigmoid sinus

乳突导静脉
mastoid emissary vein

髁导静脉
condylar emissary vein

椎外静脉丛
external vertebral
venous plexus

120. 枕部静脉
Veins of the occiput

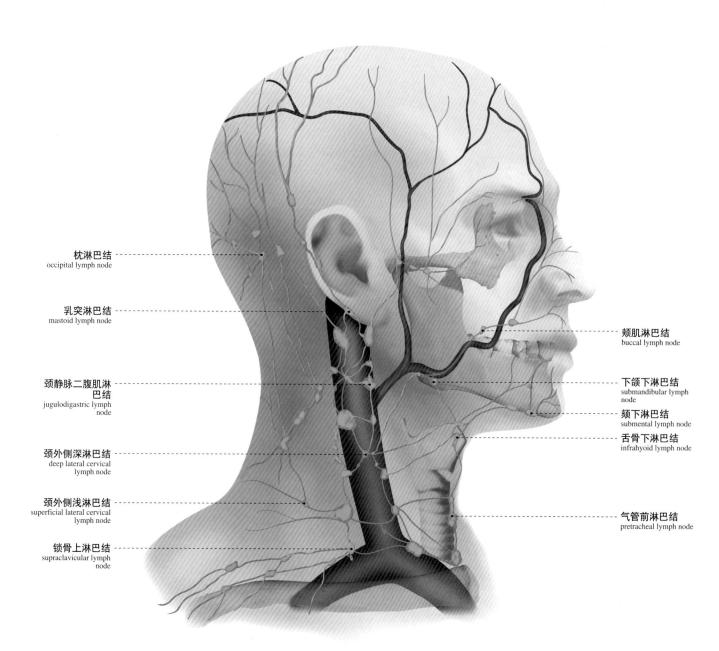

枕淋巴结
occipital lymph node

乳突淋巴结
mastoid lymph node

颈静脉二腹肌淋巴结
jugulodigastric lymph node

颈外侧深淋巴结
deep lateral cervical lymph node

颈外侧浅淋巴结
superficial lateral cervical lymph node

锁骨上淋巴结
supraclavicular lymph node

颊肌淋巴结
buccal lymph node

下颌下淋巴结
submandibular lymph node

颏下淋巴结
submental lymph node

舌骨下淋巴结
infrahyoid lymph node

气管前淋巴结
pretracheal lymph node

121. 头颈部淋巴管和淋巴结（侧面观）
Lymphatic vessels and lymph nodes of the head and neck (lateral aspect)

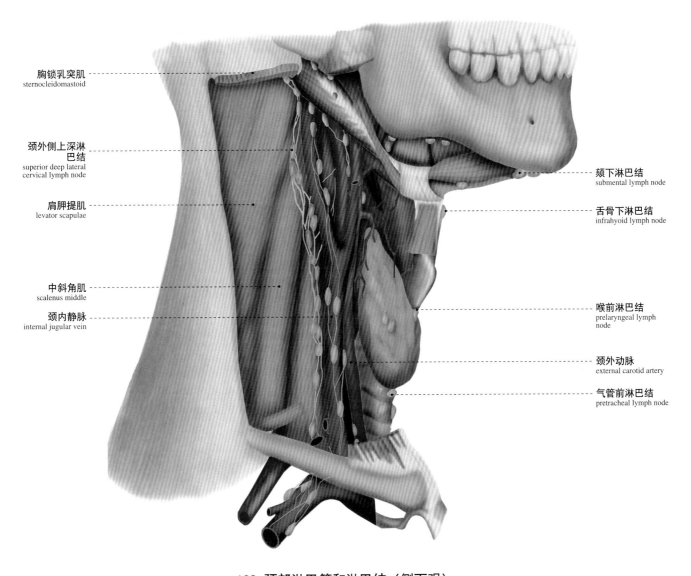

胸锁乳突肌
sternocleidomastoid

颈外侧上深淋巴结
superior deep lateral
cervical lymph node

肩胛提肌
levator scapulae

中斜角肌
scalenus middle

颈内静脉
internal jugular vein

颏下淋巴结
submental lymph node

舌骨下淋巴结
infrahyoid lymph node

喉前淋巴结
prelaryngeal lymph
node

颈外动脉
external carotid artery

气管前淋巴结
pretracheal lymph node

122. 颈部淋巴管和淋巴结（侧面观）
Lymphatic vessels and lymph nodes of the neck (lateral aspect)

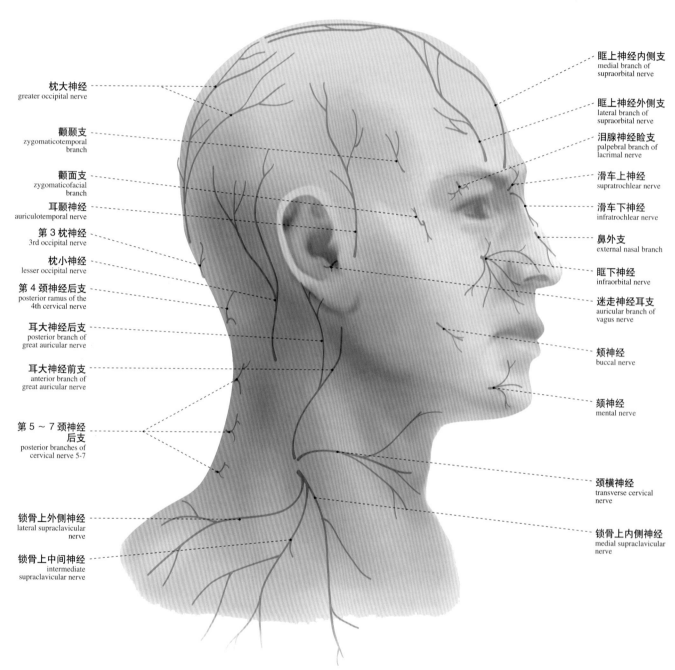

枕大神经
greater occipital nerve

颧颞支
zygomaticotemporal branch

颧面支
zygomaticofacial branch

耳颞神经
auriculotemporal nerve

第3枕神经
3rd occipital nerve

枕小神经
lesser occipital nerve

第4颈神经后支
posterior ramus of the 4th cervical nerve

耳大神经后支
posterior branch of great auricular nerve

耳大神经前支
anterior branch of great auricular nerve

第5～7颈神经后支
posterior branches of cervical nerve 5-7

锁骨上外侧神经
lateral supraclavicular nerve

锁骨上中间神经
intermediate supraclavicular nerve

眶上神经内侧支
medial branch of supraorbital nerve

眶上神经外侧支
lateral branch of supraorbital nerve

泪腺神经睑支
palpebral branch of lacrimal nerve

滑车上神经
supratrochlear nerve

滑车下神经
infratrochlear nerve

鼻外支
external nasal branch

眶下神经
infraorbital nerve

迷走神经耳支
auricular branch of vagus nerve

颊神经
buccal nerve

颏神经
mental nerve

颈横神经
transverse cervical nerve

锁骨上内侧神经
medial supraclavicular nerve

123. 头颈部皮神经
Cutaneous nerve of the head and neck

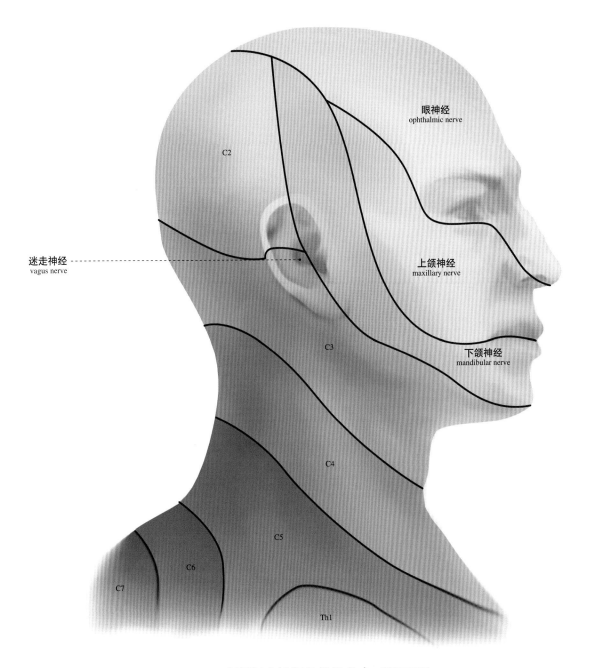

眼神经
ophthalmic nerve

C2

迷走神经
vagus nerve

上颌神经
maxillary nerve

下颌神经
mandibular nerve

C3

C4

C5

C6

C7

Th1

124. 头颈部皮神经节段性分布（侧面观）
Segmental distribution of cutaneous nerve of the head and neck (lateral aspect)

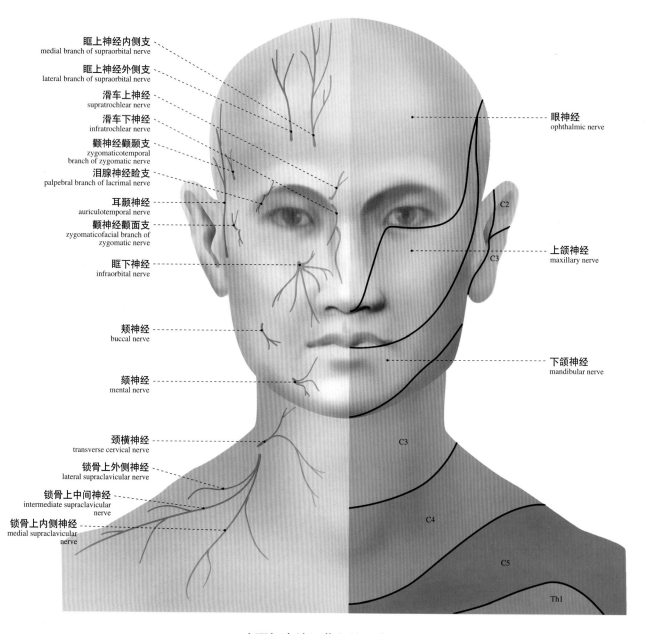

眶上神经内侧支
medial branch of supraorbital nerve

眶上神经外侧支
lateral branch of supraorbital nerve

滑车上神经
supratrochlear nerve

滑车下神经
infratrochlear nerve

颧神经颧颞支
zygomaticotemporal
branch of zygomatic nerve

泪腺神经睑支
palpebral branch of lacrimal nerve

耳颞神经
auriculotemporal nerve

颧神经颧面支
zygomaticofacial branch of
zygomatic nerve

眶下神经
infraorbital nerve

颊神经
buccal nerve

颏神经
mental nerve

颈横神经
transverse cervical nerve

锁骨上外侧神经
lateral supraclavicular nerve

锁骨上中间神经
intermediate supraclavicular
nerve

锁骨上内侧神经
medial supraclavicular
nerve

眼神经
ophthalmic nerve

上颌神经
maxillary nerve

下颌神经
mandibular nerve

C2

C3

C3

C4

C5

Th1

125. 头颈部皮神经节段性分布（前面观）
Cutaneous and segmental innervation of the head and neck (anterior aspect)

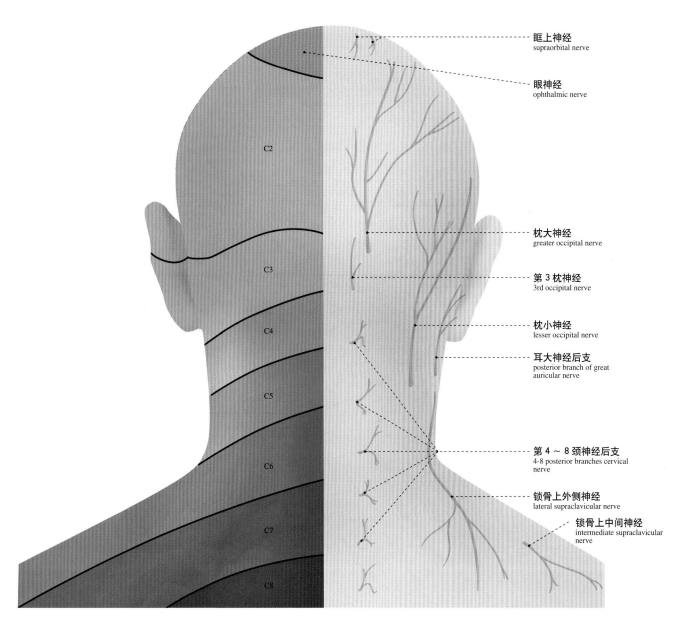

眶上神经
supraorbital nerve

眼神经
ophthalmic nerve

枕大神经
greater occipital nerve

第 3 枕神经
3rd occipital nerve

枕小神经
lesser occipital nerve

耳大神经后支
posterior branch of great auricular nerve

第 4 ～ 8 颈神经后支
4-8 posterior branches cervical nerve

锁骨上外侧神经
lateral supraclavicular nerve

锁骨上中间神经
intermediate supraclavicular nerve

126. 头颈部皮神经节段性分布（后面观）
Cutaneous and segmental innervation of the head and neck (posterior aspect)

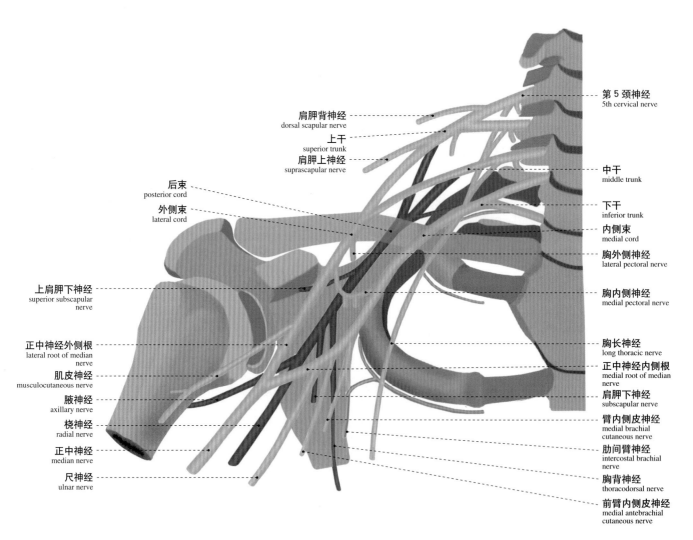

肩胛背神经
dorsal scapular nerve

上干
superior trunk

肩胛上神经
suprascapular nerve

第 5 颈神经
5th cervical nerve

中干
middle trunk

下干
inferior trunk

内侧束
medial cord

胸外侧神经
lateral pectoral nerve

后束
posterior cord

外侧束
lateral cord

胸内侧神经
medial pectoral nerve

上肩胛下神经
superior subscapular
nerve

胸长神经
long thoracic nerve

正中神经外侧根
lateral root of median
nerve

正中神经内侧根
medial root of median
nerve

肌皮神经
musculocutaneous nerve

肩胛下神经
subscapular nerve

腋神经
axillary nerve

臂内侧皮神经
medial brachial
cutaneous nerve

桡神经
radial nerve

肋间臂神经
intercostal brachial
nerve

正中神经
median nerve

胸背神经
thoracodorsal nerve

尺神经
ulnar nerve

前臂内侧皮神经
medial antebrachial
cutaneous nerve

127. 臂丛的组成和分支

Constitution and branches of the brachial plexus

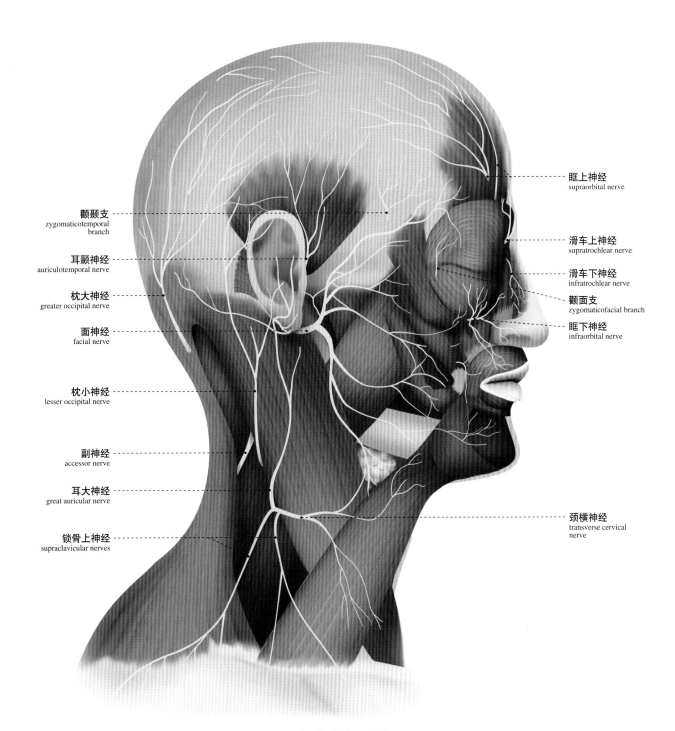

颧颞支
zygomaticotemporal
branch

耳颞神经
auriculotemporal nerve

枕大神经
greater occipital nerve

面神经
facial nerve

枕小神经
lesser occipital nerve

副神经
accessor nerve

耳大神经
great auricular nerve

锁骨上神经
supraclavicular nerves

眶上神经
supraorbital nerve

滑车上神经
supratrochlear nerve

滑车下神经
infratrochlear nerve

颧面支
zygomaticofacial branch

眶下神经
infraorbital nerve

颈横神经
transverse cervical
nerve

128. 头颈部感觉神经分布
Distribution of sensory nerves of the head and neck

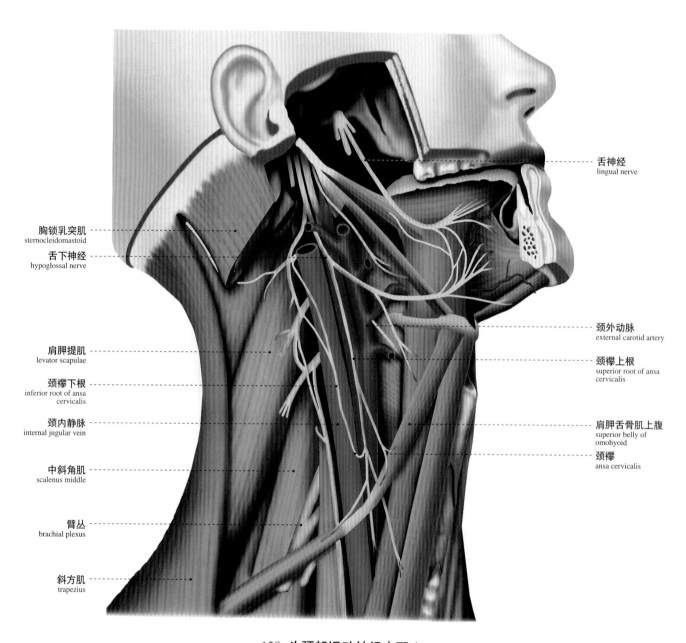

胸锁乳突肌
sternocleidomastoid

舌下神经
hypoglossal nerve

肩胛提肌
levator scapulae

颈襻下根
inferior root of ansa cervicalis

颈内静脉
internal jugular vein

中斜角肌
scalenus middle

臂丛
brachial plexus

斜方肌
trapezius

舌神经
lingual nerve

颈外动脉
external carotid artery

颈襻上根
superior root of ansa cervicalis

肩胛舌骨肌上腹
superior belly of omohyoid

颈襻
ansa cervicalis

129. 头颈部运动神经支配 1
Motor innervation of the head and neck 1

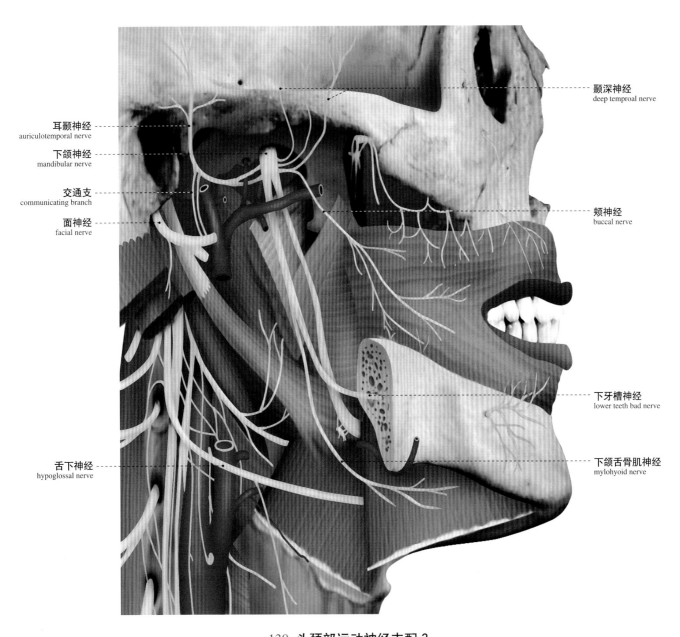

耳颞神经
auriculotemporal nerve

下颌神经
mandibular nerve

交通支
communicating branch

面神经
facial nerve

舌下神经
hypoglossal nerve

颞深神经
deep temproal nerve

颊神经
buccal nerve

下牙槽神经
lower teeth bad nerve

下颌舌骨肌神经
mylohyoid nerve

130. 头颈部运动神经支配 2
Motor innervation of the head and neck 2

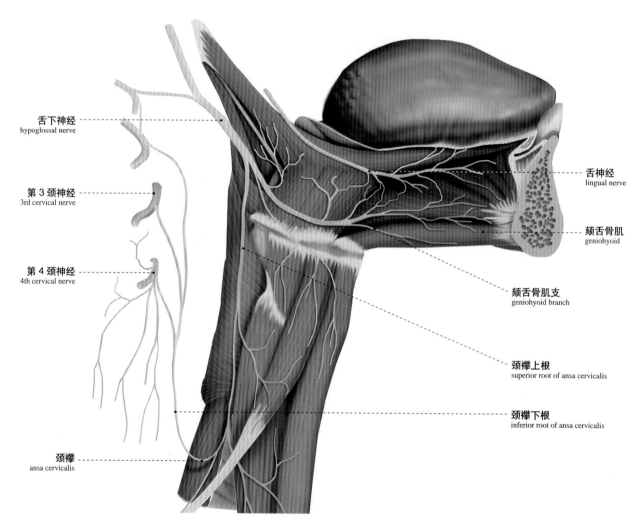

舌下神经
hypoglossal nerve

第 3 颈神经
3rd cervical nerve

第 4 颈神经
4th cervical nerve

颈襻
ansa cervicalis

舌神经
lingual nerve

颏舌骨肌
geniohyoid

颏舌骨肌支
geniohyoid branch

颈襻上根
superior root of ansa cervicalis

颈襻下根
inferior root of ansa cervicalis

131. 头颈部运动神经支配 3
Motor innervation of the head and neck 3

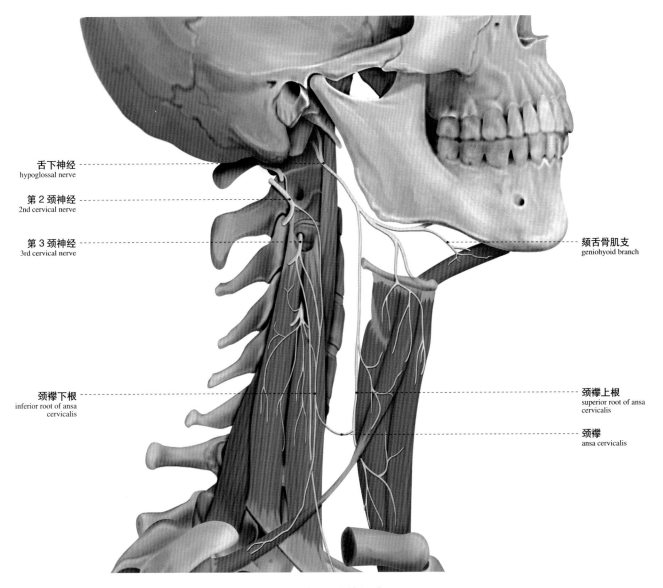

舌下神经
hypoglossal nerve

第 2 颈神经
2nd cervical nerve

第 3 颈神经
3rd cervical nerve

颏舌骨肌支
geniohyoid branch

颈襻下根
inferior root of ansa
cervicalis

颈襻上根
superior root of ansa
cervicalis

颈襻
ansa cervicalis

132. 头颈部运动神经支配 4

Motor innervation of the head and neck 4

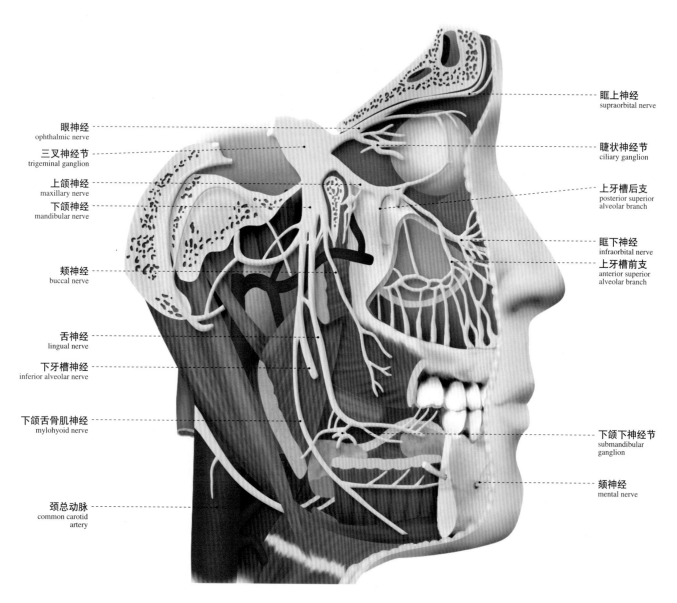

眼神经
ophthalmic nerve

三叉神经节
trigeminal ganglion

上颌神经
maxillary nerve

下颌神经
mandibular nerve

颊神经
buccal nerve

舌神经
lingual nerve

下牙槽神经
inferior alveolar nerve

下颌舌骨肌神经
mylohyoid nerve

颈总动脉
common carotid artery

眶上神经
supraorbital nerve

睫状神经节
ciliary ganglion

上牙槽后支
posterior superior alveolar branch

眶下神经
infraorbital nerve

上牙槽前支
anterior superior alveolar branch

下颌下神经节
submandibular ganglion

颏神经
mental nerve

133. 三叉神经及其分支
Trigeminal nerve and its branches

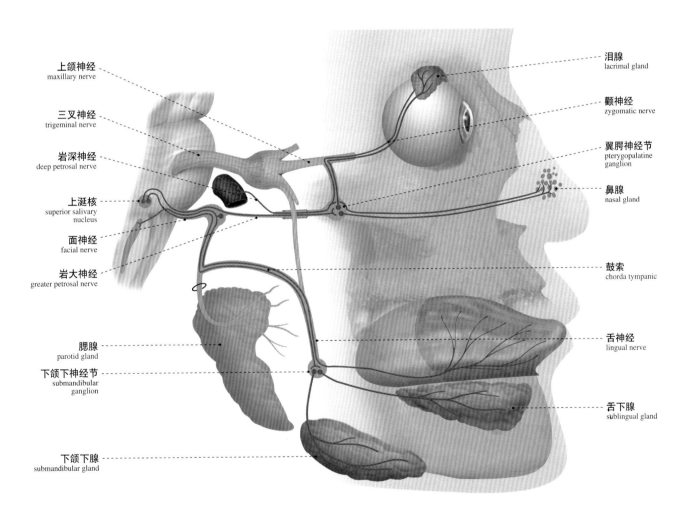

上颌神经
maxillary nerve

三叉神经
trigeminal nerve

岩深神经
deep petrosal nerve

上涎核
superior salivary nucleus

面神经
facial nerve

岩大神经
greater petrosal nerve

腮腺
parotid gland

下颌下神经节
submandibular ganglion

下颌下腺
submandibular gland

泪腺
lacrimal gland

颧神经
zygomatic nerve

翼腭神经节
pterygopalatine ganglion

鼻腺
nasal gland

鼓索
chorda tympanic

舌神经
lingual nerve

舌下腺
sublingual gland

134. 面神经的副交感纤维
Parasympathetic fibers of the facial nerve

第二章

面 部

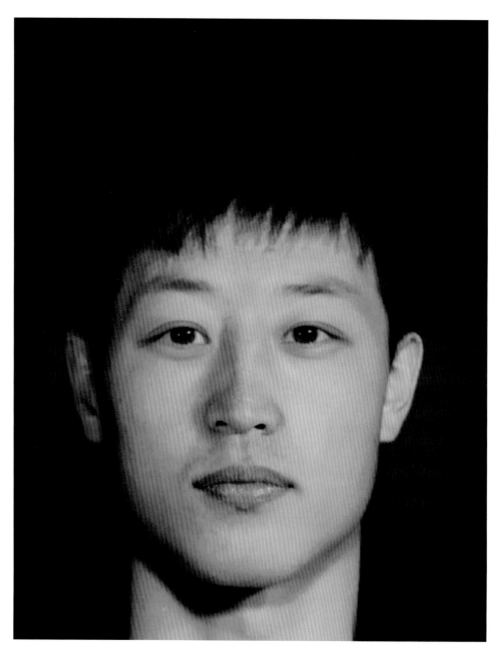

135. 面部体表（前面观）
Facial surface (anterior aspect)

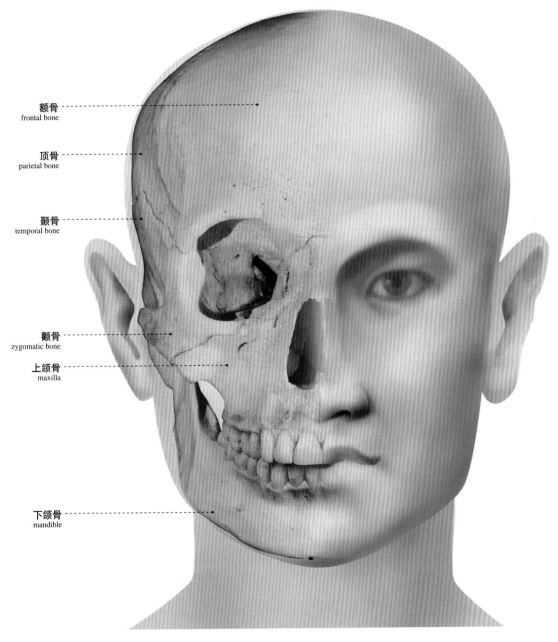

额骨
frontal bone

顶骨
parietal bone

颞骨
temporal bone

颧骨
zygomatic bone

上颌骨
maxilla

下颌骨
mandible

136. 面部骨骼与面部体表对照（前面观）
Comparison of the facial bones and the facial surface (anterior aspect)

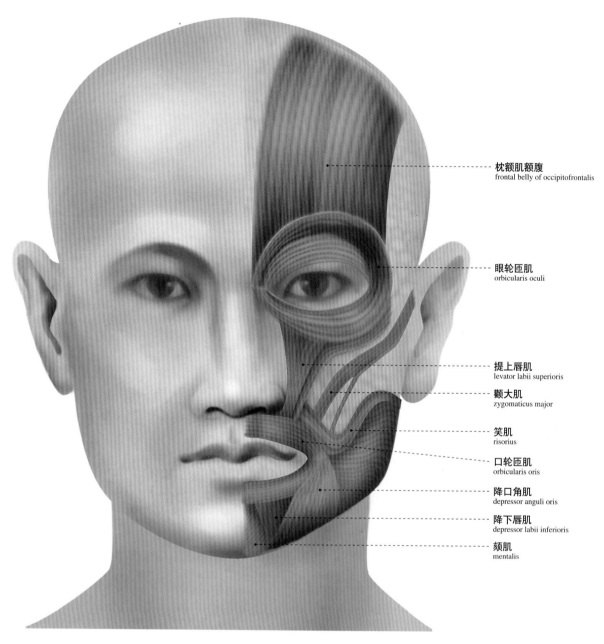

枕额肌额腹
frontal belly of occipitofrontalis

眼轮匝肌
orbicularis oculi

提上唇肌
levator labii superioris

颧大肌
zygomaticus major

笑肌
risorius

口轮匝肌
orbicularis oris

降口角肌
depressor anguli oris

降下唇肌
depressor labii inferioris

颏肌
mentalis

137. 面部肌肉与面部体表对照（前面观）
Comparison of the facial muscles and the facial surface (anterior aspect)

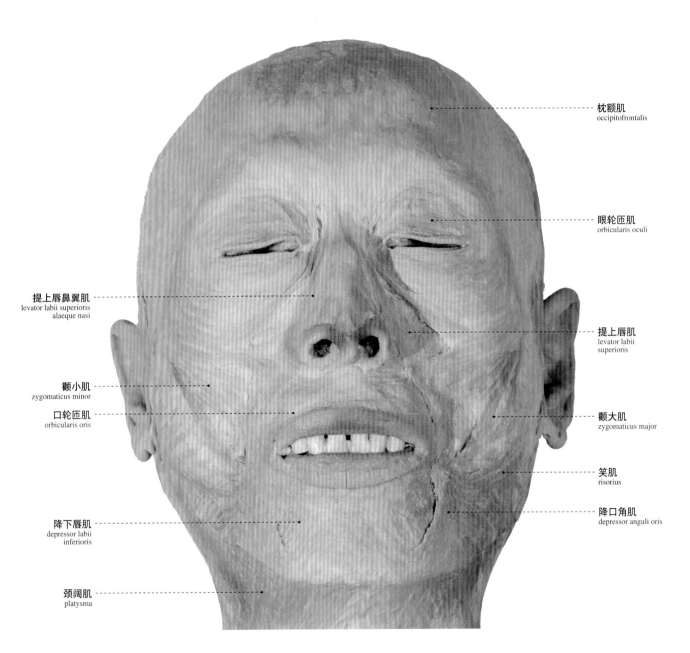

枕额肌
occipitofrontalis

眼轮匝肌
orbicularis oculi

提上唇鼻翼肌
levator labii superioris
alaeque nasi

提上唇肌
levator labii
superioris

颧小肌
zygomaticus minor

颧大肌
zygomaticus major

口轮匝肌
orbicularis oris

笑肌
risorius

降口角肌
depressor anguli oris

降下唇肌
depressor labii
inferioris

颈阔肌
platysma

138. 面部肌肉（前面观）
Muscles of the face (anterior aspect)

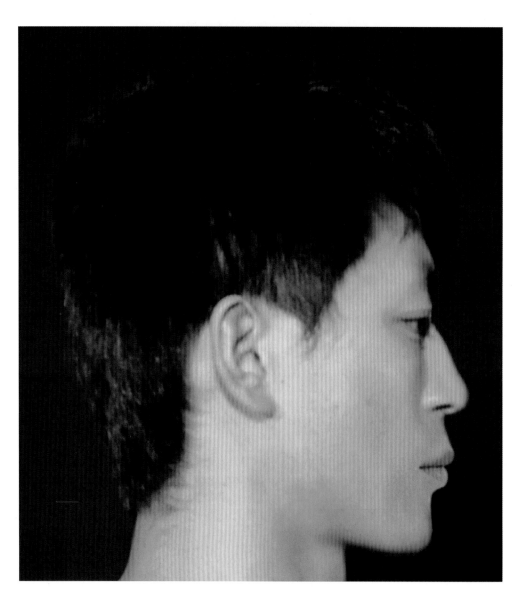

139. 面部体表（侧面观）
Facial surface (lateral aspect)

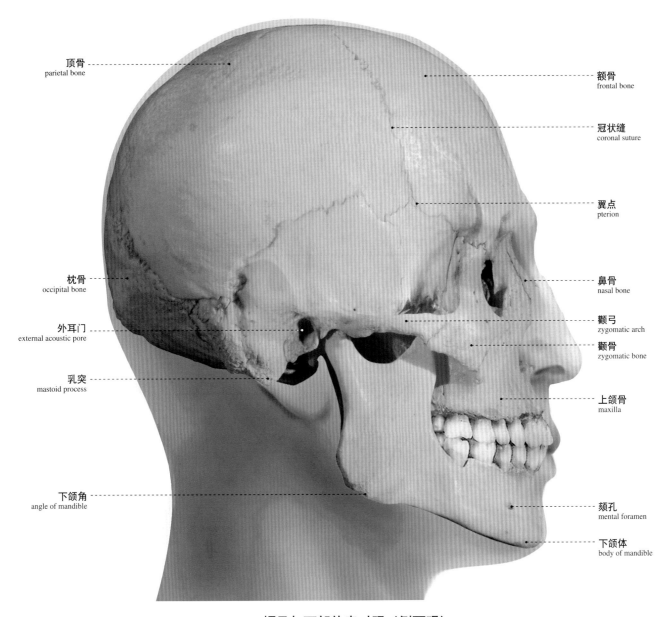

顶骨
parietal bone

额骨
frontal bone

冠状缝
coronal suture

翼点
pterion

枕骨
occipital bone

鼻骨
nasal bone

外耳门
external acoustic pore

颧弓
zygomatic arch

颧骨
zygomatic bone

乳突
mastoid process

上颌骨
maxilla

下颌角
angle of mandible

颏孔
mental foramen

下颌体
body of mandible

140. 颅骨与面部体表对照（侧面观）
Comparison of the skull and the facial surface (lateral aspect)

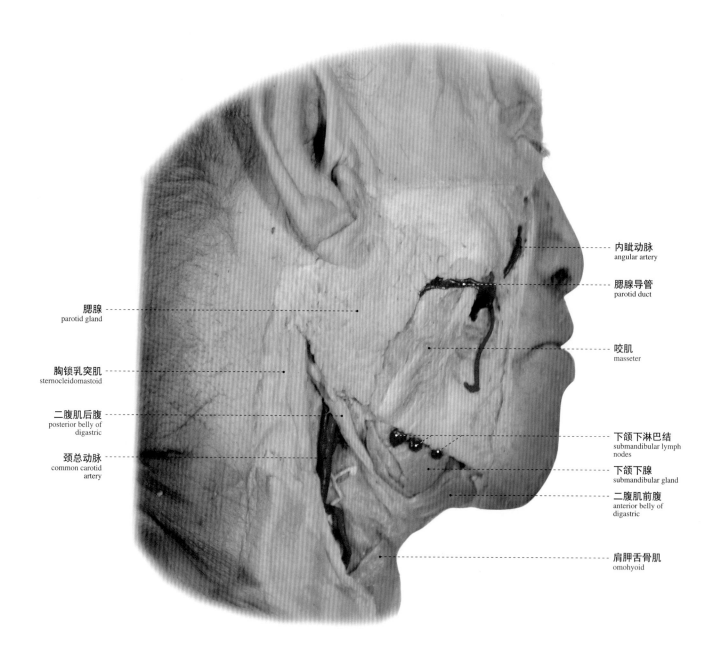

内眦动脉
angular artery

腮腺导管
parotid duct

咬肌
masseter

下颌下淋巴结
submandibular lymph nodes

下颌下腺
submandibular gland

二腹肌前腹
anterior belly of digastric

肩胛舌骨肌
omohyoid

腮腺
parotid gland

胸锁乳突肌
sternocleidomastoid

二腹肌后腹
posterior belly of digastric

颈总动脉
common carotid artery

141. 面部局部解剖（侧面观 1）
Facial topography (lateral aspect 1)

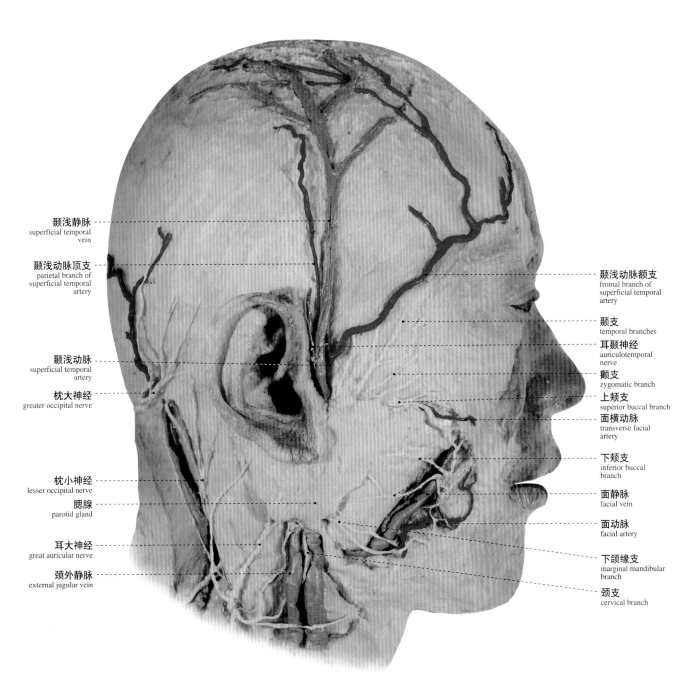

颞浅静脉
superficial temporal vein

颞浅动脉顶支
parietal branch of superficial temporal artery

颞浅动脉
superficial temporal artery

枕大神经
greater occipital nerve

枕小神经
lesser occipital nerve

腮腺
parotid gland

耳大神经
great auricular nerve

颈外静脉
external jugular vein

颞浅动脉额支
frontal branch of superficial temporal artery

颞支
temporal branches

耳颞神经
auriculotemporal nerve

颧支
zygomatic branch

上颊支
superior buccal branch

面横动脉
transverse facial artery

下颊支
inferior buccal branch

面静脉
facial vein

面动脉
facial artery

下颌缘支
marginal mandibular branch

颈支
cervical branch

142. 面部局部解剖（侧面观 2）
Facial topography (lateral aspect 2)

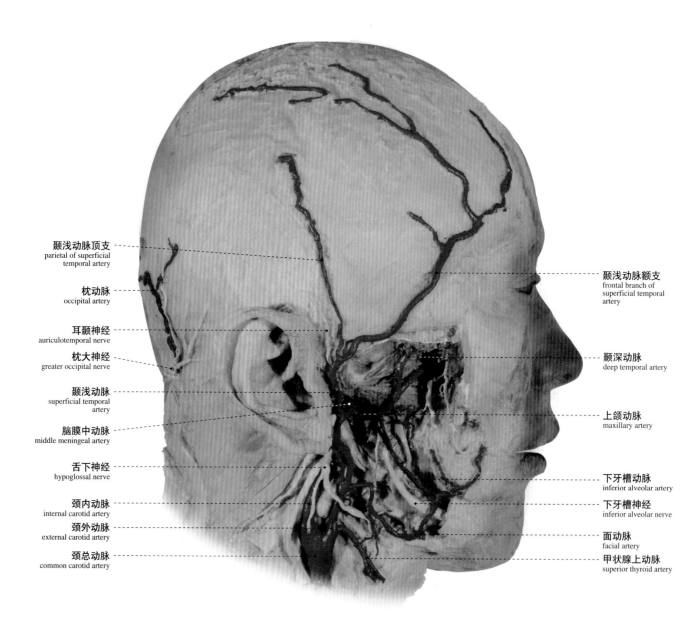

颞浅动脉顶支
parietal of superficial
temporal artery

枕动脉
occipital artery

耳颞神经
auriculotemporal nerve

枕大神经
greater occipital nerve

颞浅动脉
superficial temporal
artery

脑膜中动脉
middle meningeal artery

舌下神经
hypoglossal nerve

颈内动脉
internal carotid artery

颈外动脉
external carotid artery

颈总动脉
common carotid artery

颞浅动脉额支
frontal branch of
superficial temporal
artery

颞深动脉
deep temporal artery

上颌动脉
maxillary artery

下牙槽动脉
inferior alveolar artery

下牙槽神经
inferior alveolar nerve

面动脉
facial artery

甲状腺上动脉
superior thyroid artery

143. 面部局部解剖（侧面观 3）
Facial topography (lateral aspect 3)

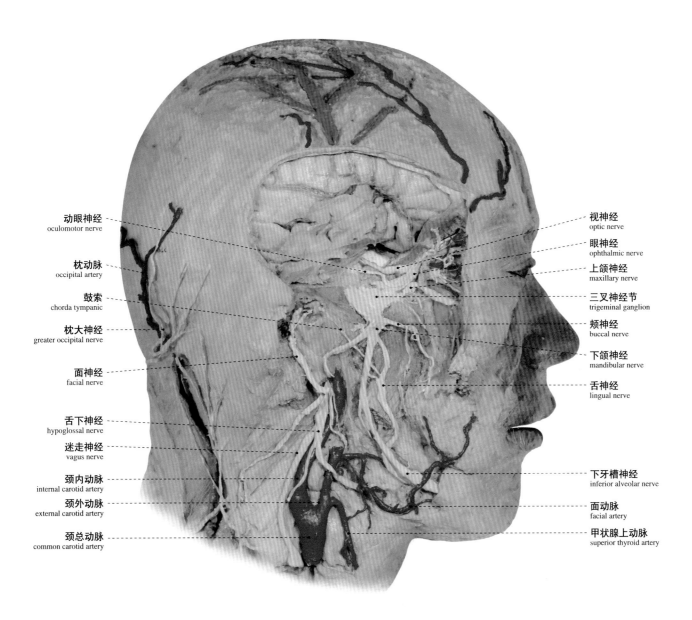

动眼神经
oculomotor nerve

枕动脉
occipital artery

鼓索
chorda tympanic

枕大神经
greater occipital nerve

面神经
facial nerve

舌下神经
hypoglossal nerve

迷走神经
vagus nerve

颈内动脉
internal carotid artery

颈外动脉
external carotid artery

颈总动脉
common carotid artery

视神经
optic nerve

眼神经
ophthalmic nerve

上颌神经
maxillary nerve

三叉神经节
trigeminal ganglion

颊神经
buccal nerve

下颌神经
mandibular nerve

舌神经
lingual nerve

下牙槽神经
inferior alveolar nerve

面动脉
facial artery

甲状腺上动脉
superior thyroid artery

144. 面部局部解剖（侧面观 4）
Facial topography (lateral aspect 4)

颈 部

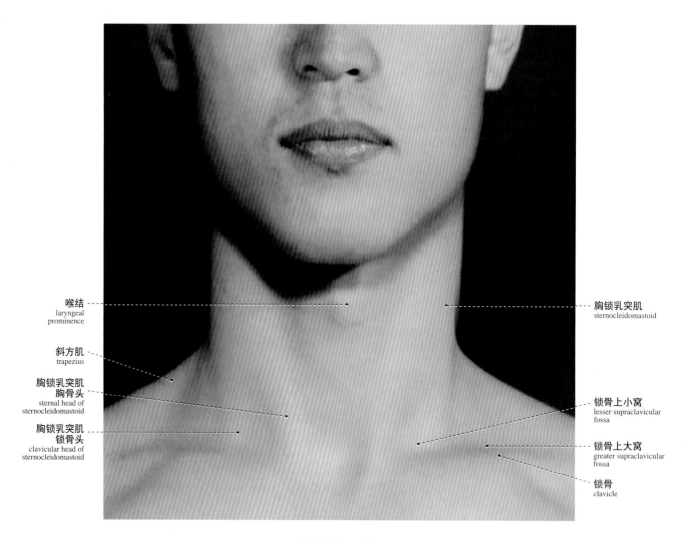

喉结
laryngeal prominence

斜方肌
trapezius

胸锁乳突肌
胸骨头
sternal head of sternocleidomastoid

胸锁乳突肌
锁骨头
clavicular head of sternocleidomastoid

胸锁乳突肌
sternocleidomastoid

锁骨上小窝
lesser supraclavicular fossa

锁骨上大窝
greater supraclavicular fossa

锁骨
clavicle

145. 颈部体表（前面观）
Neck surface (anterior aspect)

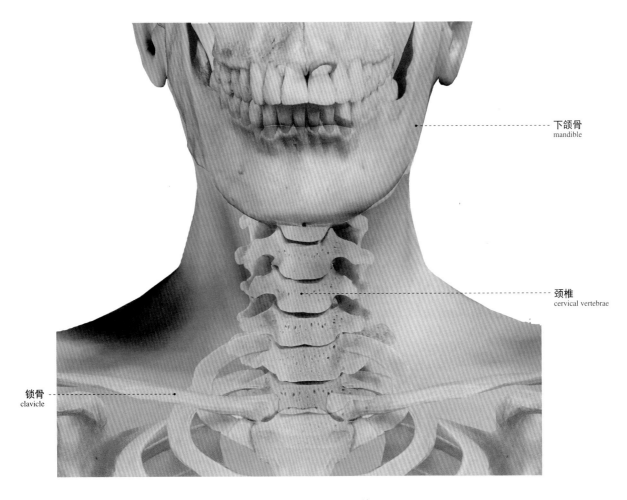

下颌骨
mandible

颈椎
cervical vertebrae

锁骨
clavicle

146. 颈部骨骼与体表对照（前面观）
Comparison of the neck bones and the neck surface (anterior aspect)

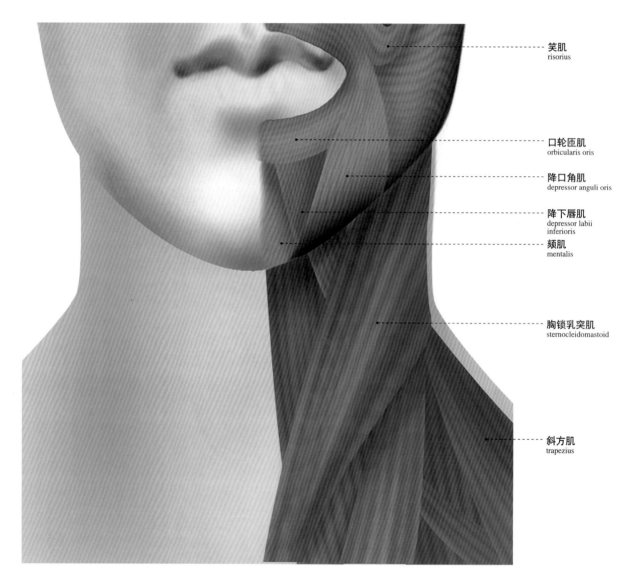

笑肌
risorius

口轮匝肌
orbicularis oris

降口角肌
depressor anguli oris

降下唇肌
depressor labii inferioris

颏肌
mentalis

胸锁乳突肌
sternocleidomastoid

斜方肌
trapezius

147. 颈部肌肉与颈部体表对照（前面观）
Comparison of the neck muscles and the neck surface (anterior aspect)

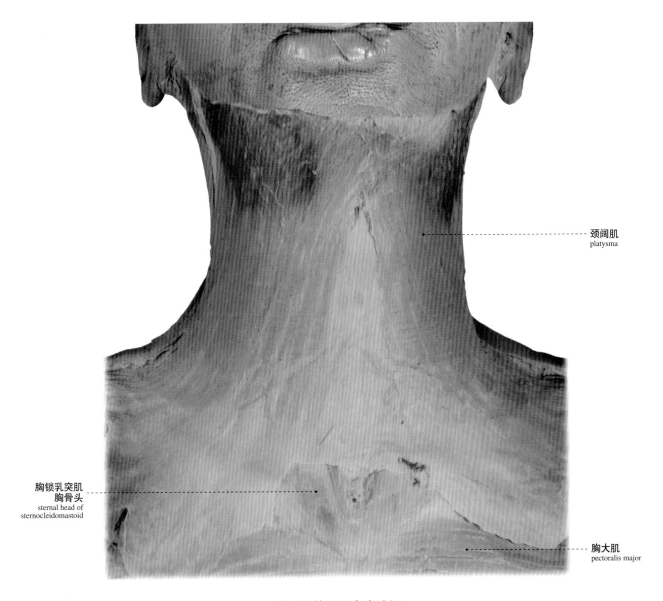

颈阔肌
platysma

胸锁乳突肌
胸骨头
sternal head of
sternocleidomastoid

胸大肌
pectoralis major

148. 颈前区局部解剖 1
Topography of anterior region of the neck 1

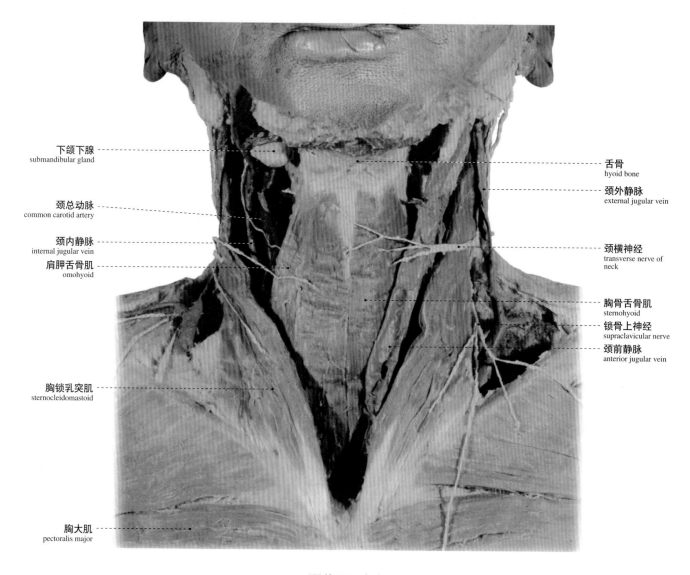

下颌下腺
submandibular gland

颈总动脉
common carotid artery

颈内静脉
internal jugular vein

肩胛舌骨肌
omohyoid

胸锁乳突肌
sternocleidomastoid

胸大肌
pectoralis major

舌骨
hyoid bone

颈外静脉
external jugular vein

颈横神经
transverse nerve of neck

胸骨舌骨肌
sternohyoid

锁骨上神经
supraclavicular nerve

颈前静脉
anterior jugular vein

149. 颈前区局部解剖 2
Topography of anterior region of the neck 2

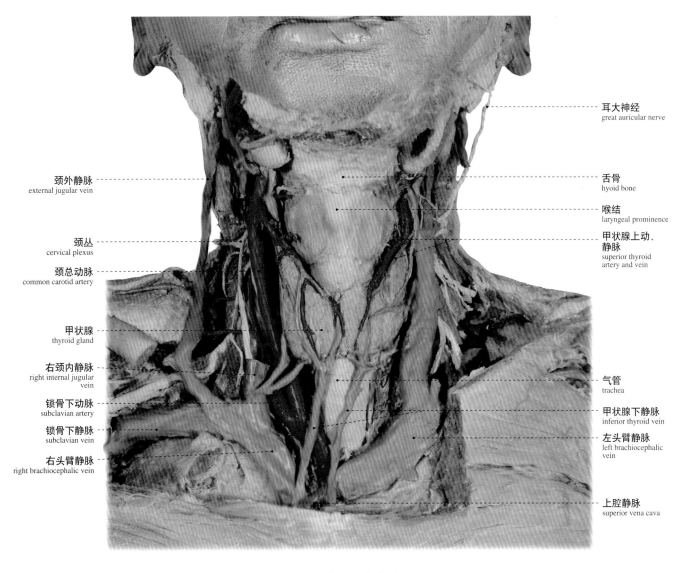

颈外静脉
external jugular vein

颈丛
cervical plexus

颈总动脉
common carotid artery

甲状腺
thyroid gland

右颈内静脉
right internal jugular vein

锁骨下动脉
subclavian artery

锁骨下静脉
subclavian vein

右头臂静脉
right brachiocephalic vein

耳大神经
great auricular nerve

舌骨
hyoid bone

喉结
laryngeal prominence

甲状腺上动、静脉
superior thyroid artery and vein

气管
trachea

甲状腺下静脉
inferior thyroid vein

左头臂静脉
left brachiocephalic vein

上腔静脉
superior vena cava

150. 颈前区局部解剖 3
Topography of anterior region of the neck 3

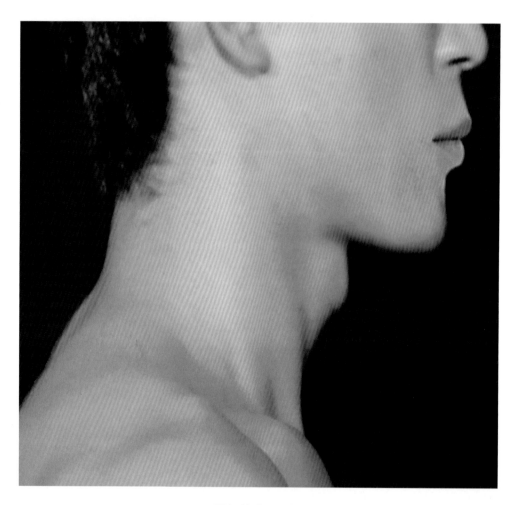

151. 颈部体表（侧面观）
Neck surface (lateral aspect)

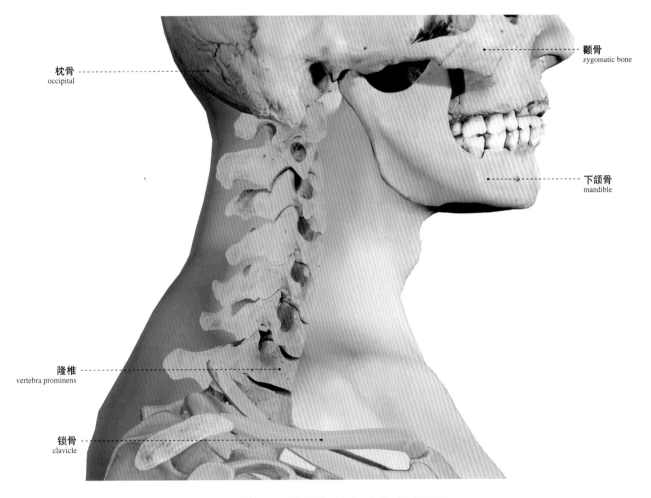

枕骨
occipital

颧骨
zygomatic bone

下颌骨
mandible

隆椎
vertebra prominens

锁骨
clavicle

152. 颈部骨骼与颈部体表对照（侧面观）
Comparison of the neck bones and the neck surface (lateral aspect)

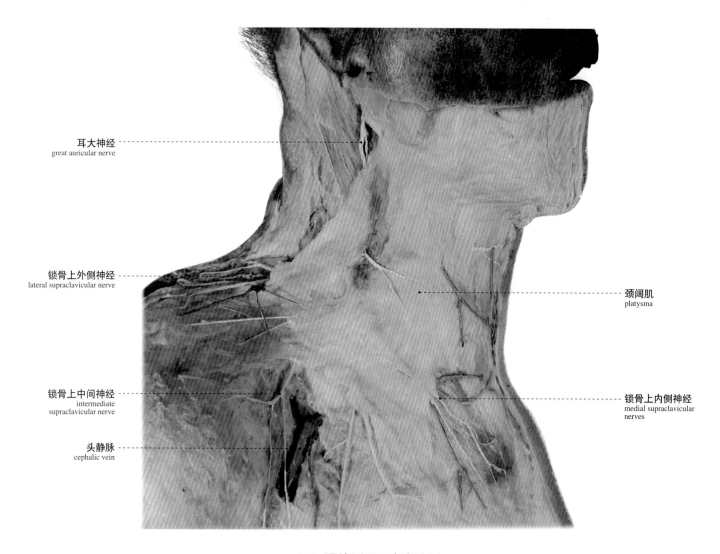

耳大神经
great auricular nerve

锁骨上外侧神经
lateral supraclavicular nerve

锁骨上中间神经
intermediate
supraclavicular nerve

头静脉
cephalic vein

颈阔肌
platysma

锁骨上内侧神经
medial supraclavicular
nerves

153. 颈外侧区局部解剖 1

Topography of lateral region of the neck 1

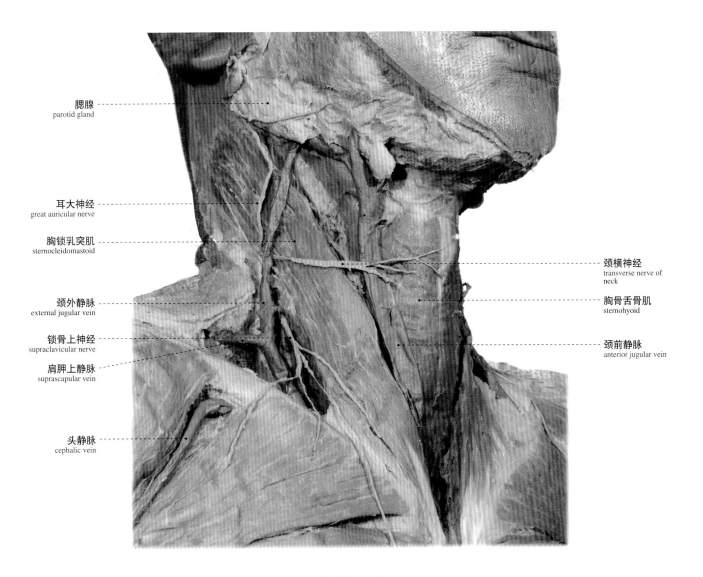

腮腺
parotid gland

耳大神经
great auricular nerve

胸锁乳突肌
sternocleidomastoid

颈外静脉
external jugular vein

锁骨上神经
supraclavicular nerve

肩胛上静脉
suprascapular vein

头静脉
cephalic vein

颈横神经
transverse nerve of neck

胸骨舌骨肌
sternohyoid

颈前静脉
anterior jugular vein

154. 颈外侧区局部解剖 2
Topography of lateral region of the neck 2

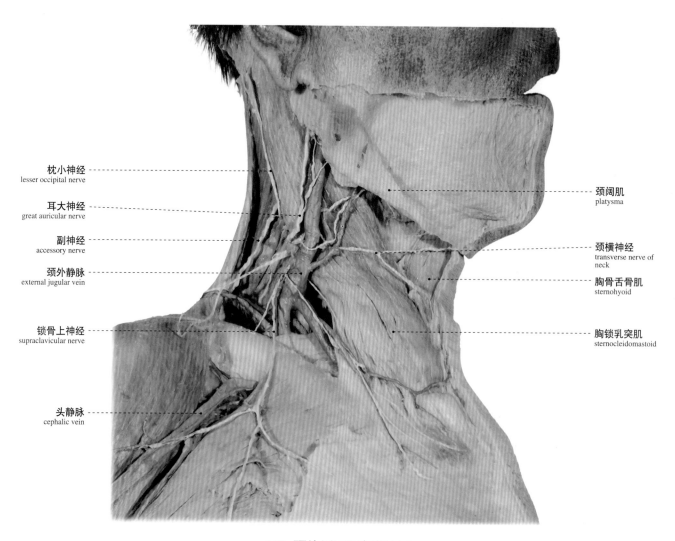

枕小神经
lesser occipital nerve

耳大神经
great auricular nerve

副神经
accessory nerve

颈外静脉
external jugular vein

锁骨上神经
supraclavicular nerve

头静脉
cephalic vein

颈阔肌
platysma

颈横神经
transverse nerve of neck

胸骨舌骨肌
sternohyoid

胸锁乳突肌
sternocleidomastoid

155. 颈外侧区局部解剖 3
Topography of lateral region of the neck 3

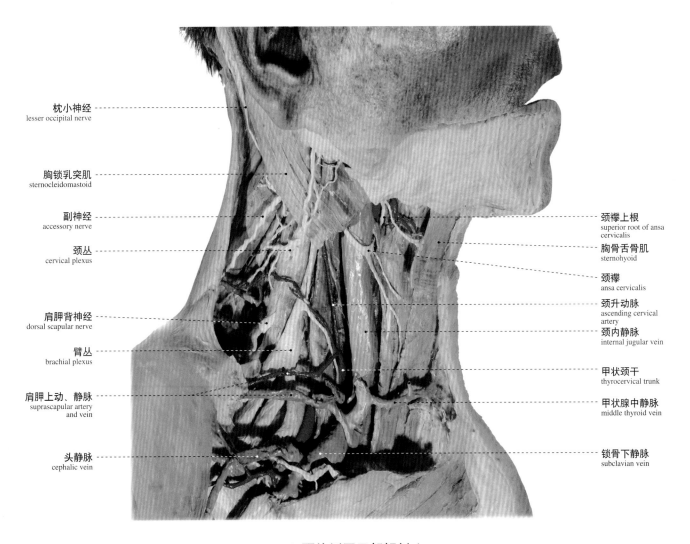

枕小神经
lesser occipital nerve

胸锁乳突肌
sternocleidomastoid

副神经
accessory nerve

颈丛
cervical plexus

肩胛背神经
dorsal scapular nerve

臂丛
brachial plexus

肩胛上动、静脉
suprascapular artery
and vein

头静脉
cephalic vein

颈襻上根
superior root of ansa
cervicalis

胸骨舌骨肌
sternohyoid

颈襻
ansa cervicalis

颈升动脉
ascending cervical
artery

颈内静脉
internal jugular vein

甲状颈干
thyrocervical trunk

甲状腺中静脉
middle thyroid vein

锁骨下静脉
subclavian vein

156. 颈外侧区局部解剖 4
Topography of lateral region of the neck 4

第四章
颈部表面解剖

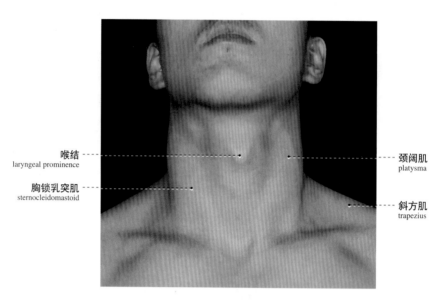

喉结
laryngeal prominence

胸锁乳突肌
sternocleidomastoid

颈阔肌
platysma

斜方肌
trapezius

157. 颈部表面解剖 1

Surface anatomy of the head and neck 1

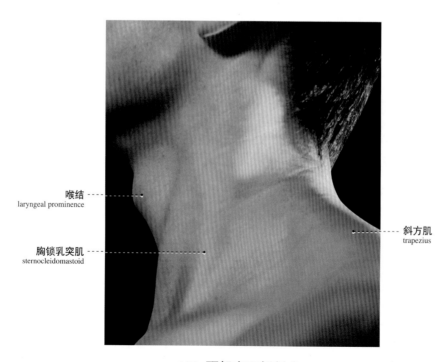

喉结
laryngeal prominence

胸锁乳突肌
sternocleidomastoid

斜方肌
trapezius

158. 颈部表面解剖 2

Surface anatomy of the head and neck 2

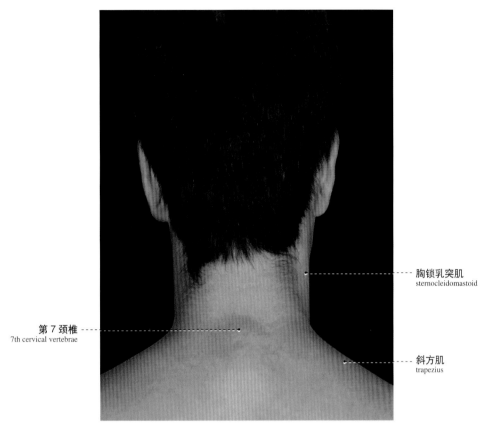

第 7 颈椎
7th cervical vertebrae

胸锁乳突肌
sternocleidomastoid

斜方肌
trapezius

159. 颈部表面解剖 3
Surface anatomy of the head and neck 3

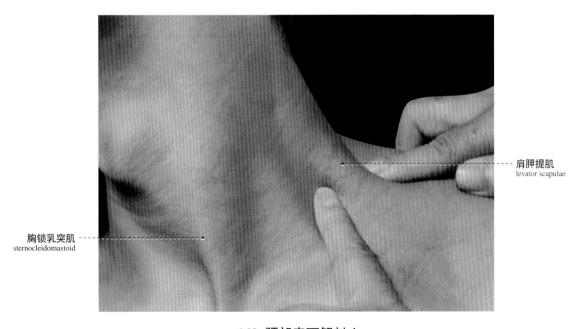

肩胛提肌
levator scapulae

胸锁乳突肌
sternocleidomastoid

160. 颈部表面解剖 4
Surface anatomy of the head and neck 4

第五章

脑

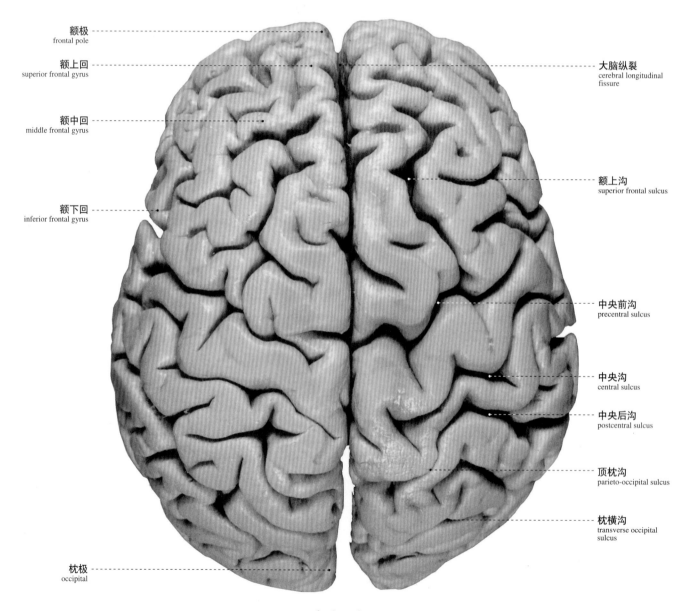

额极
frontal pole

额上回
superior frontal gyrus

额中回
middle frontal gyrus

额下回
inferior frontal gyrus

枕极
occipital

大脑纵裂
cerebral longitudinal
fissure

额上沟
superior frontal sulcus

中央前沟
precentral sulcus

中央沟
central sulcus

中央后沟
postcentral sulcus

顶枕沟
parieto-occipital sulcus

枕横沟
transverse occipital
sulcus

161. 大脑（上面观）
Cerebrum (superior aspect)

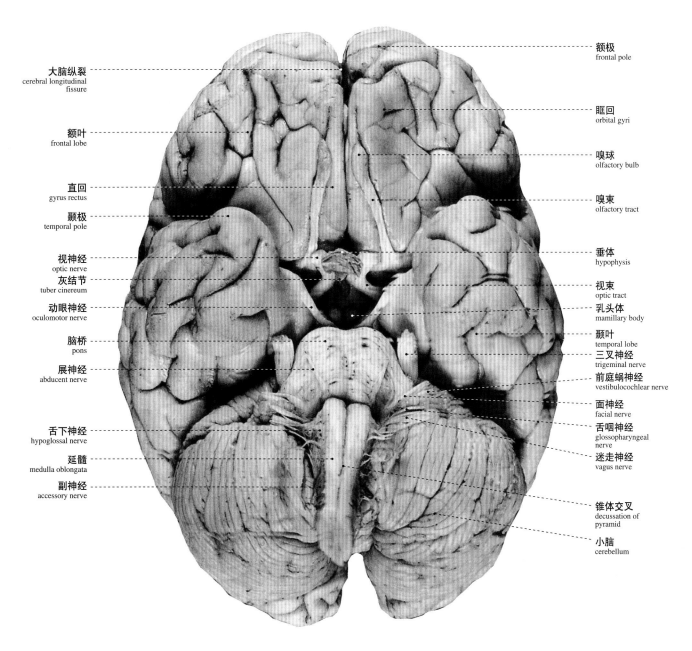

大脑纵裂
cerebral longitudinal fissure

额叶
frontal lobe

直回
gyrus rectus

颞极
temporal pole

视神经
optic nerve

灰结节
tuber cinereum

动眼神经
oculomotor nerve

脑桥
pons

展神经
abducent nerve

舌下神经
hypoglossal nerve

延髓
medulla oblongata

副神经
accessory nerve

额极
frontal pole

眶回
orbital gyri

嗅球
olfactory bulb

嗅束
olfactory tract

垂体
hypophysis

视束
optic tract

乳头体
mamillary body

颞叶
temporal lobe

三叉神经
trigeminal nerve

前庭蜗神经
vestibulocochlear nerve

面神经
facial nerve

舌咽神经
glossopharyngeal nerve

迷走神经
vagus nerve

锥体交叉
decussation of pyramid

小脑
cerebellum

162. 大脑（下面观）
Cerebrum (inferior aspect)

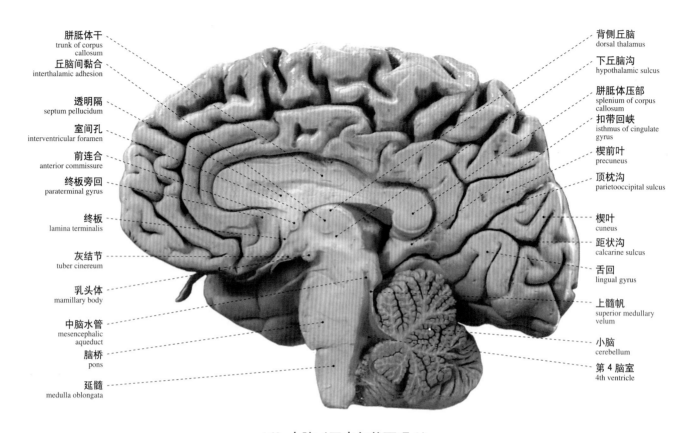

胼胝体干
trunk of corpus callosum

丘脑间黏合
interthalamic adhesion

透明隔
septum pellucidum

室间孔
interventricular foramen

前连合
anterior commissure

终板旁回
paraterminal gyrus

终板
lamina terminalis

灰结节
tuber cinereum

乳头体
mamillary body

中脑水管
mesencephalic aqueduct

脑桥
pons

延髓
medulla oblongata

背侧丘脑
dorsal thalamus

下丘脑沟
hypothalamic sulcus

胼胝体压部
splenium of corpus callosum

扣带回峡
isthmus of cingulate gyrus

楔前叶
precuneus

顶枕沟
parietooccipital sulcus

楔叶
cuneus

距状沟
calcarine sulcus

舌回
lingual gyrus

上髓帆
superior medullary velum

小脑
cerebellum

第 4 脑室
4th ventricle

163. 大脑（正中矢状面观 1）
Cerebrum (midsagittal section aspect 1)

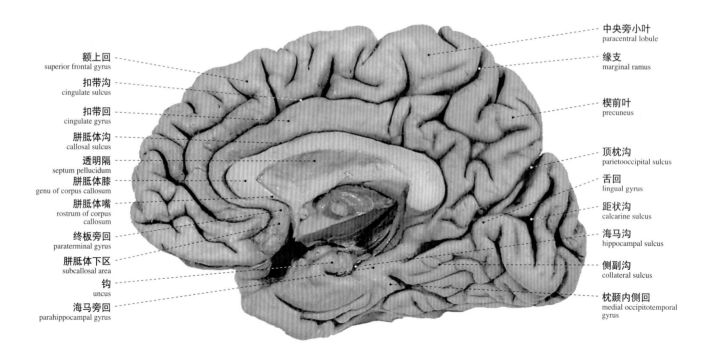

额上回
superior frontal gyrus

扣带沟
cingulate sulcus

扣带回
cingulate gyrus

胼胝体沟
callosal sulcus

透明隔
septum pellucidum

胼胝体膝
genu of corpus callosum

胼胝体嘴
rostrum of corpus callosum

终板旁回
paraterminal gyrus

胼胝体下区
subcallosal area

钩
uncus

海马旁回
parahippocampal gyrus

中央旁小叶
paracentral lobule

缘支
marginal ramus

楔前叶
precuneus

顶枕沟
parietooccipital sulcus

舌回
lingual gyrus

距状沟
calcarine sulcus

海马沟
hippocampal sulcus

侧副沟
collateral sulcus

枕颞内侧回
medial occipitotemporal gyrus

164. 大脑（正中矢状面观 2）
Cerebrum (midsagittal section aspect 2)

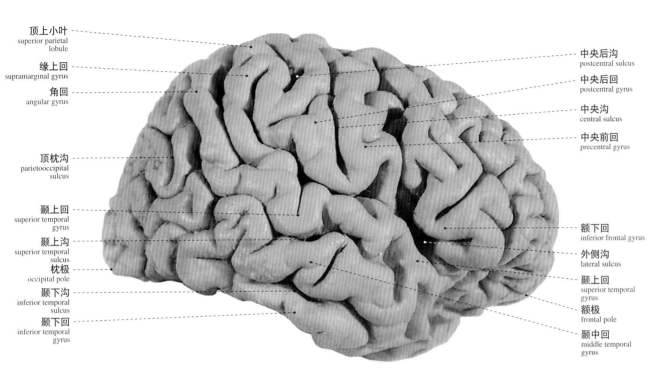

顶上小叶
superior parietal lobule

缘上回
supramarginal gyrus

角回
angular gyrus

顶枕沟
parietooccipital sulcus

颞上回
superior temporal gyrus

颞上沟
superior temporal sulcus

枕极
occipital pole

颞下沟
inferior temporal sulcus

颞下回
inferior temporal gyrus

中央后沟
postcentral sulcus

中央后回
postcentral gyrus

中央沟
central sulcus

中央前回
precentral gyrus

额下回
inferior frontal gyrus

外侧沟
lateral sulcus

颞上回
superior temporal gyrus

额极
frontal pole

颞中回
middle temporal gyrus

165. 大脑（外侧面观）
Cerebrum (lateral aspect)

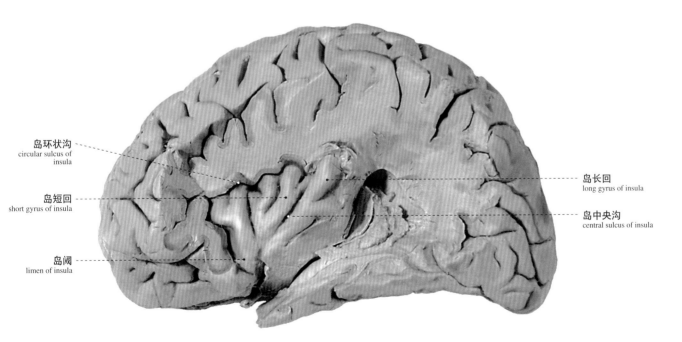

岛环状沟
circular sulcus of insula

岛短回
short gyrus of insula

岛阈
limen of insula

岛长回
long gyrus of insula

岛中央沟
central sulcus of insula

166. 岛叶
Insular lobe

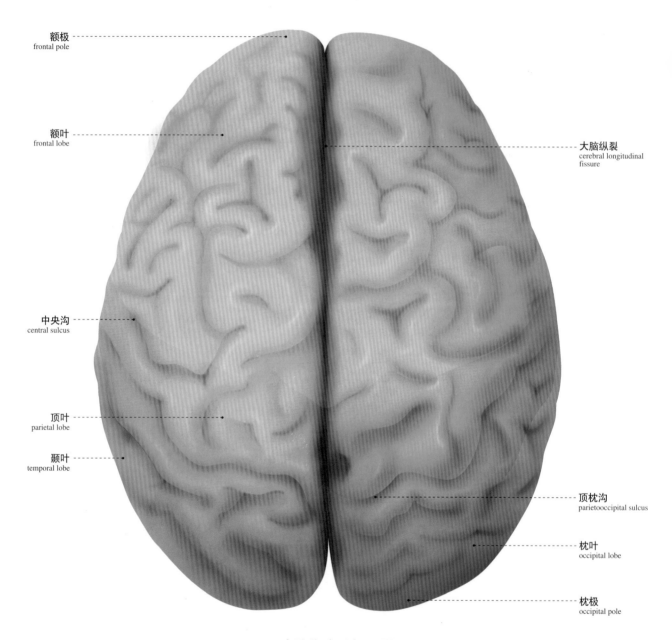

额极
frontal pole

额叶
frontal lobe

大脑纵裂
cerebral longitudinal
fissure

中央沟
central sulcus

顶叶
parietal lobe

颞叶
temporal lobe

顶枕沟
parietooccipital sulcus

枕叶
occipital lobe

枕极
occipital pole

167. 大脑分叶（上面观）
Division of the cerebrum into lobes (superior aspect)

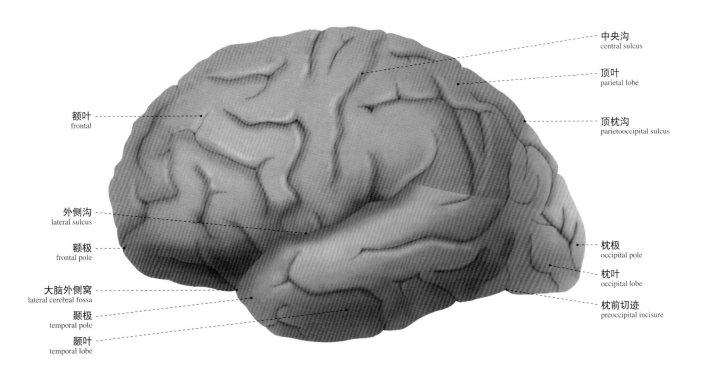

中央沟
central sulcus

顶叶
parietal lobe

顶枕沟
parietooccipital sulcus

额叶
frontal

外侧沟
lateral sulcus

额极
frontal pole

大脑外侧窝
lateral cerebral fossa

颞极
temporal pole

颞叶
temporal lobe

枕极
occipital pole

枕叶
occipital lobe

枕前切迹
preoccipital incisure

168. 大脑分叶（外侧面观）
Division of the cerebrum into lobes (lateral aspect)

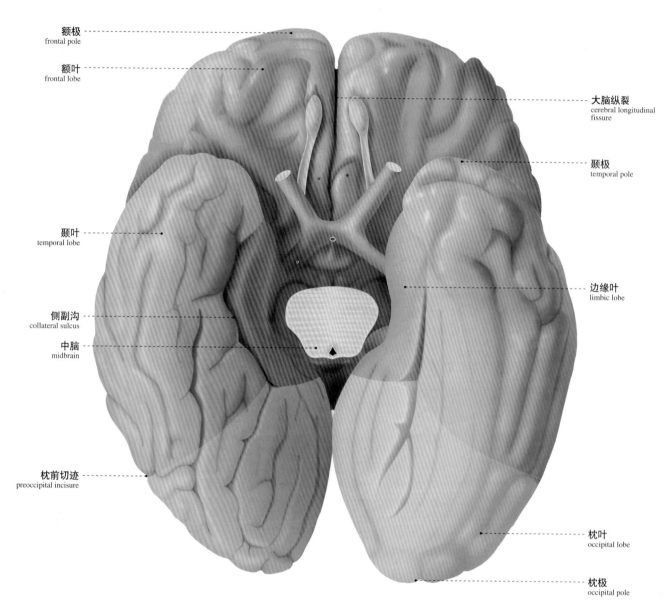

额极
frontal pole

额叶
frontal lobe

大脑纵裂
cerebral longitudinal fissure

颞极
temporal pole

颞叶
temporal lobe

边缘叶
limbic lobe

侧副沟
collateral sulcus

中脑
midbrain

枕前切迹
preoccipital incisure

枕叶
occipital lobe

枕极
occipital pole

169. 大脑分叶（下面观）

Division of the cerebrum into lobes (inferior aspect)

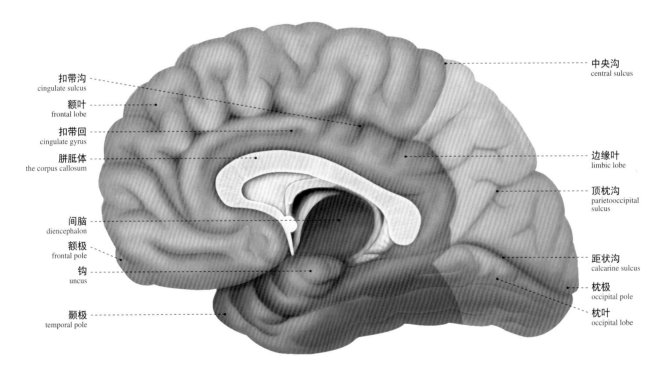

扣带沟
cingulate sulcus

额叶
frontal lobe

扣带回
cingulate gyrus

胼胝体
the corpus callosum

间脑
diencephalon

额极
frontal pole

钩
uncus

颞极
temporal pole

中央沟
central sulcus

边缘叶
limbic lobe

顶枕沟
parietooccipital
sulcus

距状沟
calcarine sulcus

枕极
occipital pole

枕叶
occipital lobe

170. 大脑分叶（正中矢状面观）
Division of the cerebrum into lobes (midsagittal section aspect)

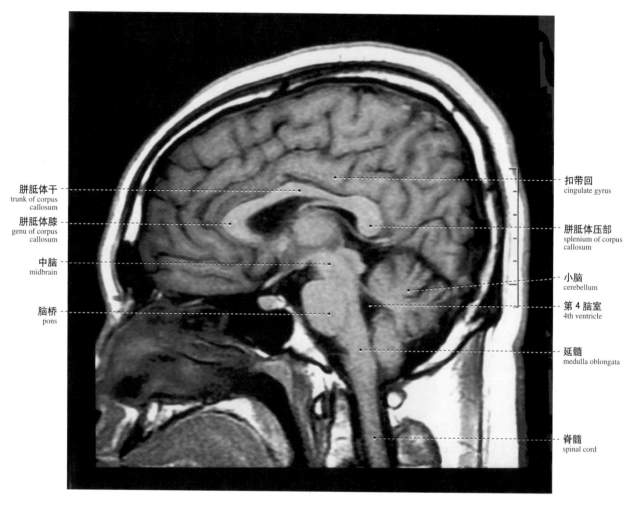

胼胝体干
trunk of corpus callosum

胼胝体膝
genu of corpus callosum

中脑
midbrain

脑桥
pons

扣带回
cingulate gyrus

胼胝体压部
splenium of corpus callosum

小脑
cerebellum

第4脑室
4th ventricle

延髓
medulla oblongata

脊髓
spinal cord

171. 脑磁共振成像（矢状位）
MRI of the brain (sagittal view)

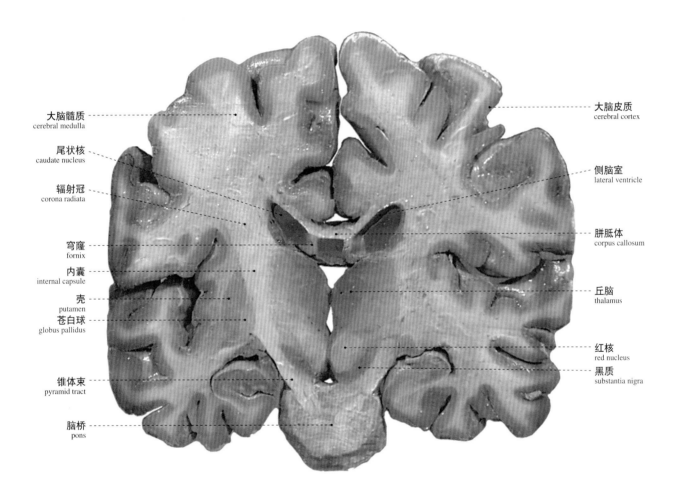

大脑髓质
cerebral medulla

尾状核
caudate nucleus

辐射冠
corona radiata

穹窿
fornix

内囊
internal capsule

壳
putamen

苍白球
globus pallidus

锥体束
pyramid tract

脑桥
pons

大脑皮质
cerebral cortex

侧脑室
lateral ventricle

胼胝体
corpus callosum

丘脑
thalamus

红核
red nucleus

黑质
substantia nigra

172. 大脑（冠状切面）
Cerebrum (coronal section)

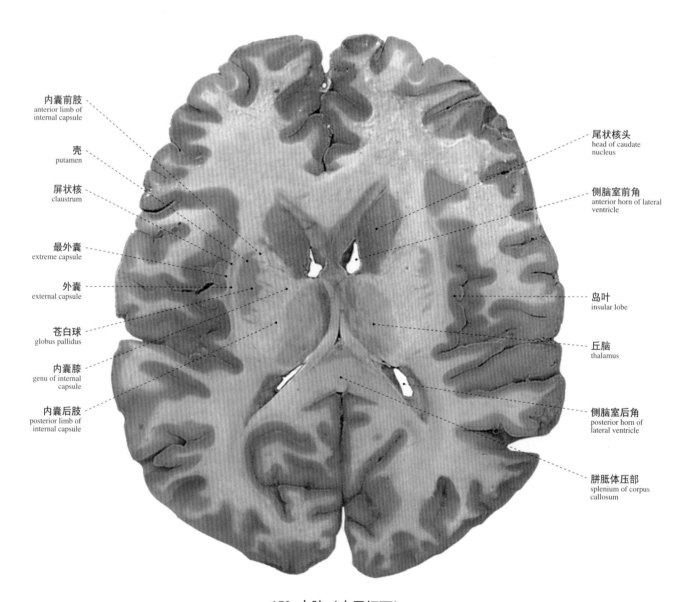

内囊前肢
anterior limb of
internal capsule

壳
putamen

屏状核
claustrum

最外囊
extreme capsule

外囊
external capsule

苍白球
globus pallidus

内囊膝
genu of internal
capsule

内囊后肢
posterior limb of
internal capsule

尾状核头
head of caudate
nucleus

侧脑室前角
anterior horn of lateral
ventricle

岛叶
insular lobe

丘脑
thalamus

侧脑室后角
posterior horn of
lateral ventricle

胼胝体压部
splenium of corpus
callosum

173. 大脑（水平切面）
Cerebrum (horizontal section)

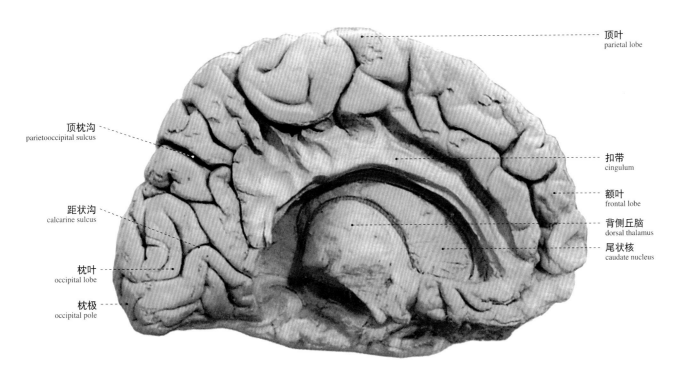

顶叶
parietal lobe

顶枕沟
parietooccipital sulcus

扣带
cingulum

额叶
frontal lobe

距状沟
calcarine sulcus

背侧丘脑
dorsal thalamus

尾状核
caudate nucleus

枕叶
occipital lobe

枕极
occipital pole

174. 基底核
Basal nuclei

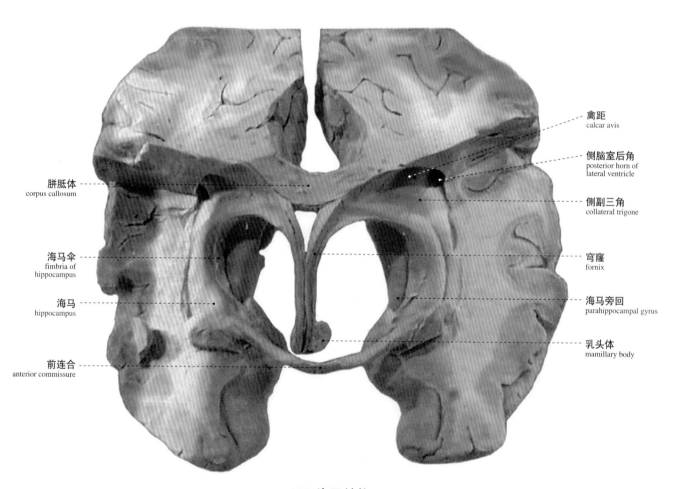

禽距
calcar avis

侧脑室后角
posterior horn of
lateral ventricle

胼胝体
corpus callosum

侧副三角
collateral trigone

海马伞
fimbria of
hippocampus

穹窿
fornix

海马
hippocampus

海马旁回
parahippocampal gyrus

乳头体
mamillary body

前连合
anterior commissure

175. 海马结构
Hippocampal formation

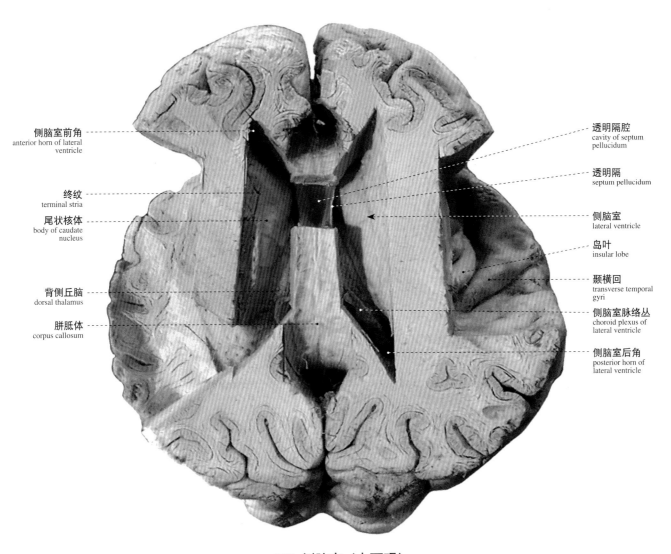

侧脑室前角
anterior horn of lateral
ventricle

终纹
terminal stria

尾状核体
body of caudate
nucleus

背侧丘脑
dorsal thalamus

胼胝体
corpus callosum

透明隔腔
cavity of septum
pellucidum

透明隔
septum pellucidum

侧脑室
lateral ventricle

岛叶
insular lobe

颞横回
transverse temporal
gyri

侧脑室脉络丛
choroid plexus of
lateral ventricle

侧脑室后角
posterior horn of
lateral ventricle

176. 侧脑室（上面观）
Lateral ventricles (superior aspect)

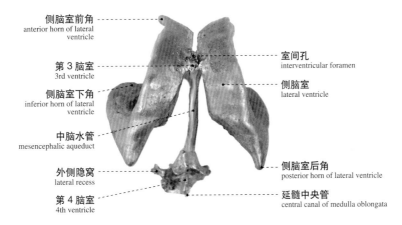

侧脑室前角
anterior horn of lateral
ventricle

第 3 脑室
3rd ventricle

侧脑室下角
inferior horn of lateral
ventricle

中脑水管
mesencephalic aqueduct

外侧隐窝
lateral recess

第 4 脑室
4th ventricle

室间孔
interventricular foramen

侧脑室
lateral ventricle

侧脑室后角
posterior horn of
lateral ventricle

延髓中央管
central canal of medulla oblongata

177. 脑室的铸型（后面观）
Ventricular cast (posterior aspect)

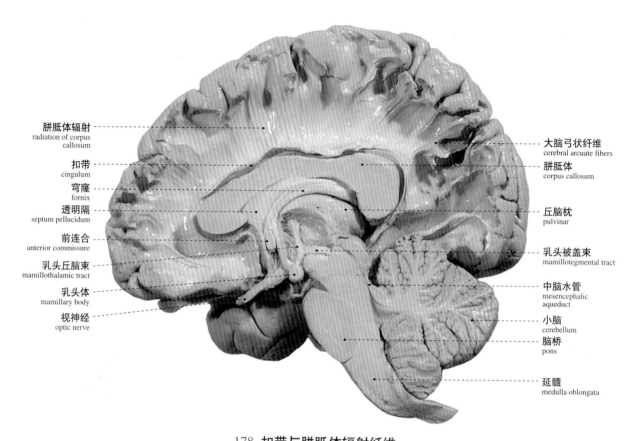

胼胝体辐射
radiation of corpus callosum

扣带
cingulum

穹窿
fornix

透明隔
septum pellucidum

前连合
anterior commissure

乳头丘脑束
mamillothalamic tract

乳头体
mamillary body

视神经
optic nerve

大脑弓状纤维
cerebral arcuate fibers

胼胝体
corpus callosum

丘脑枕
pulvinar

乳头被盖束
mamillotegmental tract

中脑水管
mesencephalic aqueduct

小脑
cerebellum

脑桥
pons

延髓
medulla oblongata

178. 扣带与胼胝体辐射纤维

Fibers of the cingulum and radiation of the corpus callosum

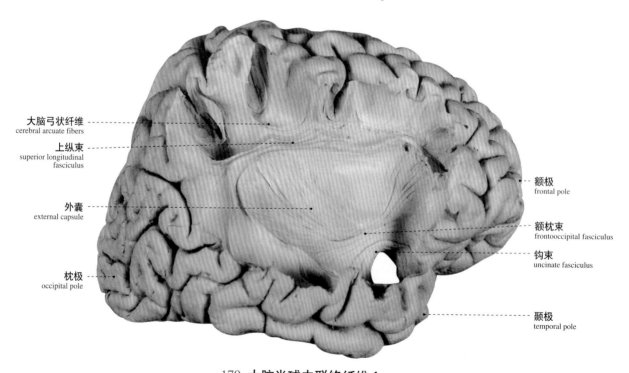

大脑弓状纤维
cerebral arcuate fibers

上纵束
superior longitudinal fasciculus

外囊
external capsule

枕极
occipital pole

额极
frontal pole

额枕束
frontooccipital fasciculus

钩束
uncinate fasciculus

颞极
temporal pole

179. 大脑半球内联络纤维 1

Association fibers in the cerebral hemisphere 1

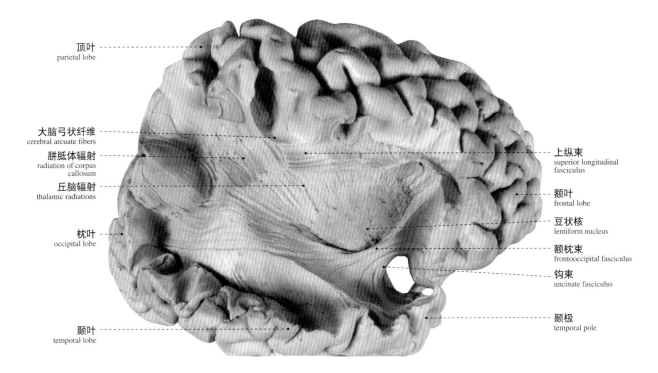

顶叶
parietal lobe

大脑弓状纤维
cerebral arcuate fibers

胼胝体辐射
radiation of corpus callosum

丘脑辐射
thalamic radiations

枕叶
occipital lobe

颞叶
temporal lobe

上纵束
superior longitudinal fasciculus

额叶
frontal lobe

豆状核
lentiform nucleus

额枕束
frontooccipital fasciculus

钩束
uncinate fasciculus

颞极
temporal pole

180. 大脑半球内联络纤维 2
Association fibers in the cerebral hemisphere 2

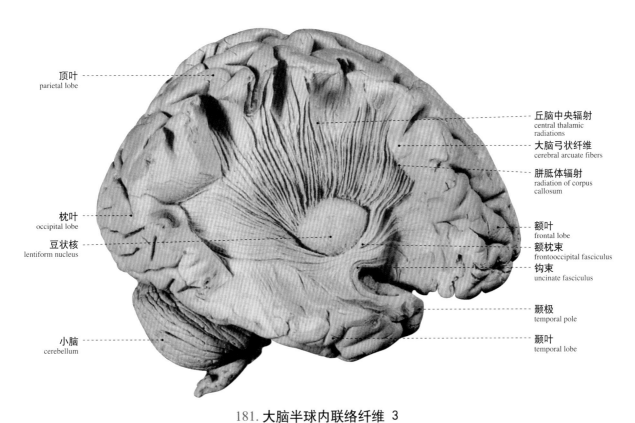

顶叶
parietal lobe

枕叶
occipital lobe

豆状核
lentiform nucleus

小脑
cerebellum

丘脑中央辐射
central thalamic radiations

大脑弓状纤维
cerebral arcuate fibers

胼胝体辐射
radiation of corpus callosum

额叶
frontal lobe

额枕束
frontooccipital fasciculus

钩束
uncinate fasciculus

颞极
temporal pole

颞叶
temporal lobe

181. 大脑半球内联络纤维 3
Association fibers in the cerebral hemisphere 3

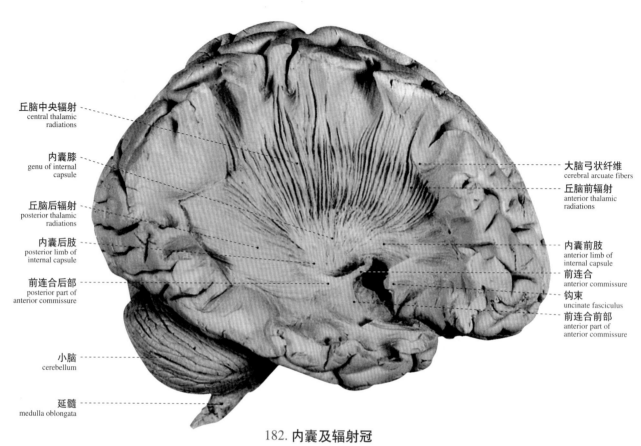

丘脑中央辐射
central thalamic
radiations

内囊膝
genu of internal
capsule

丘脑后辐射
posterior thalamic
radiations

内囊后肢
posterior limb of
internal capsule

前连合后部
posterior part of
anterior commissure

小脑
cerebellum

延髓
medulla oblongata

大脑弓状纤维
cerebral arcuate fibers

丘脑前辐射
anterior thalamic
radiations

内囊前肢
anterior limb of
internal capsule

前连合
anterior commissure

钩束
uncinate fasciculus

前连合前部
anterior part of
anterior commissure

182. 内囊及辐射冠

Internal capsule and the corona radiata

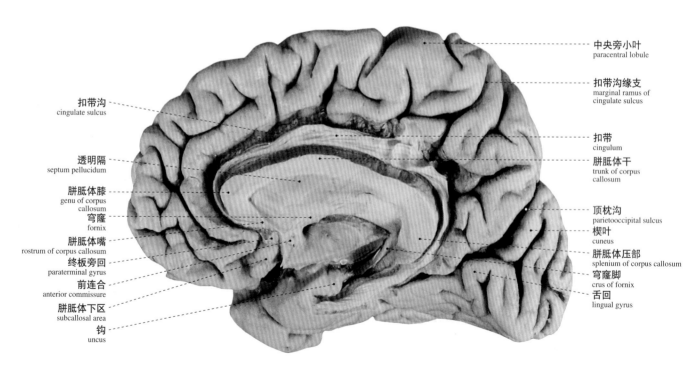

扣带沟
cingulate sulcus

透明隔
septum pellucidum

胼胝体膝
genu of corpus
callosum

穹窿
fornix

胼胝体嘴
rostrum of corpus callosum

终板旁回
paraterminal gyrus

前连合
anterior commissure

胼胝体下区
subcallosal area

钩
uncus

中央旁小叶
paracentral lobule

扣带沟缘支
marginal ramus of
cingulate sulcus

扣带
cingulum

胼胝体干
trunk of corpus
callosum

顶枕沟
parietooccipital sulcus

楔叶
cuneus

胼胝体压部
splenium of corpus callosum

穹窿脚
crus of fornix

舌回
lingual gyrus

183. 扣带

Cingulum

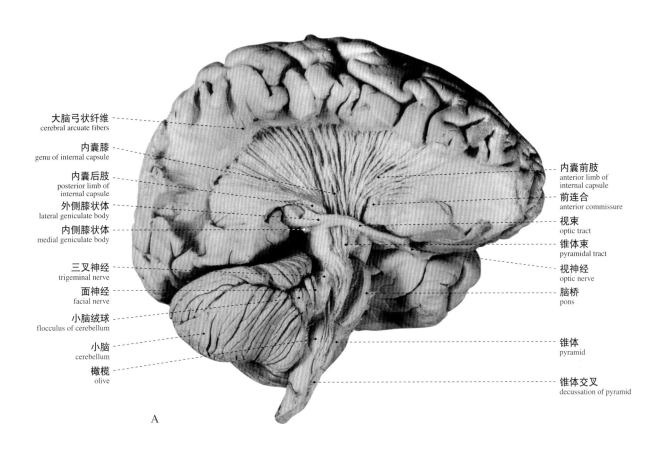

大脑弓状纤维
cerebral arcuate fibers

内囊膝
genu of internal capsule

内囊后肢
posterior limb of
internal capsule

外侧膝状体
lateral geniculate body

内侧膝状体
medial geniculate body

三叉神经
trigeminal nerve

面神经
facial nerve

小脑绒球
flocculus of cerebellum

小脑
cerebellum

橄榄
olive

内囊前肢
anterior limb of
internal capsule

前连合
anterior commissure

视束
optic tract

锥体束
pyramidal tract

视神经
optic nerve

脑桥
pons

锥体
pyramid

锥体交叉
decussation of pyramid

A

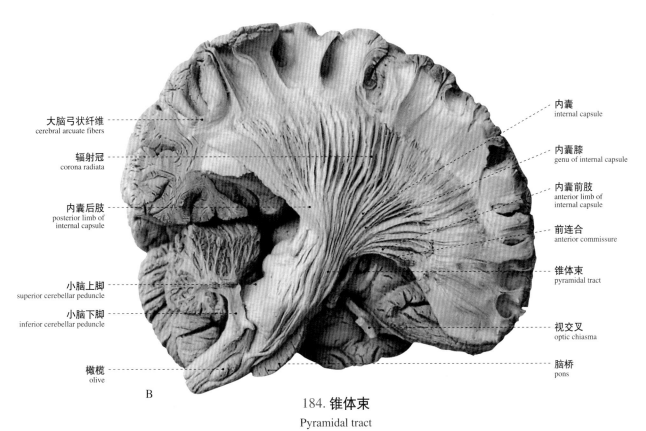

大脑弓状纤维
cerebral arcuate fibers

辐射冠
corona radiata

内囊后肢
posterior limb of
internal capsule

小脑上脚
superior cerebellar peduncle

小脑下脚
inferior cerebellar peduncle

橄榄
olive

内囊
internal capsule

内囊膝
genu of internal capsule

内囊前肢
anterior limb of
internal capsule

前连合
anterior commissure

锥体束
pyramidal tract

视交叉
optic chiasma

脑桥
pons

B

184. 锥体束
Pyramidal tract

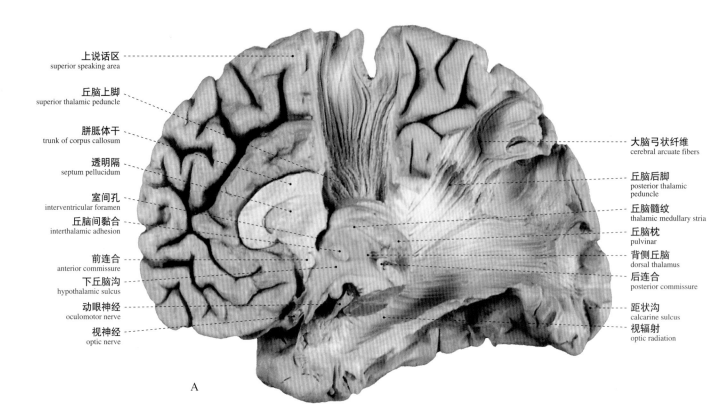

上说话区
superior speaking area

丘脑上脚
superior thalamic peduncle

胼胝体干
trunk of corpus callosum

透明隔
septum pellucidum

室间孔
interventricular foramen

丘脑间黏合
interthalamic adhesion

前连合
anterior commissure

下丘脑沟
hypothalamic sulcus

动眼神经
oculomotor nerve

视神经
optic nerve

大脑弓状纤维
cerebral arcuate fibers

丘脑后脚
posterior thalamic peduncle

丘脑髓纹
thalamic medullary stria

丘脑枕
pulvinar

背侧丘脑
dorsal thalamus

后连合
posterior commissure

距状沟
calcarine sulcus

视辐射
optic radiation

A

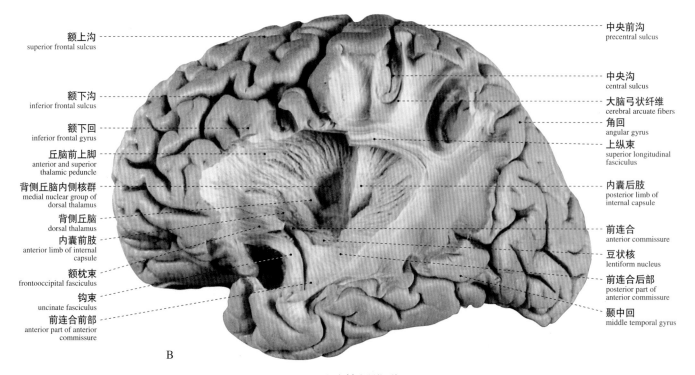

额上沟
superior frontal sulcus

额下沟
inferior frontal sulcus

额下回
inferior frontal gyrus

丘脑前上脚
anterior and superior thalamic peduncle

背侧丘脑内侧核群
medial nuclear group of dorsal thalamus

背侧丘脑
dorsal thalamus

内囊前肢
anterior limb of internal capsule

额枕束
frontooccipital fasciculus

钩束
uncinate fasciculus

前连合前部
anterior part of anterior commissure

中央前沟
precentral sulcus

中央沟
central sulcus

大脑弓状纤维
cerebral arcuate fibers

角回
angular gyrus

上纵束
superior longitudinal fasciculus

内囊后肢
posterior limb of internal capsule

前连合
anterior commissure

豆状核
lentiform nucleus

前连合后部
posterior part of anterior commissure

颞中回
middle temporal gyrus

B

185. 丘脑的纤维联系
Fibrous connection of the thalamus

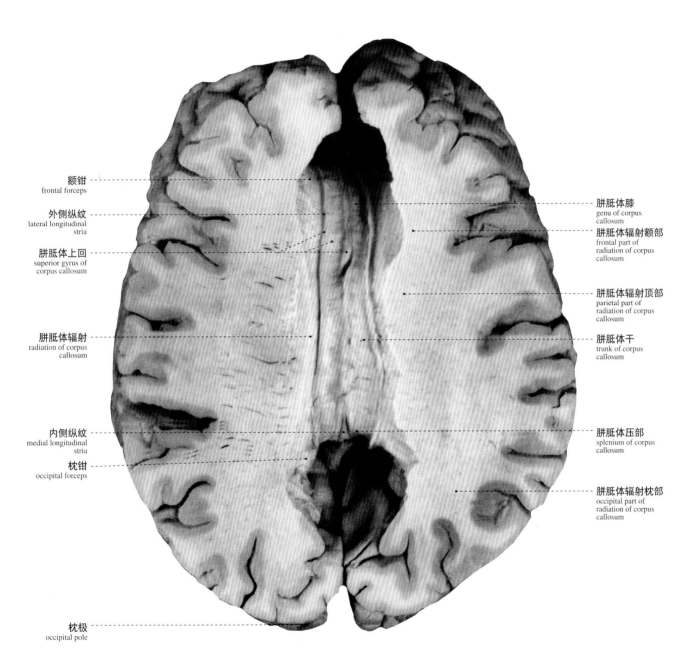

额钳
frontal forceps

外侧纵纹
lateral longitudinal
stria

胼胝体上回
superior gyrus of
corpus callosum

胼胝体辐射
radiation of corpus
callosum

内侧纵纹
medial longitudinal
stria

枕钳
occipital forceps

枕极
occipital pole

胼胝体膝
genu of corpus
callosum

胼胝体辐射额部
frontal part of
radiation of corpus
callosum

胼胝体辐射顶部
parietal part of
radiation of corpus
callosum

胼胝体干
trunk of corpus
callosum

胼胝体压部
splenium of corpus
callosum

胼胝体辐射枕部
occipital part of
radiation of corpus
callosum

186. 胼胝体（上面观 1）
Corpus callosum (superior aspect 1)

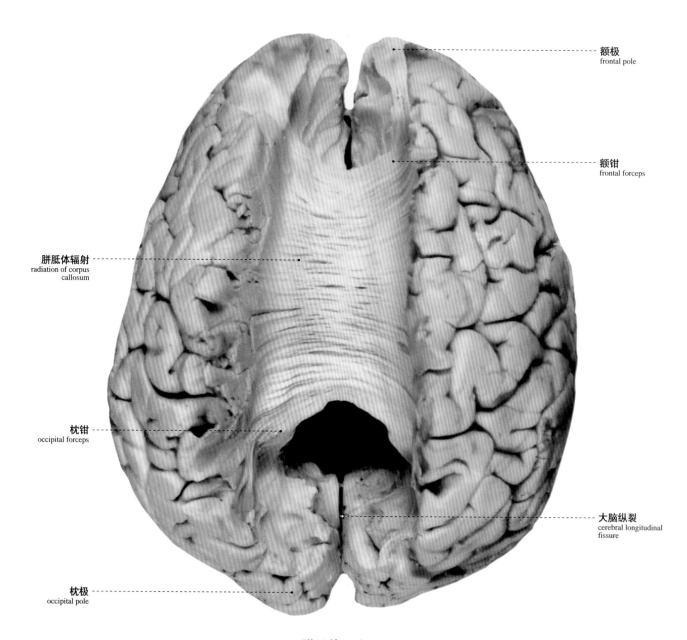

额极
frontal pole

额钳
frontal forceps

胼胝体辐射
radiation of corpus
callosum

枕钳
occipital forceps

大脑纵裂
cerebral longitudinal
fissure

枕极
occipital pole

187. 胼胝体（上面观 2）
Corpus callosum (superior aspect 2)

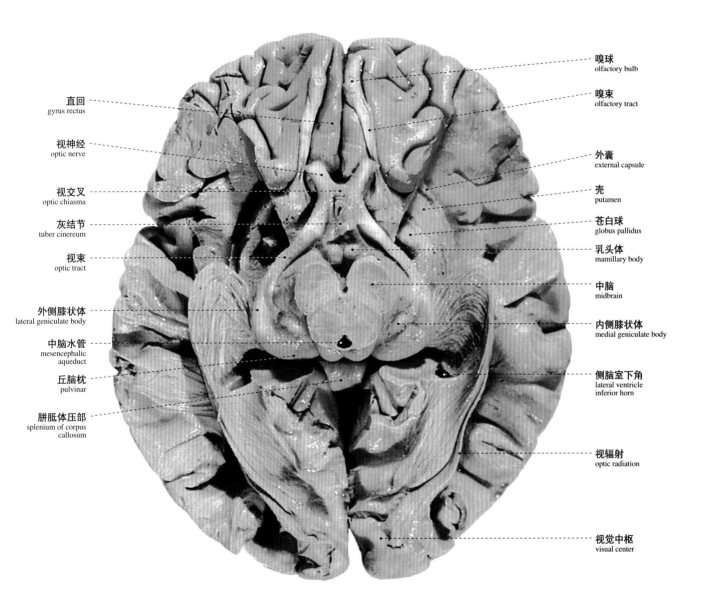

直回
gyrus rectus

视神经
optic nerve

视交叉
optic chiasma

灰结节
tuber cinereum

视束
optic tract

外侧膝状体
lateral geniculate body

中脑水管
mesencephalic aqueduct

丘脑枕
pulvinar

胼胝体压部
splenium of corpus callosum

嗅球
olfactory bulb

嗅束
olfactory tract

外囊
external capsule

壳
putamen

苍白球
globus pallidus

乳头体
mamillary body

中脑
midbrain

内侧膝状体
medial geniculate body

侧脑室下角
lateral ventricle inferior horn

视辐射
optic radiation

视觉中枢
visual center

188. 视束及视辐射
Optic tract and the optic radiation

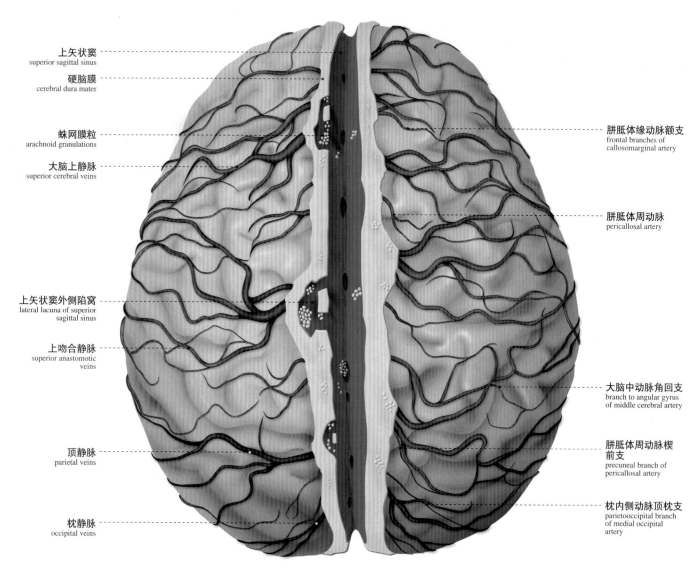

上矢状窦
superior sagittal sinus

硬脑膜
cerebral dura mater

蛛网膜粒
arachnoid granulations

大脑上静脉
superior cerebral veins

上矢状窦外侧陷窝
lateral lacuna of superior
sagittal sinus

上吻合静脉
superior anastomotic
veins

顶静脉
parietal veins

枕静脉
occipital veins

胼胝体缘动脉额支
frontal branches of
callosomarginal artery

胼胝体周动脉
pericallosal artery

大脑中动脉角回支
branch to angular gyrus
of middle cerebral artery

胼胝体周动脉楔
前支
precuneal branch of
pericallosal artery

枕内侧动脉顶枕支
parietooccipital branch
of medial occipital
artery

189. 大脑的浅动脉和静脉
Superficial arteries and veins of the cerebrum

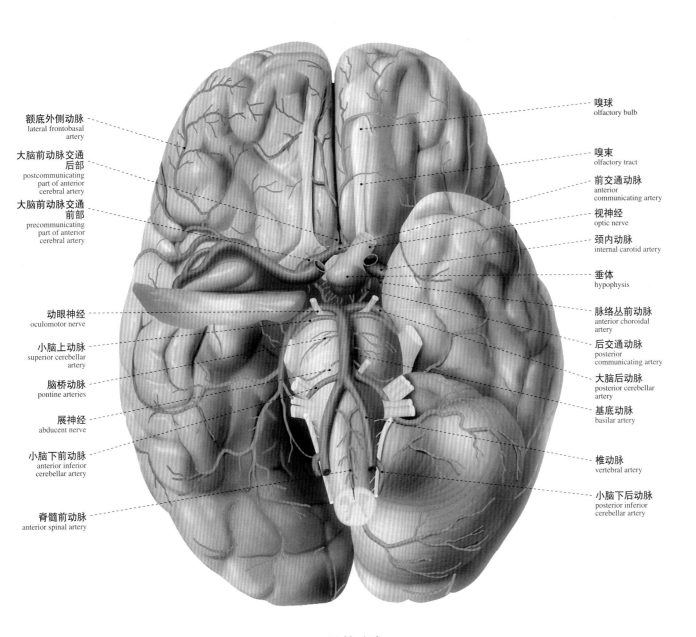

额底外侧动脉
lateral frontobasal artery

大脑前动脉交通后部
postcommunicating part of anterior cerebral artery

大脑前动脉交通前部
precommunicating part of anterior cerebral artery

动眼神经
oculomotor nerve

小脑上动脉
superior cerebellar artery

脑桥动脉
pontine arteries

展神经
abducent nerve

小脑下前动脉
anterior inferior cerebellar artery

脊髓前动脉
anterior spinal artery

嗅球
olfactory bulb

嗅束
olfactory tract

前交通动脉
anterior communicating artery

视神经
optic nerve

颈内动脉
internal carotid artery

垂体
hypophysis

脉络丛前动脉
anterior choroidal artery

后交通动脉
posterior communicating artery

大脑后动脉
posterior cerebellar artery

基底动脉
basilar artery

椎动脉
vertebral artery

小脑下后动脉
posterior inferior cerebellar artery

190. 脑的动脉
Cerebral arteries

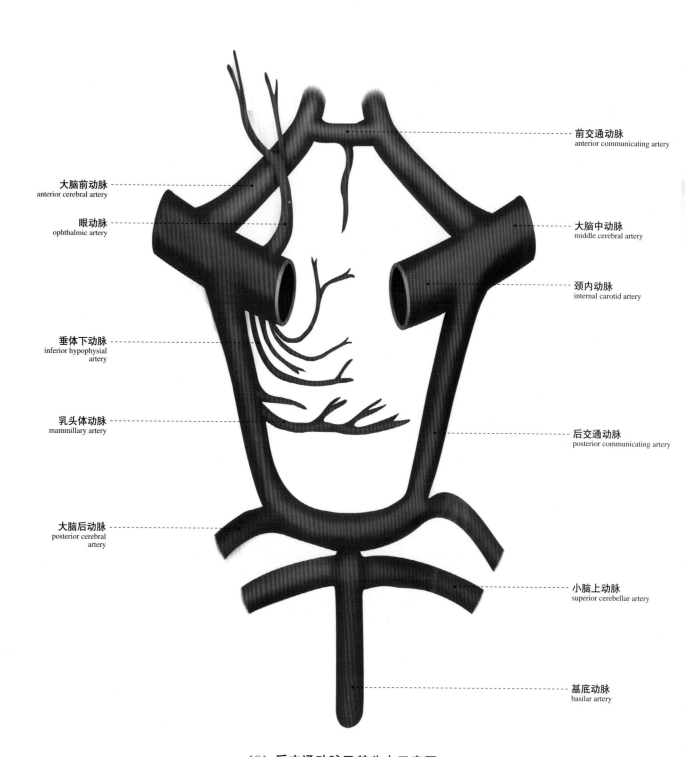

大脑前动脉
anterior cerebral artery

眼动脉
ophthalmic artery

垂体下动脉
inferior hypophysial
artery

乳头体动脉
mammillary artery

大脑后动脉
posterior cerebral
artery

前交通动脉
anterior communicating artery

大脑中动脉
middle cerebral artery

颈内动脉
internal carotid artery

后交通动脉
posterior communicating artery

小脑上动脉
superior cerebellar artery

基底动脉
basilar artery

191. 后交通动脉及其分支示意图
Diagram of the posterior communicating artery and its branches

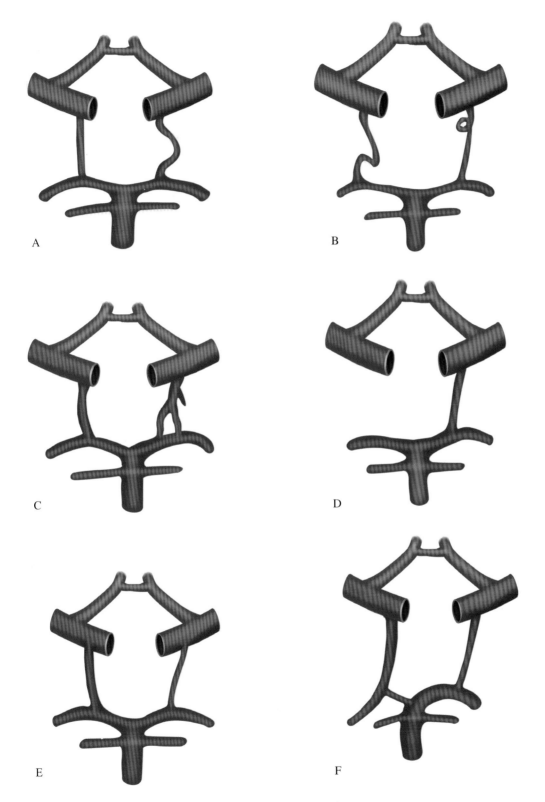

192. 后交通动脉变异示意图

Diagram of the variation of the posterior communicating artery

A. 右侧平直，左侧弯曲型；B. 右侧弯曲，左侧襻状型；C. 左侧后部丛状型；D. 右侧交通动脉缺如；E. 左侧后交通动脉细小；
F. 右侧大脑后动脉起自后交通动脉

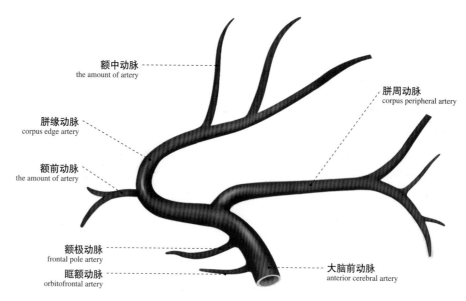

额中动脉
the amount of artery

胼周动脉
corpus peripheral artery

胼缘动脉
corpus edge artery

额前动脉
the amount of artery

额极动脉
frontal pole artery

眶额动脉
orbitofrontal artery

大脑前动脉
anterior cerebral artery

A

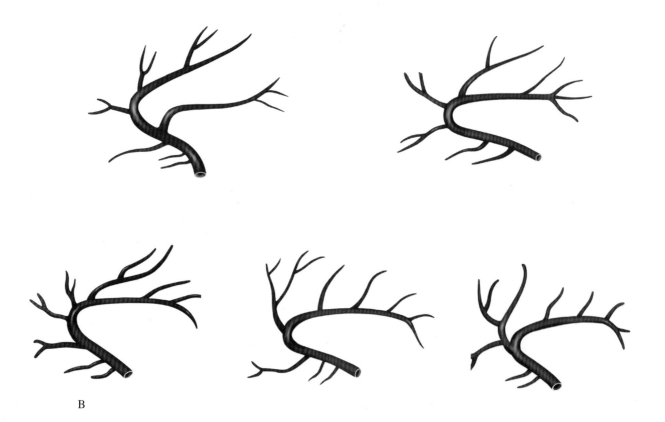

B

193. 大脑前动脉远侧段双干型的各种亚型
Various subtypes of the distal segment of the anterior cerebral artery double dry-type

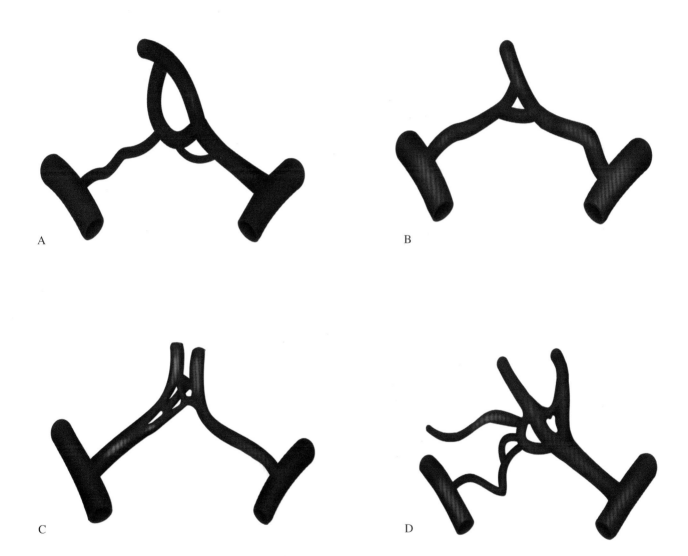

194. 大脑前动脉远侧段及前交通动脉变异示意图
Diagram for the variation of the distal segment of the anterior cerebral artery and the anterior communicating artery

A. 右侧大脑前动脉近侧段细小，增粗的前交通动脉起自左大脑前动脉；B. 双侧大脑前动脉近侧段走行异常，前交通动脉基本正常；C. 双侧大脑前动脉近侧段走行基本正常，前交通动脉呈丛状分布；D. 右侧大脑前动脉近侧段细小，左侧大脑前动脉增粗代偿，前交通动脉呈丛状分布

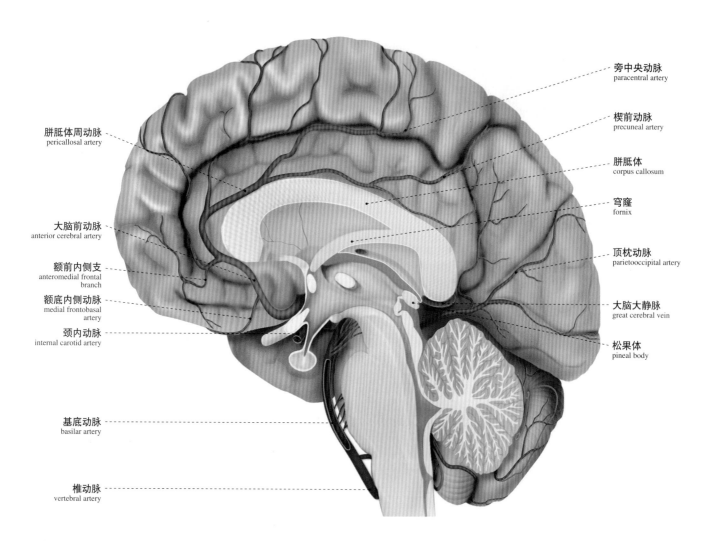

胼胝体周动脉
pericallosal artery

大脑前动脉
anterior cerebral artery

额前内侧支
anteromedial frontal
branch

额底内侧动脉
medial frontobasal
artery

颈内动脉
internal carotid artery

基底动脉
basilar artery

椎动脉
vertebral artery

旁中央动脉
paracentral artery

楔前动脉
precuneal artery

胼胝体
corpus callosum

穹窿
fornix

顶枕动脉
parietooccipital artery

大脑大静脉
great cerebral vein

松果体
pineal body

195. 大脑动脉（正中矢状断面观 1）
Arteries of the cerebrum (midsagittal section aspect 1)

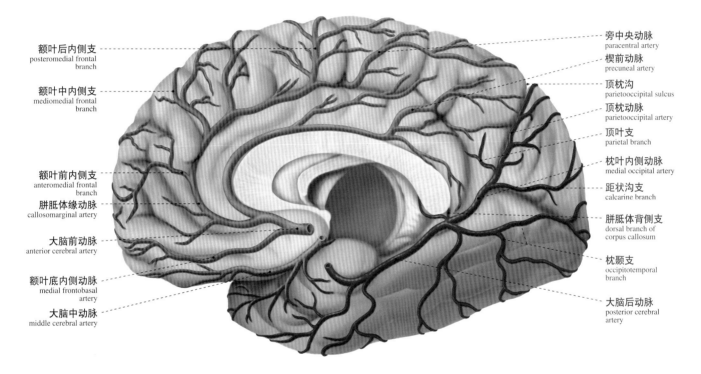

额叶后内侧支
posteromedial frontal branch

额叶中内侧支
mediomedial frontal branch

额叶前内侧支
anteromedial frontal branch

胼胝体缘动脉
callosomarginal artery

大脑前动脉
anterior cerebral artery

额叶底内侧动脉
medial frontobasal artery

大脑中动脉
middle cerebral artery

旁中央动脉
paracentral artery

楔前动脉
precuneal artery

顶枕沟
parietooccipital sulcus

顶枕动脉
parietooccipital artery

顶叶支
parietal branch

枕叶内侧动脉
medial occipital artery

距状沟支
calcarine branch

胼胝体背侧支
dorsal branch of corpus callosum

枕颞支
occipitotemporal branch

大脑后动脉
posterior cerebral artery

196. 大脑动脉（正中矢状断面观 2）
Arteries of the cerebrum (midsagittal section aspect 2)

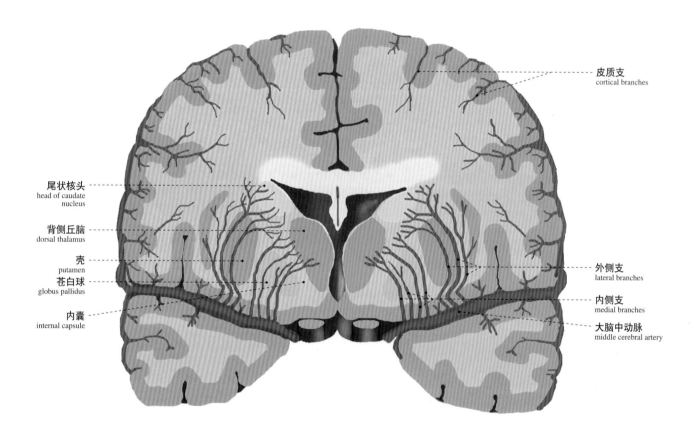

皮质支
cortical branches

尾状核头
head of caudate
nucleus

背侧丘脑
dorsal thalamus

壳
putamen

苍白球
globus pallidus

内囊
internal capsule

外侧支
lateral branches

内侧支
medial branches

大脑中动脉
middle cerebral artery

197. 大脑动脉的皮质支和中央支
Cortical and the central branches of the cerebral arteries

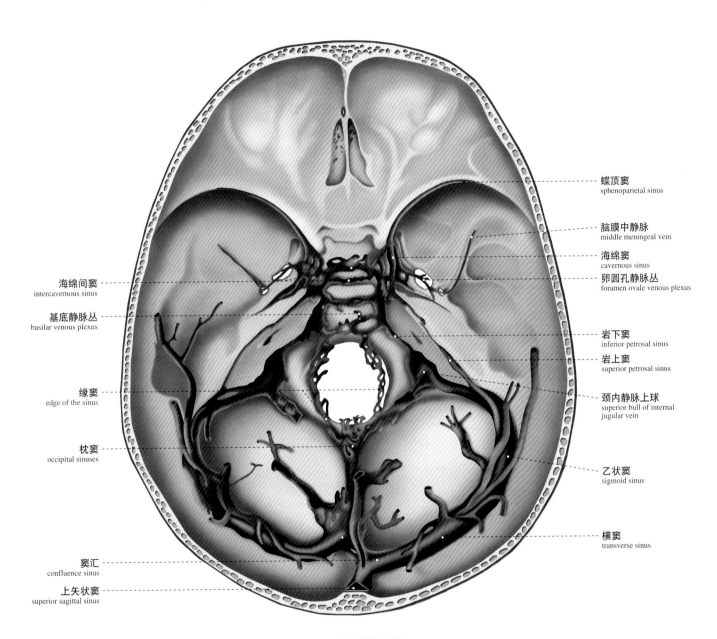

蝶顶窦
sphenoparietal sinus

脑膜中静脉
middle meningeal vein

海绵窦
cavernous sinus

卵圆孔静脉丛
foramen ovale venous plexus

海绵间窦
intercavernous sinus

基底静脉丛
basilar venous plexus

岩下窦
inferior petrosal sinus

岩上窦
superior petrosal sinus

缘窦
edge of the sinus

颈内静脉上球
superior bull of internal jugular vein

枕窦
occipital sinuses

乙状窦
sigmoid sinus

横窦
transverse sinus

窦汇
confluence sinus

上矢状窦
superior sagittal sinus

198. 硬脑膜静脉窦
Dural venous sinus

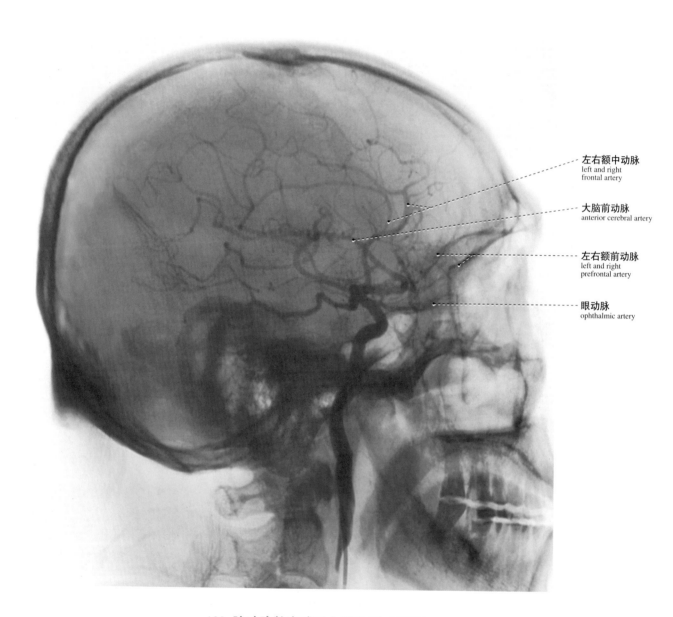

左右额中动脉
left and right
frontal artery

大脑前动脉
anterior cerebral artery

左右额前动脉
left and right
prefrontal artery

眼动脉
ophthalmic artery

199. 脑动脉数字减影血管造影（侧位）
DSA of cerebral arteries (lateral view)

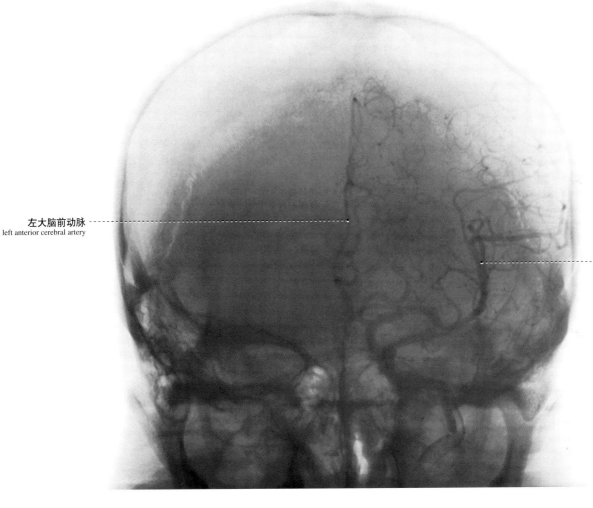

左大脑前动脉
left anterior cerebral artery

左大脑中动脉
left middle cerebral artery

200. 脑动脉数字减影血管造影（前后位）
DSA of cerebral arteries (anteroposterior view)

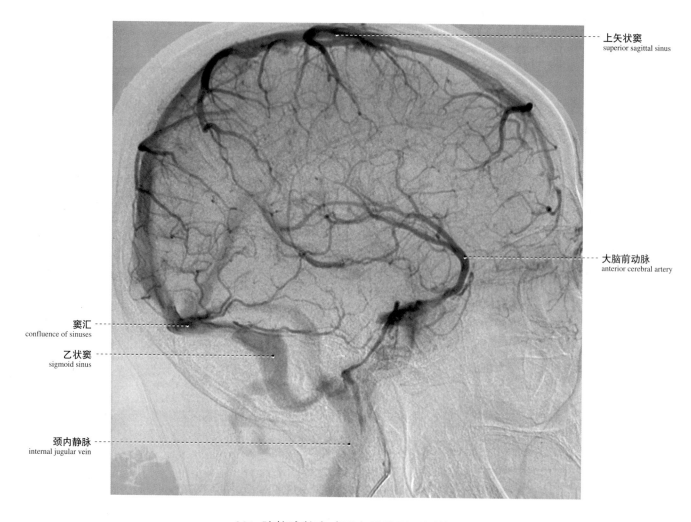

上矢状窦
superior sagittal sinus

大脑前动脉
anterior cerebral artery

窦汇
confluence of sinuses

乙状窦
sigmoid sinus

颈内静脉
internal jugular vein

201. 脑静脉数字减影血管造影（侧位）
Digital subtraction angiography of cerebral viens (lateral view)

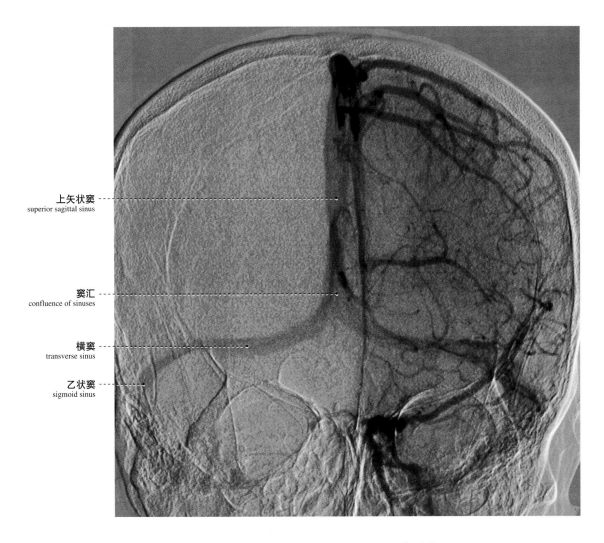

上矢状窦
superior sagittal sinus

窦汇
confluence of sinuses

横窦
transverse sinus

乙状窦
sigmoid sinus

202. 脑静脉数字减影血管造影（前后位）
Digital subtraction angiography of cerebral viens (anteroposterior view)

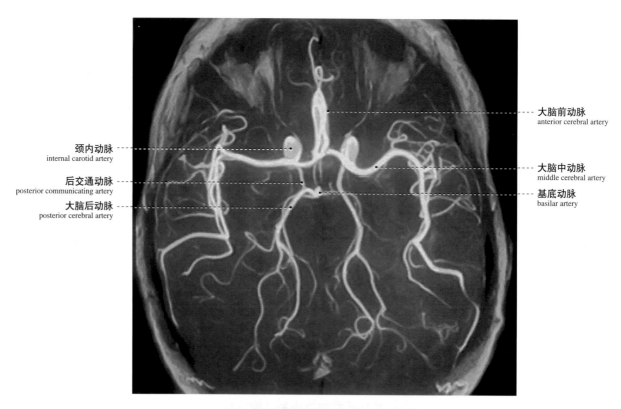

颈内动脉
internal carotid artery

后交通动脉
posterior communicating artery

大脑后动脉
posterior cerebral artery

大脑前动脉
anterior cerebral artery

大脑中动脉
middle cerebral artery

基底动脉
basilar artery

203. 脑磁共振动脉造影（上面观）
MRA of cerebral arteries (superior view)

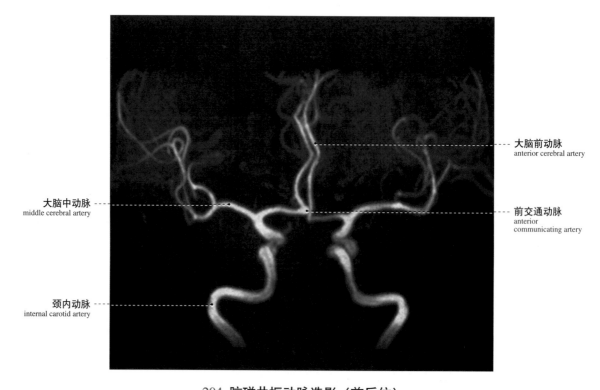

大脑中动脉
middle cerebral artery

颈内动脉
internal carotid artery

大脑前动脉
anterior cerebral artery

前交通动脉
anterior communicating artery

204. 脑磁共振动脉造影（前后位）
MRA of cerebral arteries (anteroposterior view)

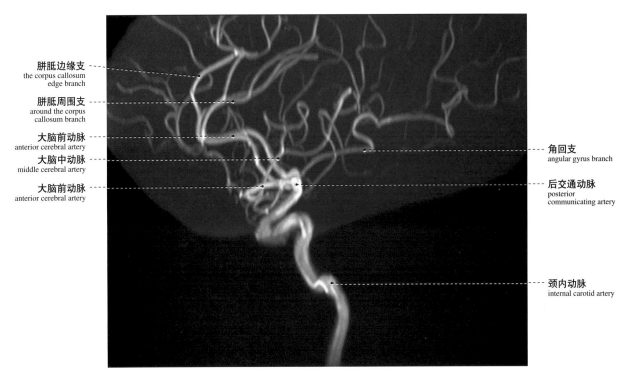

胼胝边缘支
the corpus callosum
edge branch

胼胝周围支
around the corpus
callosum branch

大脑前动脉
anterior cerebral artery

大脑中动脉
middle cerebral artery

大脑前动脉
anterior cerebral artery

角回支
angular gyrus branch

后交通动脉
posterior
communicating artery

颈内动脉
internal carotid artery

205. 脑磁共振动脉造影（侧位）
MRA of brain artery (lateral view)

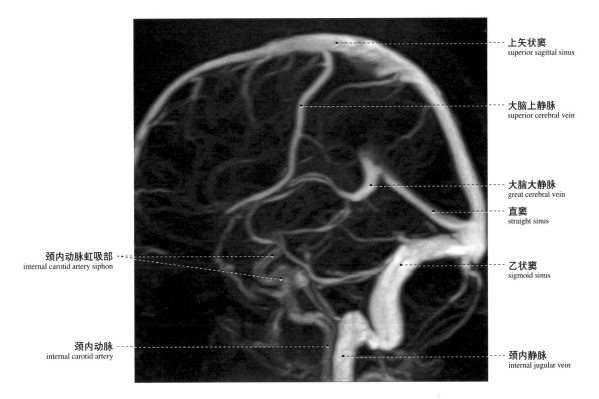

颈内动脉虹吸部
internal carotid artery siphon

颈内动脉
internal carotid artery

上矢状窦
superior sagittal sinus

大脑上静脉
superior cerebral vein

大脑大静脉
great cerebral vein

直窦
straight sinus

乙状窦
sigmoid sinus

颈内静脉
internal jugular vein

206. 脑磁共振静脉造影（侧位）
MRV of brain veins (lateral view)

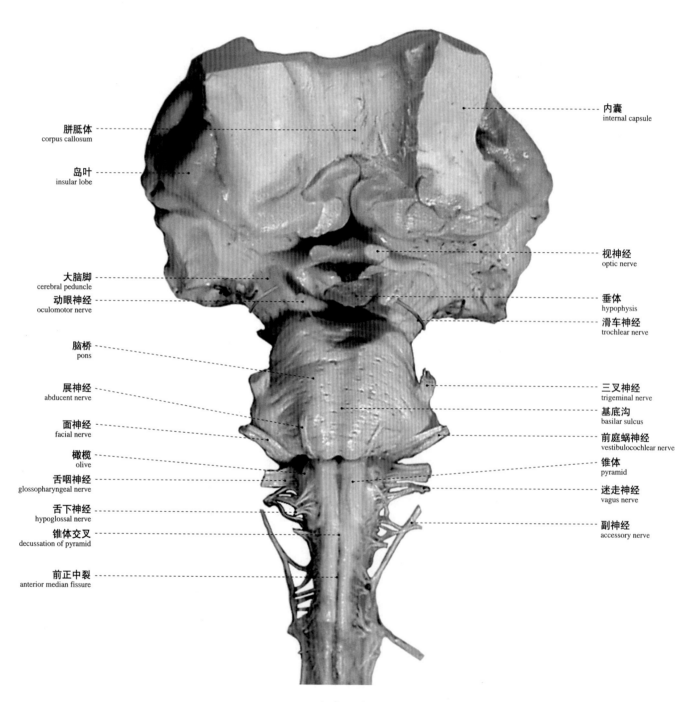

胼胝体
corpus callosum

岛叶
insular lobe

大脑脚
cerebral peduncle

动眼神经
oculomotor nerve

脑桥
pons

展神经
abducent nerve

面神经
facial nerve

橄榄
olive

舌咽神经
glossopharyngeal nerve

舌下神经
hypoglossal nerve

锥体交叉
decussation of pyramid

前正中裂
anterior median fissure

内囊
internal capsule

视神经
optic nerve

垂体
hypophysis

滑车神经
trochlear nerve

三叉神经
trigeminal nerve

基底沟
basilar sulcus

前庭蜗神经
vestibulocochlear nerve

锥体
pyramid

迷走神经
vagus nerve

副神经
accessory nerve

207. 脑干（腹面观）
Brain stem (ventral aspect)

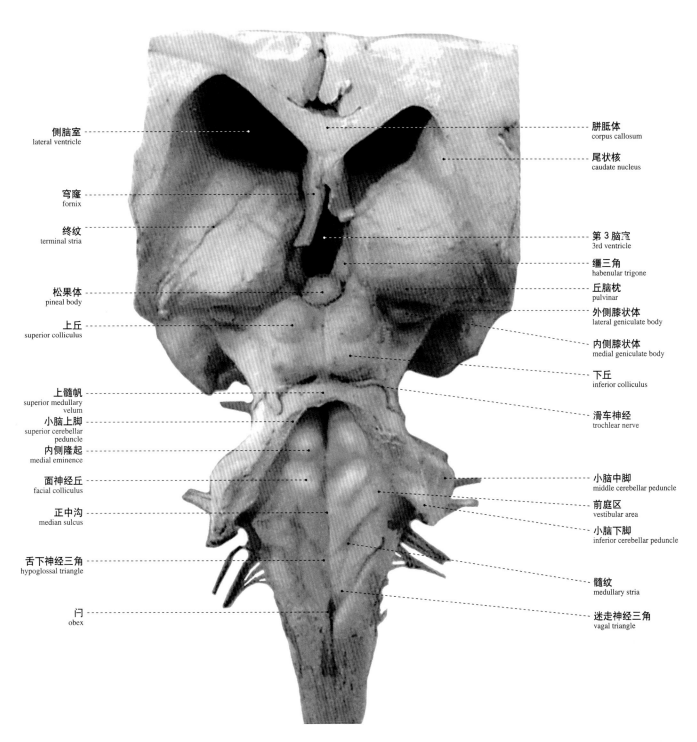

侧脑室
lateral ventricle

穹窿
fornix

终纹
terminal stria

松果体
pineal body

上丘
superior colliculus

上髓帆
superior medullary velum

小脑上脚
superior cerebellar peduncle

内侧隆起
medial eminence

面神经丘
facial colliculus

正中沟
median sulcus

舌下神经三角
hypoglossal triangle

闩
obex

胼胝体
corpus callosum

尾状核
caudate nucleus

第 3 脑室
3rd ventricle

缰三角
habenular trigone

丘脑枕
pulvinar

外侧膝状体
lateral geniculate body

内侧膝状体
medial geniculate body

下丘
inferior colliculus

滑车神经
trochlear nerve

小脑中脚
middle cerebellar peduncle

前庭区
vestibular area

小脑下脚
inferior cerebellar peduncle

髓纹
medullary stria

迷走神经三角
vagal triangle

208. 脑干（背面观）
Brain stem (dorsal aspect)

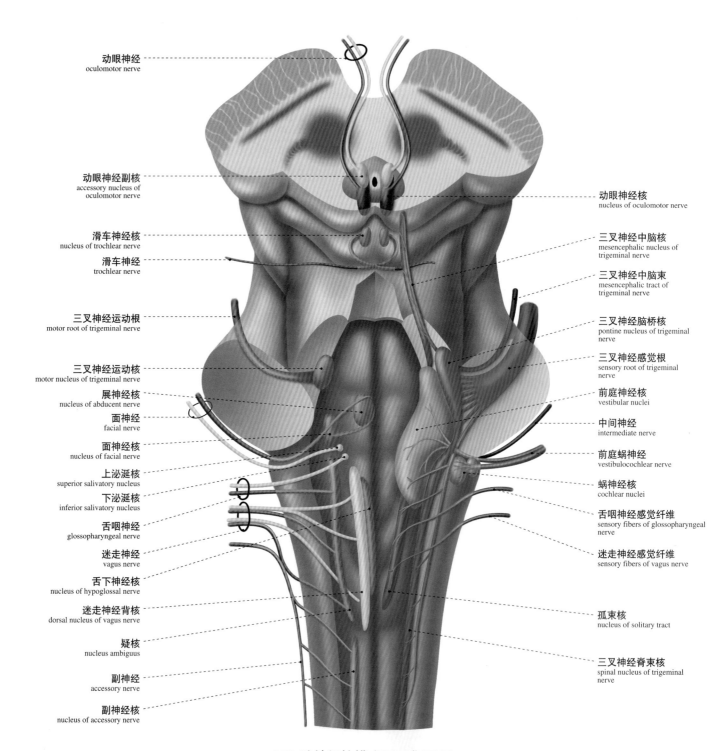

动眼神经
oculomotor nerve

动眼神经副核
accessory nucleus of
oculomotor nerve

滑车神经核
nucleus of trochlear nerve

滑车神经
trochlear nerve

三叉神经运动根
motor root of trigeminal nerve

三叉神经运动核
motor nucleus of trigeminal nerve

展神经核
nucleus of abducent nerve

面神经
facial nerve

面神经核
nucleus of facial nerve

上泌涎核
superior salivatory nucleus

下泌涎核
inferior salivatory nucleus

舌咽神经
glossopharyngeal nerve

迷走神经
vagus nerve

舌下神经核
nucleus of hypoglossal nerve

迷走神经背核
dorsal nucleus of vagus nerve

疑核
nucleus ambiguus

副神经
accessory nerve

副神经核
nucleus of accessory nerve

动眼神经核
nucleus of oculomotor nerve

三叉神经中脑核
mesencephalic nucleus of
trigeminal nerve

三叉神经中脑束
mesencephalic tract of
trigeminal nerve

三叉神经脑桥核
pontine nucleus of trigeminal
nerve

三叉神经感觉根
sensory root of trigeminal
nerve

前庭神经核
vestibular nuclei

中间神经
intermediate nerve

前庭蜗神经
vestibulocochlear nerve

蜗神经核
cochlear nuclei

舌咽神经感觉纤维
sensory fibers of glossopharyngeal
nerve

迷走神经感觉纤维
sensory fibers of vagus nerve

孤束核
nucleus of solitary tract

三叉神经脊束核
spinal nucleus of trigeminal
nerve

209. 脑神经核模式图（背面观）
Diagram of the nuclei of the cranial nerves (dorsal aspect)

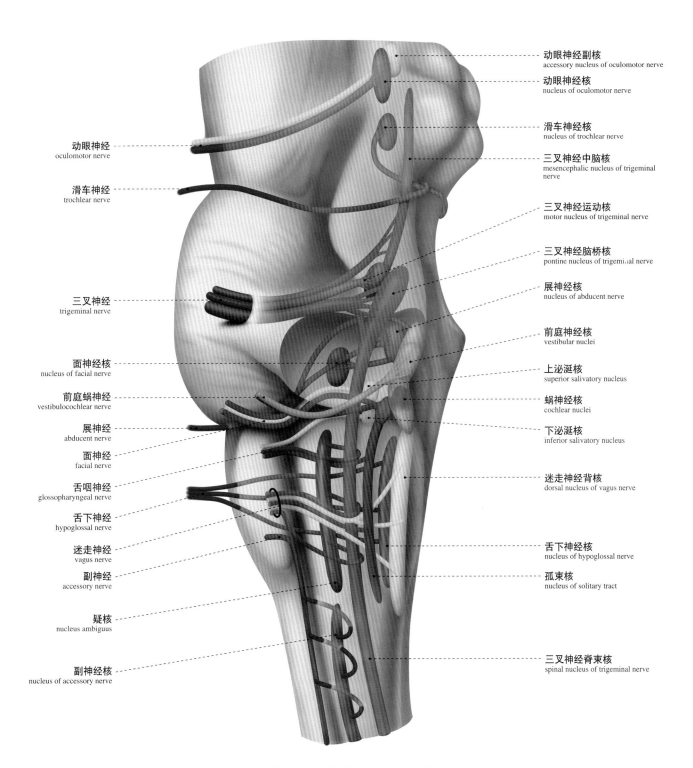

动眼神经副核
accessory nucleus of oculomotor nerve

动眼神经核
nucleus of oculomotor nerve

滑车神经核
nucleus of trochlear nerve

三叉神经中脑核
mesencephalic nucleus of trigeminal nerve

三叉神经运动核
motor nucleus of trigeminal nerve

三叉神经脑桥核
pontine nucleus of trigeminal nerve

展神经核
nucleus of abducent nerve

前庭神经核
vestibular nuclei

上泌涎核
superior salivatory nucleus

蜗神经核
cochlear nuclei

下泌涎核
inferior salivatory nucleus

迷走神经背核
dorsal nucleus of vagus nerve

舌下神经核
nucleus of hypoglossal nerve

孤束核
nucleus of solitary tract

三叉神经脊束核
spinal nucleus of trigeminal nerve

动眼神经
oculomotor nerve

滑车神经
trochlear nerve

三叉神经
trigeminal nerve

面神经核
nucleus of facial nerve

前庭蜗神经
vestibulocochlear nerve

展神经
abducent nerve

面神经
facial nerve

舌咽神经
glossopharyngeal nerve

舌下神经
hypoglossal nerve

迷走神经
vagus nerve

副神经
accessory nerve

疑核
nucleus ambiguus

副神经核
nucleus of accessory nerve

210. 脑神经核模式图（外侧面观）
Diagram of the nuclei of the cranial nerves (lateral aspect)

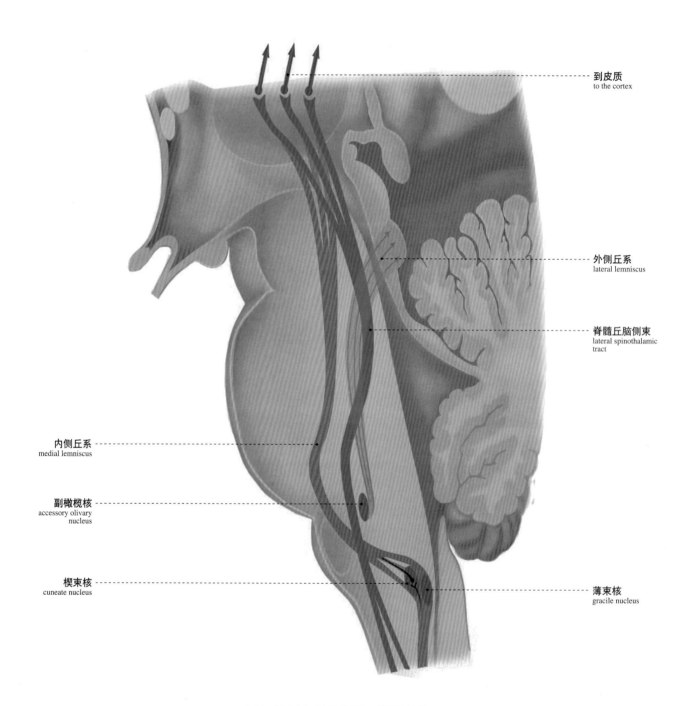

到皮质
to the cortex

外侧丘系
lateral lemniscus

脊髓丘脑侧束
lateral spinothalamic
tract

内侧丘系
medial lemniscus

副橄榄核
accessory olivary
nucleus

楔束核
cuneate nucleus

薄束核
gracile nucleus

211. 脑干上行传导路（侧面观）
Ascending tract in the brainstem (lateral aspect)

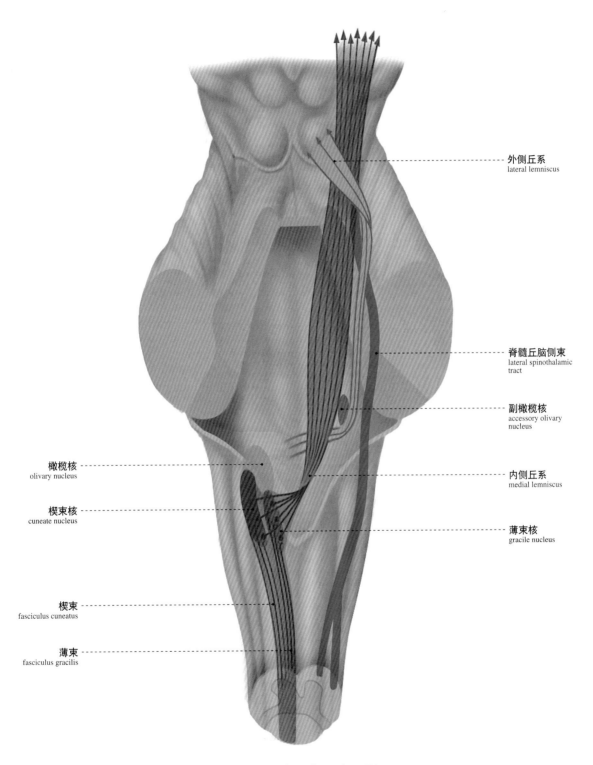

外侧丘系
lateral lemniscus

脊髓丘脑侧束
lateral spinothalamic
tract

副橄榄核
accessory olivary
nucleus

内侧丘系
medial lemniscus

薄束核
gracile nucleus

橄榄核
olivary nucleus

楔束核
cuneate nucleus

楔束
fasciculus cuneatus

薄束
fasciculus gracilis

212. 脑干上行传导路（后面观）
Ascending tract in the brainstem (posterior aspect)

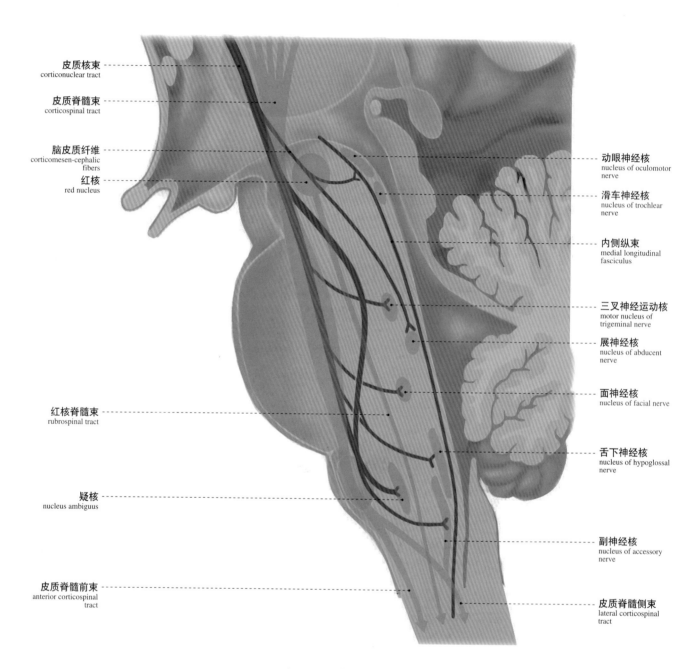

皮质核束
corticonuclear tract

皮质脊髓束
corticospinal tract

脑皮质纤维
corticomesen-cephalic fibers

红核
red nucleus

红核脊髓束
rubrospinal tract

疑核
nucleus ambiguus

皮质脊髓前束
anterior corticospinal tract

动眼神经核
nucleus of oculomotor nerve

滑车神经核
nucleus of trochlear nerve

内侧纵束
medial longitudinal fasciculus

三叉神经运动核
motor nucleus of trigeminal nerve

展神经核
nucleus of abducent nerve

面神经核
nucleus of facial nerve

舌下神经核
nucleus of hypoglossal nerve

副神经核
nucleus of accessory nerve

皮质脊髓侧束
lateral corticospinal tract

213. 脑干下行传导路（侧面观）
Descending tract in the brainstem (lateral aspect)

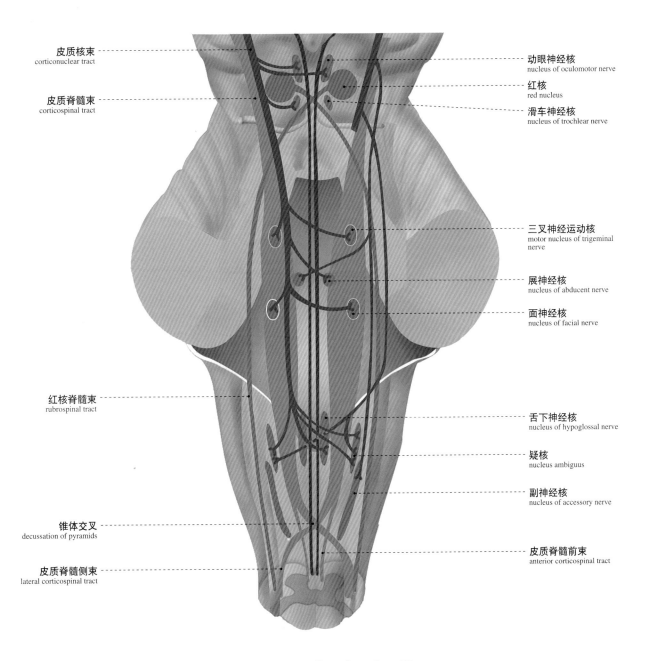

皮质核束
corticonuclear tract

皮质脊髓束
corticospinal tract

动眼神经核
nucleus of oculomotor nerve

红核
red nucleus

滑车神经核
nucleus of trochlear nerve

三叉神经运动核
motor nucleus of trigeminal nerve

展神经核
nucleus of abducent nerve

面神经核
nucleus of facial nerve

红核脊髓束
rubrospinal tract

舌下神经核
nucleus of hypoglossal nerve

疑核
nucleus ambiguus

副神经核
nucleus of accessory nerve

锥体交叉
decussation of pyramids

皮质脊髓前束
anterior corticospinal tract

皮质脊髓侧束
lateral corticospinal tract

214. 脑干下行传导路（后面观）
Descending tract in the brainstem (posterior aspect)

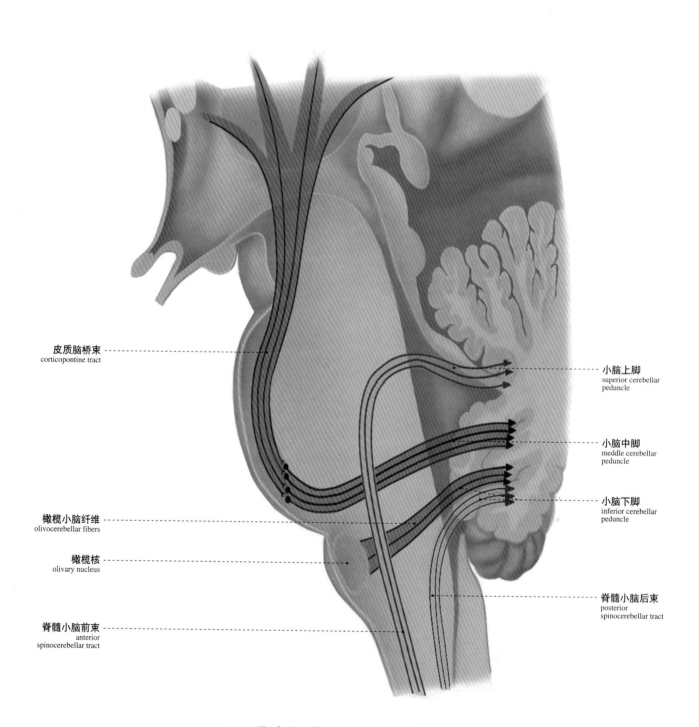

皮质脑桥束
corticopontine tract

橄榄小脑纤维
olivocerebellar fibers

橄榄核
olivary nucleus

脊髓小脑前束
anterior
spinocerebellar tract

小脑上脚
superior cerebellar
peduncle

小脑中脚
meddle cerebellar
peduncle

小脑下脚
inferior cerebellar
peduncle

脊髓小脑后束
posterior
spinocerebellar tract

215. 通过脑干的主要小脑传导路（侧面观）
Major cerebellar tracts through the brainstem (lateral aspect)

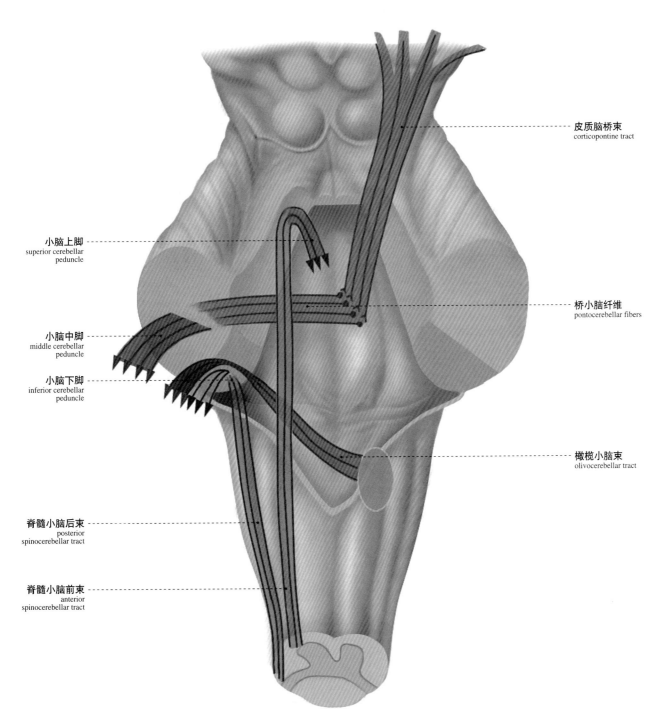

皮质脑桥束
corticopontine tract

小脑上脚
superior cerebellar
peduncle

桥小脑纤维
pontocerebellar fibers

小脑中脚
middle cerebellar
peduncle

小脑下脚
inferior cerebellar
peduncle

橄榄小脑束
olivocerebellar tract

脊髓小脑后束
posterior
spinocerebellar tract

脊髓小脑前束
anterior
spinocerebellar tract

216. 通过脑干的主要小脑传导路（背面观）
Major cerebellar tracts through the brainstem (posterior aspect)

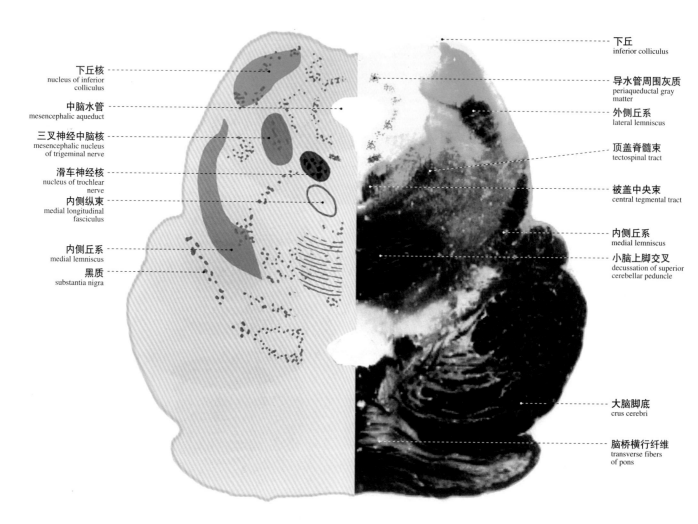

下丘核
nucleus of inferior colliculus

中脑水管
mesencephalic aqueduct

三叉神经中脑核
mesencephalic nucleus of trigeminal nerve

滑车神经核
nucleus of trochlear nerve

内侧纵束
medial longitudinal fasciculus

内侧丘系
medial lemniscus

黑质
substantia nigra

下丘
inferior colliculus

导水管周围灰质
periaqueductal gray matter

外侧丘系
lateral lemniscus

顶盖脊髓束
tectospinal tract

被盖中央束
central tegmental tract

内侧丘系
medial lemniscus

小脑上脚交叉
decussation of superior cerebellar peduncle

大脑脚底
crus cerebri

脑桥横行纤维
transverse fibers of pons

217. 中脑横切面（经下丘）
Transverse section of the midbrain (through the inferior colliculus)

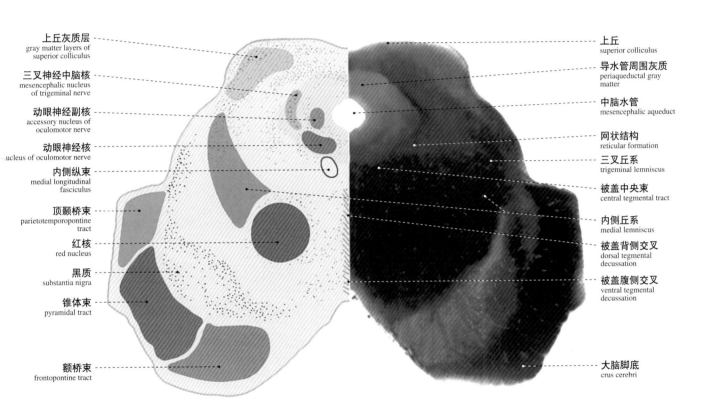

上丘灰质层
gray matter layers of
superior colliculus

三叉神经中脑核
mesencephalic nucleus
of trigeminal nerve

动眼神经副核
accessory nucleus of
oculomotor nerve

动眼神经核
nucleus of oculomotor nerve

内侧纵束
medial longitudinal
fasciculus

顶颞桥束
parietotemporopontine
tract

红核
red nucleus

黑质
substantia nigra

锥体束
pyramidal tract

额桥束
frontopontine tract

上丘
superior colliculus

导水管周围灰质
periaqueductal gray
matter

中脑水管
mesencephalic aqueduct

网状结构
reticular formation

三叉丘系
trigeminal lemniscus

被盖中央束
central tegmental tract

内侧丘系
medial lemniscus

被盖背侧交叉
dorsal tegmental
decussation

被盖腹侧交叉
ventral tegmental
decussation

大脑脚底
crus cerebri

218. 中脑横切面（经上丘）

Transverse section of the midbrain (through the superior colliculus)

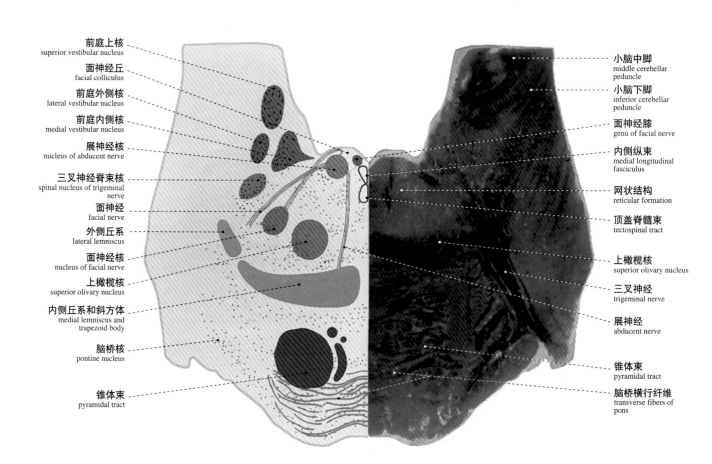

前庭上核
superior vestibular nucleus

面神经丘
facial colliculus

前庭外侧核
lateral vestibular nucleus

前庭内侧核
medial vestibular nucleus

展神经核
nucleus of abducent nerve

三叉神经脊束核
spinal nucleus of trigeminal nerve

面神经
facial nerve

外侧丘系
lateral lemniscus

面神经核
nucleus of facial nerve

上橄榄核
superior olivary nucleus

内侧丘系和斜方体
medial lemniscus and trapezoid body

脑桥核
pontine nucleus

锥体束
pyramidal tract

小脑中脚
middle cerebellar peduncle

小脑下脚
inferior cerebellar peduncle

面神经膝
genu of facial nerve

内侧纵束
medial longitudinal fasciculus

网状结构
reticular formation

顶盖脊髓束
tectospinal tract

上橄榄核
superior olivary nucleus

三叉神经
trigeminal nerve

展神经
abducent nerve

锥体束
pyramidal tract

脑桥横行纤维
transverse fibers of pons

219. 脑桥横切面（经面丘）
Transverse section of the pons (through the facial colliculus)

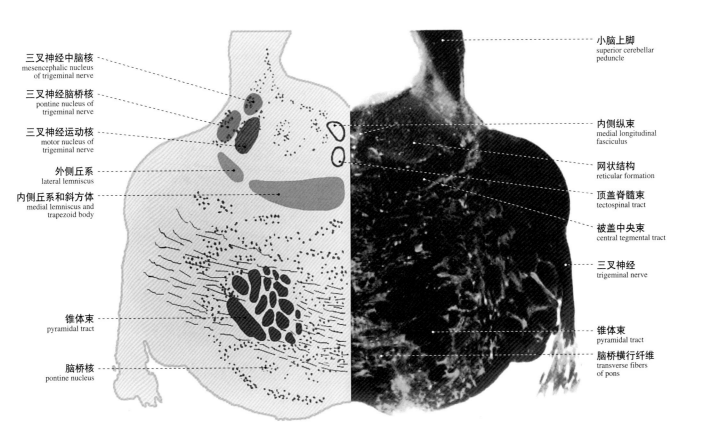

三叉神经中脑核
mesencephalic nucleus
of trigeminal nerve

三叉神经脑桥核
pontine nucleus of
trigeminal nerve

三叉神经运动核
motor nucleus of
trigeminal nerve

外侧丘系
lateral lemniscus

内侧丘系和斜方体
medial lemniscus and
trapezoid body

锥体束
pyramidal tract

脑桥核
pontine nucleus

小脑上脚
superior cerebellar
peduncle

内侧纵束
medial longitudinal
fasciculus

网状结构
reticular formation

顶盖脊髓束
tectospinal tract

被盖中央束
central tegmental tract

三叉神经
trigeminal nerve

锥体束
pyramidal tract

脑桥横行纤维
transverse fibers
of pons

220. 脑桥中部横切面
Transverse section of the middle part of the pons

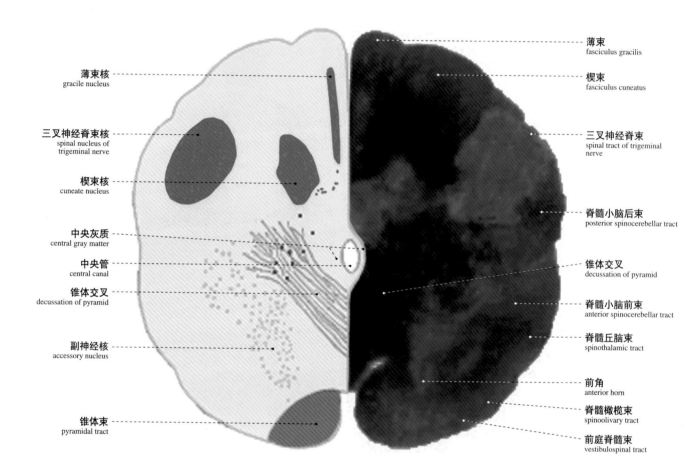

薄束核
gracile nucleus

三叉神经脊束核
spinal nucleus of
trigeminal nerve

楔束核
cuneate nucleus

中央灰质
central gray matter

中央管
central canal

锥体交叉
decussation of pyramid

副神经核
accessory nucleus

锥体束
pyramidal tract

薄束
fasciculus gracilis

楔束
fasciculus cuneatus

三叉神经脊束
spinal tract of trigeminal
nerve

脊髓小脑后束
posterior spinocerebellar tract

锥体交叉
decussation of pyramid

脊髓小脑前束
anterior spinocerebellar tract

脊髓丘脑束
spinothalamic tract

前角
anterior horn

脊髓橄榄束
spinoolivary tract

前庭脊髓束
vestibulospinal tract

221. 延髓横切面（经锥体交叉）
Transverse section of the medulla oblongata (through the pyramidal decussation)

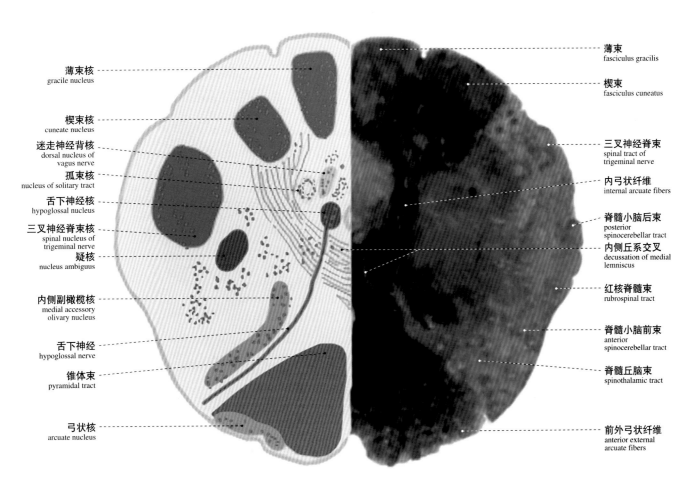

薄束核
gracile nucleus

楔束核
cuneate nucleus

迷走神经背核
dorsal nucleus of
vagus nerve

孤束核
nucleus of solitary tract

舌下神经核
hypoglossal nucleus

三叉神经脊束核
spinal nucleus of
trigeminal nerve

疑核
nucleus ambiguus

内侧副橄榄核
medial accessory
olivary nucleus

舌下神经
hypoglossal nerve

锥体束
pyramidal tract

弓状核
arcuate nucleus

薄束
fasciculus gracilis

楔束
fasciculus cuneatus

三叉神经脊束
spinal tract of
trigeminal nerve

内弓状纤维
internal arcuate fibers

脊髓小脑后束
posterior
spinocerebellar tract

内侧丘系交叉
decussation of medial
lemniscus

红核脊髓束
rubrospinal tract

脊髓小脑前束
anterior
spinocerebellar tract

脊髓丘脑束
spinothalamic tract

前外弓状纤维
anterior external
arcuate fibers

222. 延髓横切面（经内侧丘系交叉）
Transverse section of the medulla oblongata (through the decussation of the medial lemniscus)

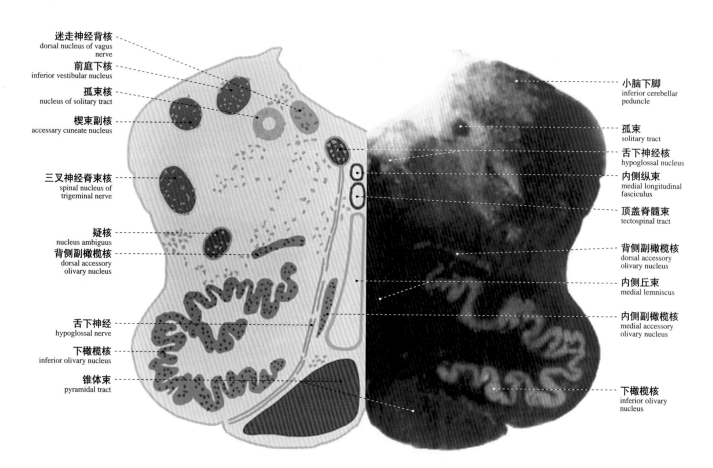

迷走神经背核
dorsal nucleus of vagus nerve

前庭下核
inferior vestibular nucleus

孤束核
nucleus of solitary tract

楔束副核
accessary cuneate nucleus

三叉神经脊束核
spinal nucleus of trigeminal nerve

疑核
nucleus ambiguus

背侧副橄榄核
dorsal accessory olivary nucleus

舌下神经
hypoglossal nerve

下橄榄核
inferior olivary nucleus

锥体束
pyramidal tract

小脑下脚
inferior cerebellar peduncle

孤束
solitary tract

舌下神经核
hypoglossal nucleus

内侧纵束
medial longitudinal fasciculus

顶盖脊髓束
tectospinal tract

背侧副橄榄核
dorsal accessory olivary nucleus

内侧丘束
medial lemniscus

内侧副橄榄核
medial accessory olivary nucleus

下橄榄核
inferior olivary nucleus

223. 延髓横切面（经橄榄中部）
Transverse section of the medulla oblongata (through the middle portion of the olive)

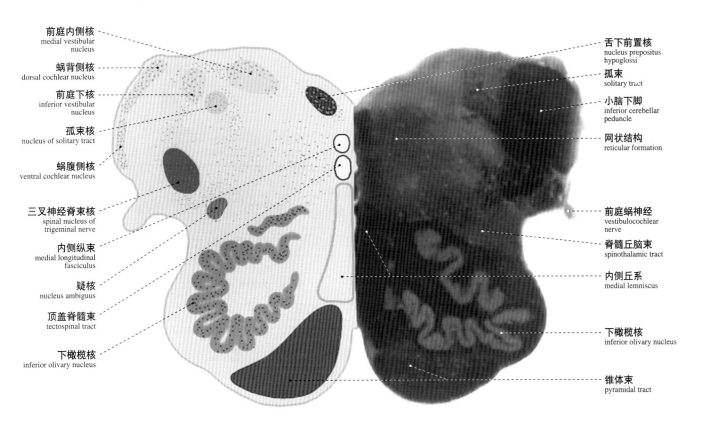

前庭内侧核
medial vestibular
nucleus

蜗背侧核
dorsal cochlear nucleus

前庭下核
inferior vestibular
nucleus

孤束核
nucleus of solitary tract

蜗腹侧核
ventral cochlear nucleus

三叉神经脊束核
spinal nucleus of
trigeminal nerve

内侧纵束
medial longitudinal
fasciculus

疑核
nucleus ambiguus

顶盖脊髓束
tectospinal tract

下橄榄核
inferior olivary nucleus

舌下前置核
nucleus prepositus
hypoglossi

孤束
solitary tract

小脑下脚
inferior cerebellar
peduncle

网状结构
reticular formation

前庭蜗神经
vestibulocochlear
nerve

脊髓丘脑束
spinothalamic tract

内侧丘系
medial lemniscus

下橄榄核
inferior olivary nucleus

锥体束
pyramidal tract

224. 延髓横切面（经橄榄上部）

Transverse section of the medulla oblongata (through the superior portion of the olive)

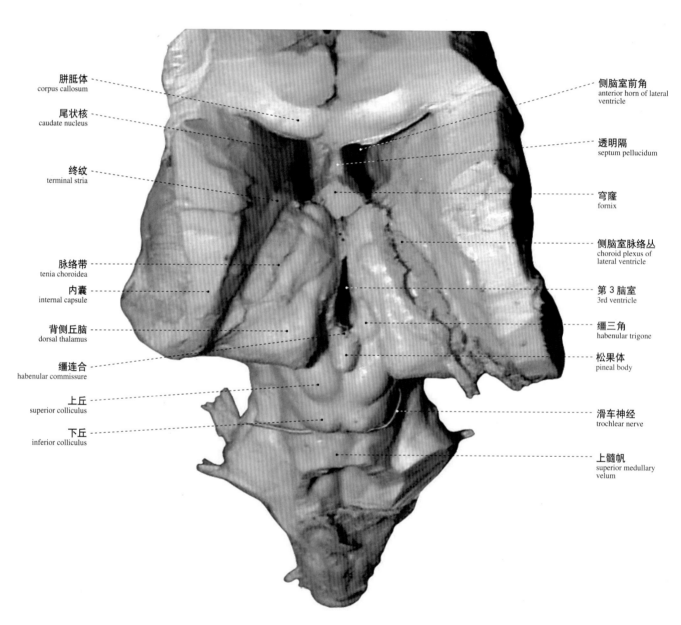

肼胝体
corpus callosum

尾状核
caudate nucleus

终纹
terminal stria

脉络带
tenia choroidea

内囊
internal capsule

背侧丘脑
dorsal thalamus

缰连合
habenular commissure

上丘
superior colliculus

下丘
inferior colliculus

侧脑室前角
anterior horn of lateral ventricle

透明隔
septum pellucidum

穹窿
fornix

侧脑室脉络丛
choroid plexus of lateral ventricle

第 3 脑室
3rd ventricle

缰三角
habenular trigone

松果体
pineal body

滑车神经
trochlear nerve

上髓帆
superior medullary velum

225. 间脑（背面观）
Diencephalon (dorsal aspect)

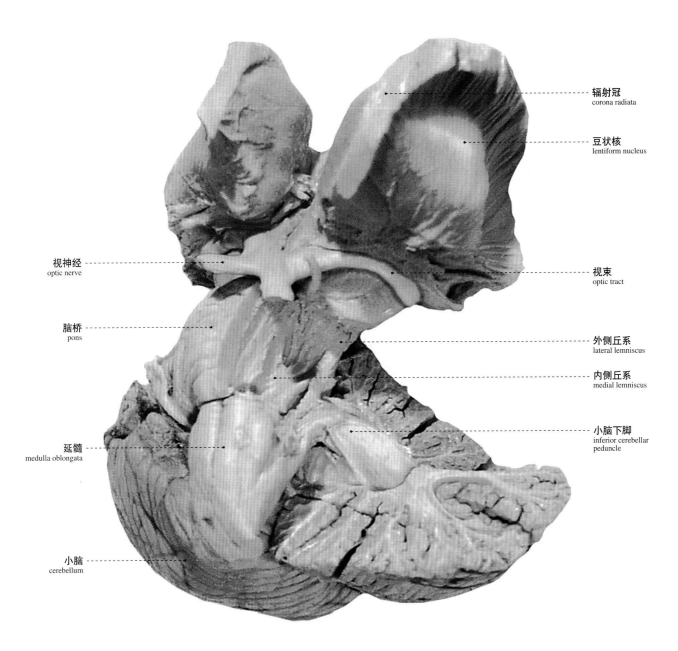

视神经
optic nerve

脑桥
pons

延髓
medulla oblongata

小脑
cerebellum

辐射冠
corona radiata

豆状核
lentiform nucleus

视束
optic tract

外侧丘系
lateral lemniscus

内侧丘系
medial lemniscus

小脑下脚
inferior cerebellar
peduncle

226. 内侧丘系和外侧丘系
Medial and lateral lemniscuses

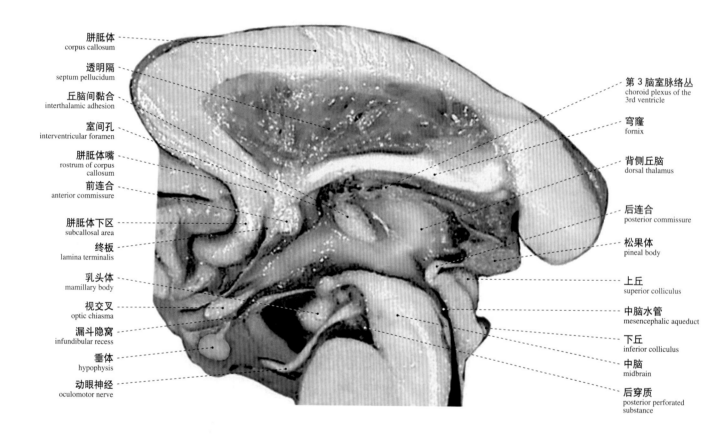

胼胝体
corpus callosum

透明隔
septum pellucidum

丘脑间黏合
interthalamic adhesion

室间孔
interventricular foramen

胼胝体嘴
rostrum of corpus callosum

前连合
anterior commissure

胼胝体下区
subcallosal area

终板
lamina terminalis

乳头体
mamillary body

视交叉
optic chiasma

漏斗隐窝
infundibular recess

垂体
hypophysis

动眼神经
oculomotor nerve

第 3 脑室脉络丛
choroid plexus of the 3rd ventricle

穹窿
fornix

背侧丘脑
dorsal thalamus

后连合
posterior commissure

松果体
pineal body

上丘
superior colliculus

中脑水管
mesencephalic aqueduct

下丘
inferior colliculus

中脑
midbrain

后穿质
posterior perforated substance

227. 间脑（内侧面观）
Diencephalon (medial aspect)

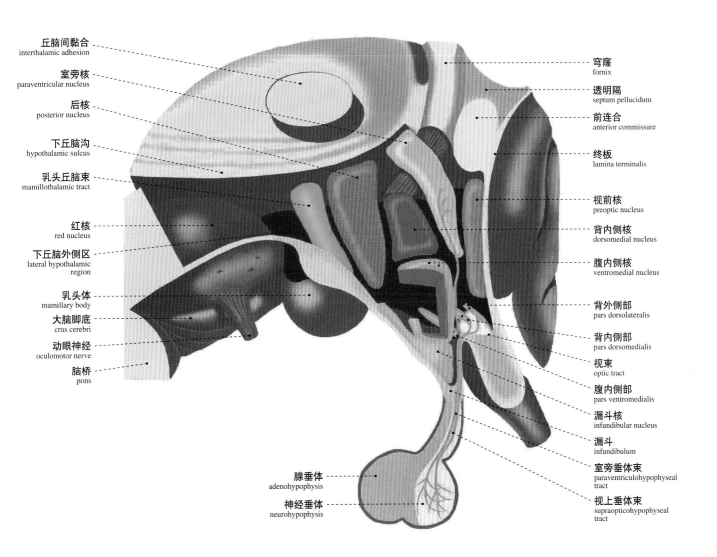

丘脑间黏合
interthalamic adhesion

室旁核
paraventricular nucleus

后核
posterior nucleus

下丘脑沟
hypothalamic sulcus

乳头丘脑束
mamillothalamic tract

红核
red nucleus

下丘脑外侧区
lateral hypothalamic
region

乳头体
mamillary body

大脑脚底
crus cerebri

动眼神经
oculomotor nerve

脑桥
pons

腺垂体
adenohypophysis

神经垂体
neurohypophysis

穹窿
fornix

透明隔
septum pellucidum

前连合
anterior commissure

终板
lamina terminalis

视前核
preoptic nucleus

背内侧核
dorsomedial nucleus

腹内侧核
ventromedial nucleus

背外侧部
pars dorsolateralis

背内侧部
pars dorsomedialis

视束
optic tract

腹内侧部
pars ventromedialis

漏斗核
infundibular nucleus

漏斗
infundibulum

室旁垂体束
paraventriculohypophyseal
tract

视上垂体束
supraopticohypophyseal
tract

228. 下丘脑核团
Hypothalamic nuclei

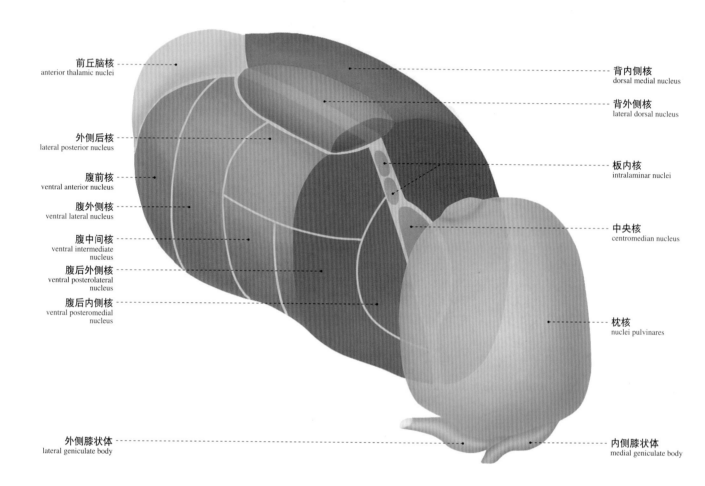

前丘脑核
anterior thalamic nuclei

外侧后核
lateral posterior nucleus

腹前核
ventral anterior nucleus

腹外侧核
ventral lateral nucleus

腹中间核
ventral intermediate
nucleus

腹后外侧核
ventral posterolateral
nucleus

腹后内侧核
ventral posteromedial
nucleus

外侧膝状体
lateral geniculate body

背内侧核
dorsal medial nucleus

背外侧核
lateral dorsal nucleus

板内核
intralaminar nuclei

中央核
centromedian nucleus

枕核
nuclei pulvinares

内侧膝状体
medial geniculate body

229. 背侧丘脑核团
Dorsal thalamus nuclei

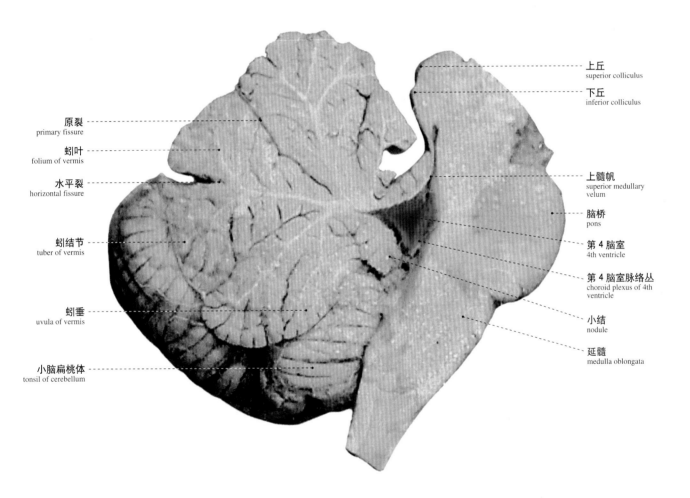

原裂
primary fissure

蚓叶
folium of vermis

水平裂
horizontal fissure

蚓结节
tuber of vermis

蚓垂
uvula of vermis

小脑扁桃体
tonsil of cerebellum

上丘
superior colliculus

下丘
inferior colliculus

上髓帆
superior medullary velum

脑桥
pons

第4脑室
4th ventricle

第4脑室脉络丛
choroid plexus of 4th ventricle

小结
nodule

延髓
medulla oblongata

230. 小脑（正中矢状切面）
Cerebellum (median sagittal section)

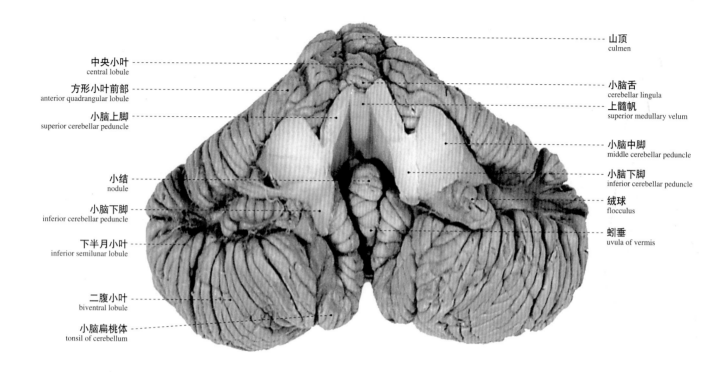

中央小叶
central lobule

方形小叶前部
anterior quadrangular lobule

小脑上脚
superior cerebellar peduncle

小结
nodule

小脑下脚
inferior cerebellar peduncle

下半月小叶
inferior semilunar lobule

二腹小叶
biventral lobule

小脑扁桃体
tonsil of cerebellum

山顶
culmen

小脑舌
cerebellar lingula

上髓帆
superior medullary velum

小脑中脚
middle cerebellar peduncle

小脑下脚
inferior cerebellar peduncle

绒球
flocculus

蚓垂
uvula of vermis

231. 小脑（前面观）
Cerebellum (anterior aspect)

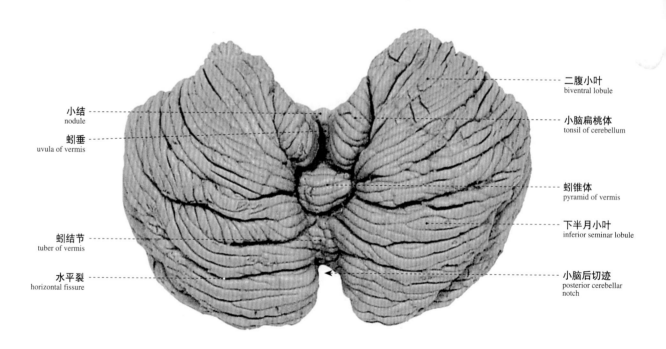

小结
nodule

蚓垂
uvula of vermis

蚓结节
tuber of vermis

水平裂
horizontal fissure

二腹小叶
biventral lobule

小脑扁桃体
tonsil of cerebellum

蚓锥体
pyramid of vermis

下半月小叶
inferior seminar lobule

小脑后切迹
posterior cerebellar notch

232. 小脑（下面观）
Cerebellum (inferior aspect)

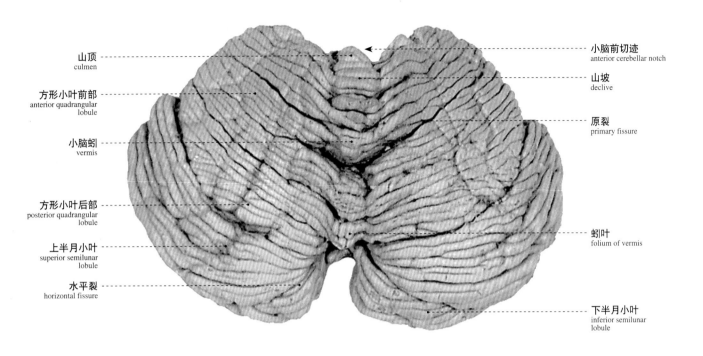

山顶
culmen

方形小叶前部
anterior quadrangular lobule

小脑蚓
vermis

方形小叶后部
posterior quadrangular lobule

上半月小叶
superior semilunar lobule

水平裂
horizontal fissure

小脑前切迹
anterior cerebellar notch

山坡
declive

原裂
primary fissure

蚓叶
folium of vermis

下半月小叶
inferior semilunar lobule

233. 小脑（上面观）
Cerebellum (superior aspect)

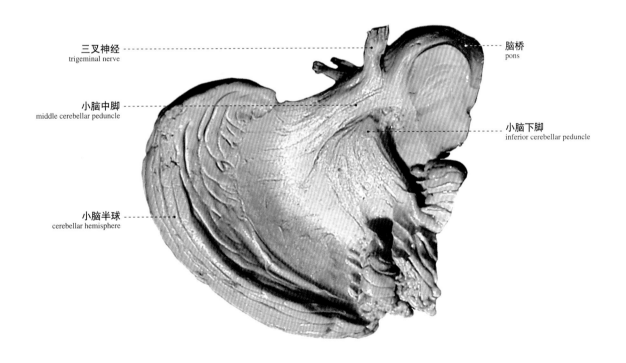

三叉神经
trigeminal nerve

小脑中脚
middle cerebellar peduncle

小脑半球
cerebellar hemisphere

脑桥
pons

小脑下脚
inferior cerebellar peduncle

234. 小脑脚
Peduncles of the cerebellum

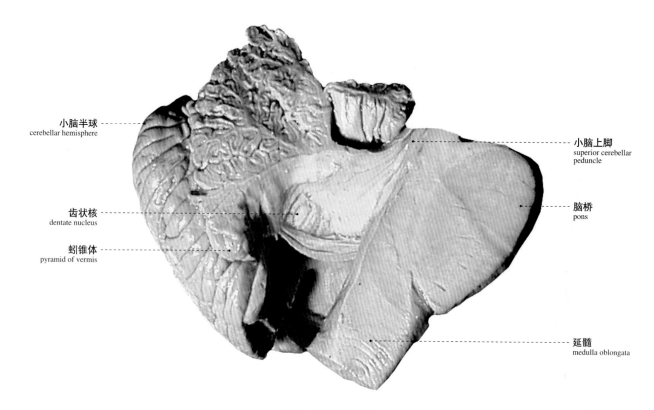

小脑半球
cerebellar hemisphere

齿状核
dentate nucleus

蚓锥体
pyramid of vermis

小脑上脚
superior cerebellar peduncle

脑桥
pons

延髓
medulla oblongata

235. 小脑齿状核
Dentate nucleus of the cerebellum

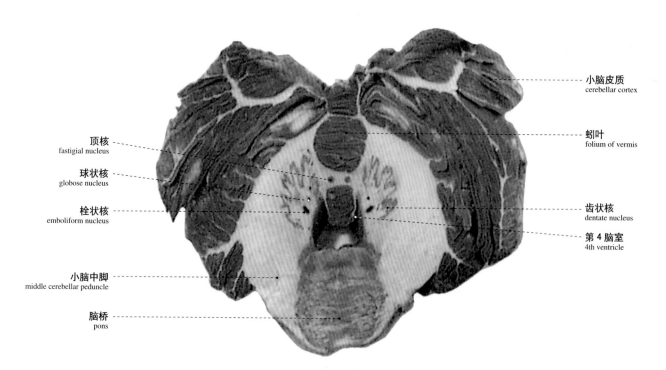

顶核
fastigial nucleus

球状核
globose nucleus

栓状核
emboliform nucleus

小脑中脚
middle cerebellar peduncle

脑桥
pons

小脑皮质
cerebellar cortex

蚓叶
folium of vermis

齿状核
dentate nucleus

第 4 脑室
4th ventricle

236. 小脑（横切面）
Cerebellum (transverse section)

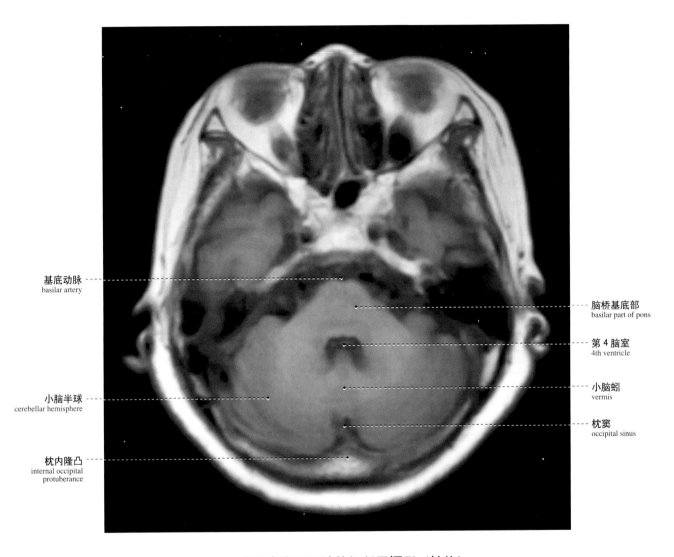

基底动脉
basilar artery

小脑半球
cerebellar hemisphere

枕内隆凸
internal occipital
protuberance

脑桥基底部
basilar part of pons

第 4 脑室
4th ventricle

小脑蚓
vermis

枕窦
occipital sinus

237. 小脑中脚层面计算机断层摄影（轴位）
CT of the middle cerebellar peduncles (axial view)

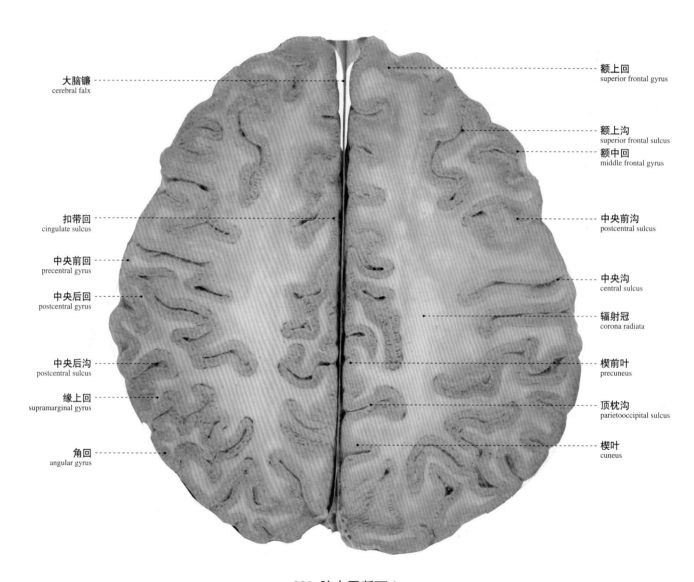

大脑镰
cerebral falx

额上回
superior frontal gyrus

额上沟
superior frontal sulcus

额中回
middle frontal gyrus

扣带回
cingulate sulcus

中央前沟
postcentral sulcus

中央前回
precentral gyrus

中央沟
central sulcus

中央后回
postcentral gyrus

辐射冠
corona radiata

中央后沟
postcentral sulcus

楔前叶
precuneus

缘上回
supramarginal gyrus

顶枕沟
parietooccipital sulcus

角回
angular gyrus

楔叶
cuneus

238. 脑水平断面 1
Horizontal section of the brain 1

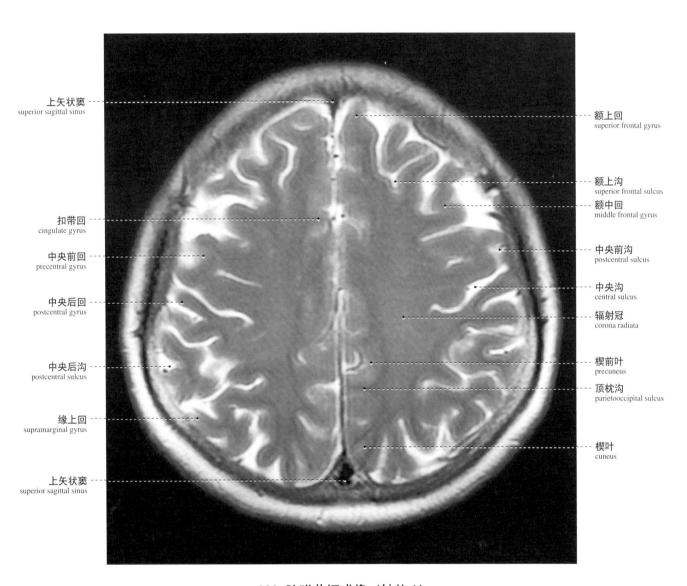

上矢状窦
superior sagittal sinus

扣带回
cingulate gyrus

中央前回
precentral gyrus

中央后回
postcentral gyrus

中央后沟
postcentral sulcus

缘上回
supramarginal gyrus

上矢状窦
superior sagittal sinus

额上回
superior frontal gyrus

额上沟
superior frontal sulcus

额中回
middle frontal gyrus

中央前沟
postcentral sulcus

中央沟
central sulcus

辐射冠
corona radiata

楔前叶
precuneus

顶枕沟
parietooccipital sulcus

楔叶
cuneus

239. 脑磁共振成像（轴位 1）
MRI of the brain (axial view 1)

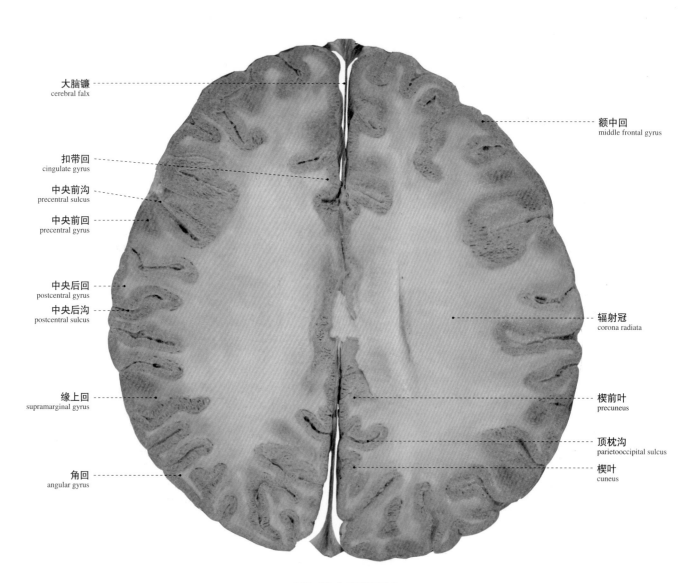

大脑镰
cerebral falx

额中回
middle frontal gyrus

扣带回
cingulate gyrus

中央前沟
precentral sulcus

中央前回
precentral gyrus

中央后回
postcentral gyrus

中央后沟
postcentral sulcus

辐射冠
corona radiata

缘上回
supramarginal gyrus

楔前叶
precuneus

顶枕沟
parietooccipital sulcus

角回
angular gyrus

楔叶
cuneus

240. 脑水平断面 2
Horizontal section of the brain 2

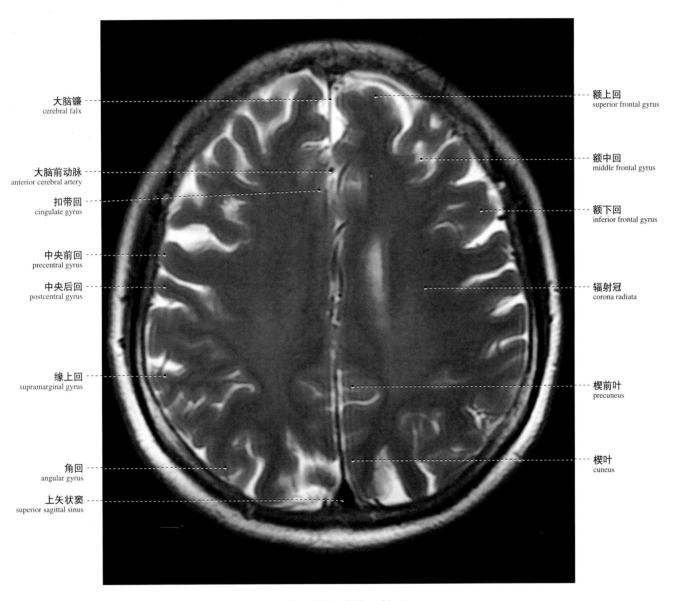

大脑镰
cerebral falx

大脑前动脉
anterior cerebral artery

扣带回
cingulate gyrus

中央前回
precentral gyrus

中央后回
postcentral gyrus

缘上回
supramarginal gyrus

角回
angular gyrus

上矢状窦
superior sagittal sinus

额上回
superior frontal gyrus

额中回
middle frontal gyrus

额下回
inferior frontal gyrus

辐射冠
corona radiata

楔前叶
precuneus

楔叶
cuneus

241. 脑磁共振成像（轴位 2）
MRI of the brain (axial view 2)

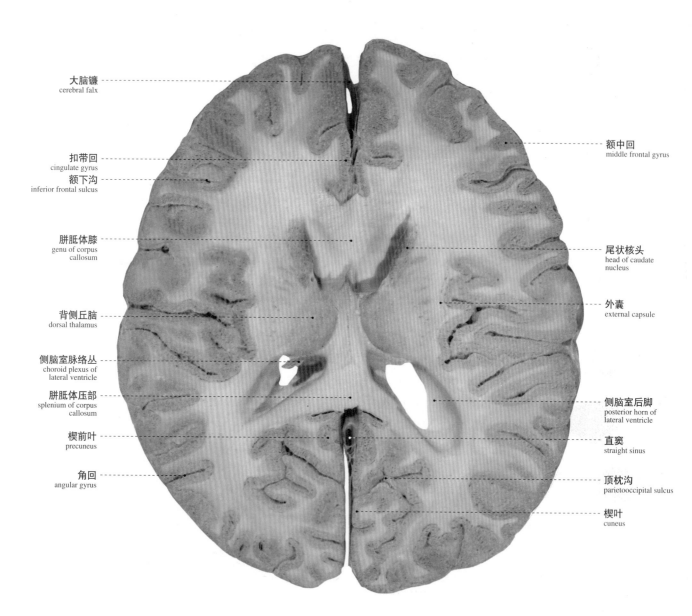

大脑镰
cerebral falx

扣带回
cingulate gyrus

额下沟
inferior frontal sulcus

胼胝体膝
genu of corpus callosum

背侧丘脑
dorsal thalamus

侧脑室脉络丛
choroid plexus of lateral ventricle

胼胝体压部
splenium of corpus callosum

楔前叶
precuneus

角回
angular gyrus

额中回
middle frontal gyrus

尾状核头
head of caudate nucleus

外囊
external capsule

侧脑室后脚
posterior horn of lateral ventricle

直窦
straight sinus

顶枕沟
parietooccipital sulcus

楔叶
cuneus

242. 脑水平断面 3
Horizontal section of the brain 3

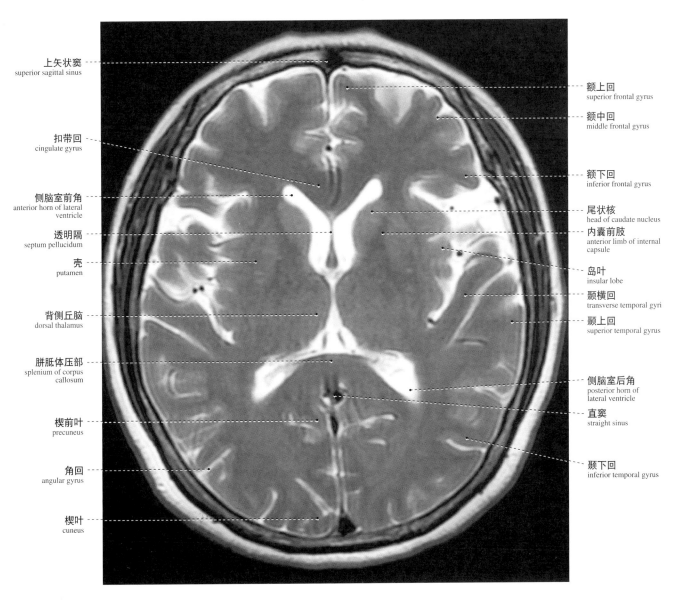

上矢状窦
superior sagittal sinus

扣带回
cingulate gyrus

侧脑室前角
anterior horn of lateral ventricle

透明隔
septum pellucidum

壳
putamen

背侧丘脑
dorsal thalamus

胼胝体压部
splenium of corpus callosum

楔前叶
precuneus

角回
angular gyrus

楔叶
cuneus

额上回
superior frontal gyrus

额中回
middle frontal gyrus

额下回
inferior frontal gyrus

尾状核
head of caudate nucleus

内囊前肢
anterior limb of internal capsule

岛叶
insular lobe

颞横回
transverse temporal gyri

颞上回
superior temporal gyrus

侧脑室后角
posterior horn of lateral ventricle

直窦
straight sinus

颞下回
inferior temporal gyrus

243. 脑磁共振成像（轴位 3）
MRI of the brain (axial view 3)

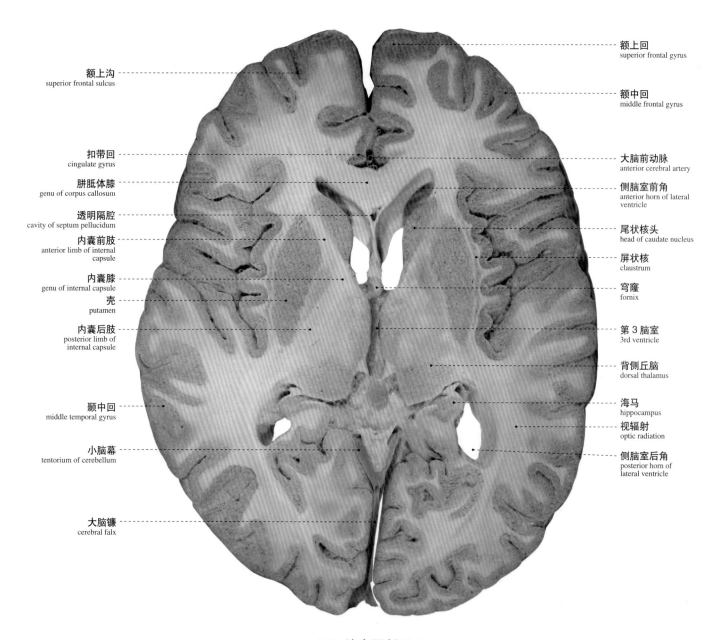

额上沟
superior frontal sulcus

扣带回
cingulate gyrus

胼胝体膝
genu of corpus callosum

透明隔腔
cavity of septum pellucidum

内囊前肢
anterior limb of internal capsule

内囊膝
genu of internal capsule

壳
putamen

内囊后肢
posterior limb of internal capsule

颞中回
middle temporal gyrus

小脑幕
tentorium of cerebellum

大脑镰
cerebral falx

额上回
superior frontal gyrus

额中回
middle frontal gyrus

大脑前动脉
anterior cerebral artery

侧脑室前角
anterior horn of lateral ventricle

尾状核头
head of caudate nucleus

屏状核
claustrum

穹窿
fornix

第3脑室
3rd ventricle

背侧丘脑
dorsal thalamus

海马
hippocampus

视辐射
optic radiation

侧脑室后角
posterior horn of lateral ventricle

244. 脑水平断面 4
Horizontal section of the brain 4

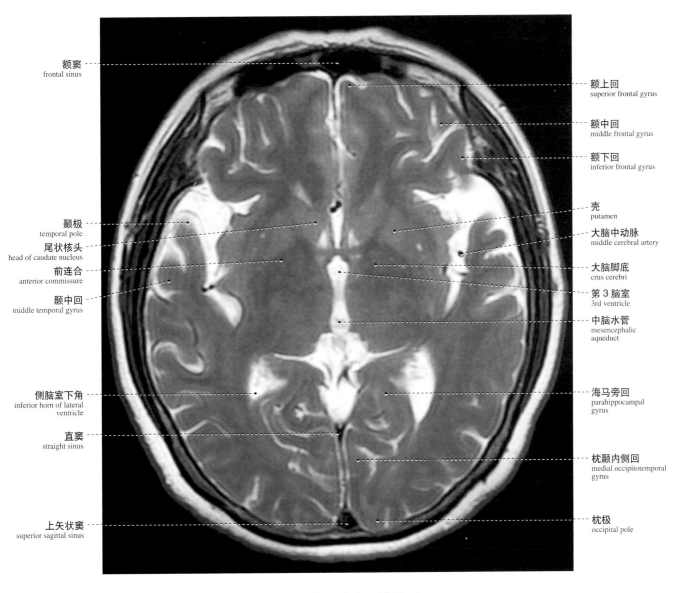

额窦
frontal sinus

额上回
superior frontal gyrus

额中回
middle frontal gyrus

额下回
inferior frontal gyrus

壳
putamen

颞极
temporal pole

大脑中动脉
middle cerebral artery

尾状核头
head of caudate nucleus

大脑脚底
crus cerebri

前连合
anterior commissure

第3脑室
3rd ventricle

颞中回
middle temporal gyrus

中脑水管
mesencephalic aqueduct

侧脑室下角
inferior horn of lateral ventricle

海马旁回
parahippocampal gyrus

直窦
straight sinus

枕颞内侧回
medial occipitotemporal gyrus

上矢状窦
superior sagittal sinus

枕极
occipital pole

245. 脑磁共振成像（轴位4）
MRI of the brain (axial view 4)

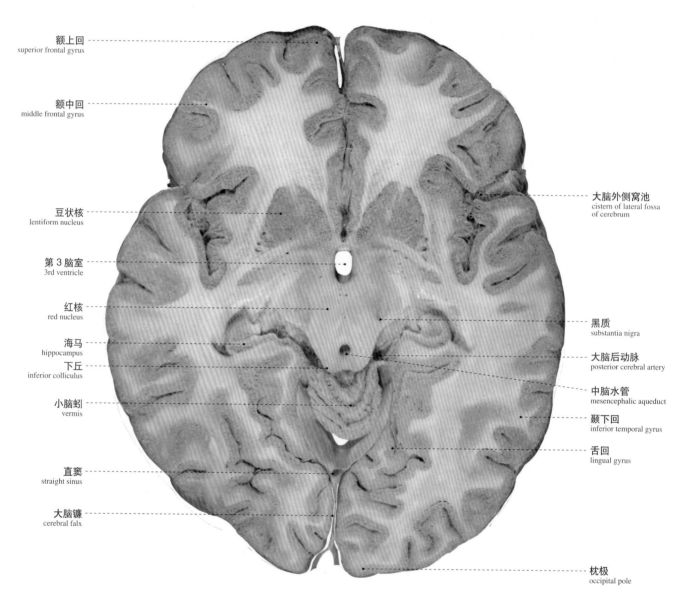

额上回
superior frontal gyrus

额中回
middle frontal gyrus

豆状核
lentiform nucleus

第 3 脑室
3rd ventricle

红核
red nucleus

海马
hippocampus

下丘
inferior colliculus

小脑蚓
vermis

直窦
straight sinus

大脑镰
cerebral falx

大脑外侧窝池
cistern of lateral fossa
of cerebrum

黑质
substantia nigra

大脑后动脉
posterior cerebral artery

中脑水管
mesencephalic aqueduct

颞下回
inferior temporal gyrus

舌回
lingual gyrus

枕极
occipital pole

246. 脑水平断面 5
Horizontal section of the brain 5

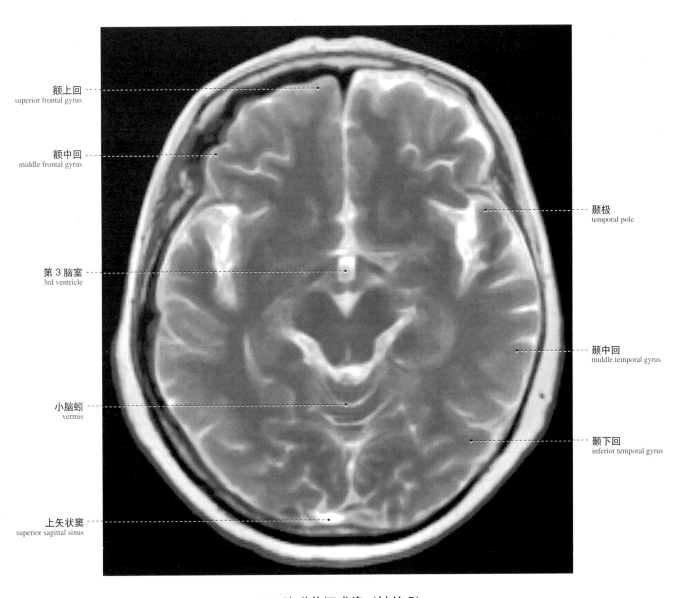

额上回
superior frontal gyrus

额中回
middle frontal gyrus

第 3 脑室
3rd ventricle

小脑蚓
vermis

上矢状窦
superior sagittal sinus

颞极
temporal pole

颞中回
middle temporal gyrus

颞下回
inferior temporal gyrus

247. 脑磁共振成像（轴位 5）
MRI of the brain (axial view 5)

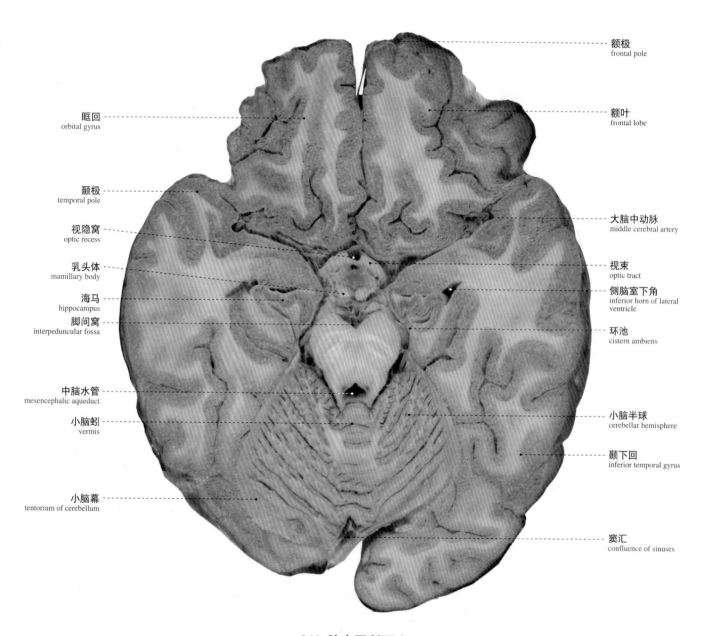

额极
frontal pole

额叶
frontal lobe

眶回
orbital gyrus

颞极
temporal pole

大脑中动脉
middle cerebral artery

视隐窝
optic recess

视束
optic tract

乳头体
mamillary body

侧脑室下角
inferior horn of lateral ventricle

海马
hippocampus

环池
cistern ambiens

脚间窝
interpeduncular fossa

中脑水管
mesencephalic aqueduct

小脑半球
cerebellar hemisphere

小脑蚓
vermis

颞下回
inferior temporal gyrus

小脑幕
tentorium of cerebellum

窦汇
confluence of sinuses

248. 脑水平断面 6
Horizontal section of the brain 6

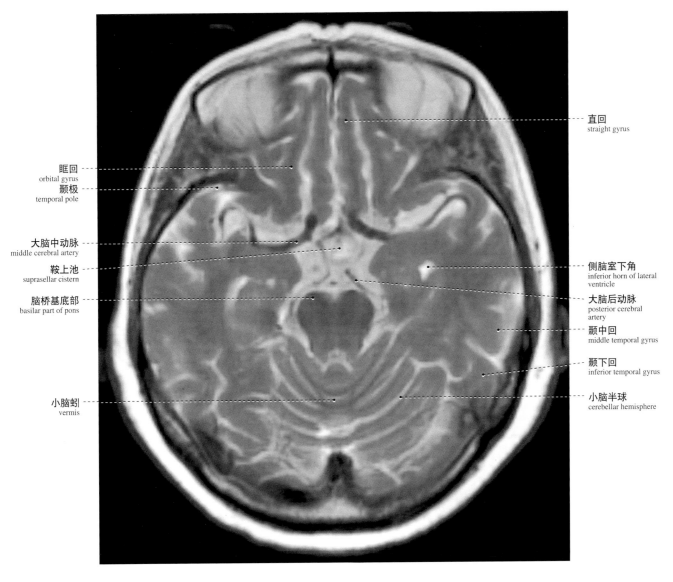

眶回
orbital gyrus

颞极
temporal pole

大脑中动脉
middle cerebral artery

鞍上池
suprasellar cistern

脑桥基底部
basilar part of pons

小脑蚓
vermis

直回
straight gyrus

侧脑室下角
inferior horn of lateral ventricle

大脑后动脉
posterior cerebral artery

颞中回
middle temporal gyrus

颞下回
inferior temporal gyrus

小脑半球
cerebellar hemisphere

249. 脑磁共振成像（轴位 6）
MRI of the brain (axial view 6)

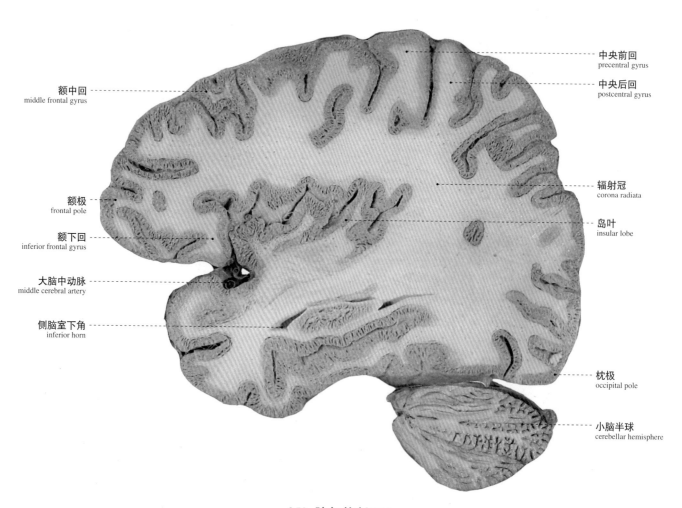

额中回
middle frontal gyrus

额极
frontal pole

额下回
inferior frontal gyrus

大脑中动脉
middle cerebral artery

侧脑室下角
inferior horn

中央前回
precentral gyrus

中央后回
postcentral gyrus

辐射冠
corona radiata

岛叶
insular lobe

枕极
occipital pole

小脑半球
cerebellar hemisphere

250. 脑矢状断面 1

Sagittal section of the brain 1

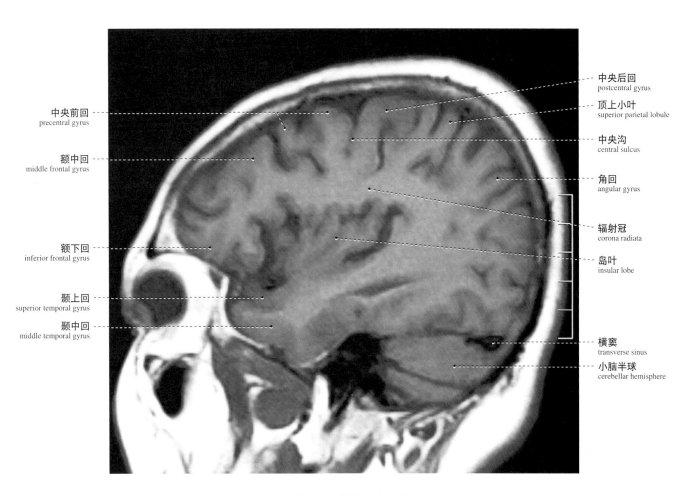

中央后回
postcentral gyrus

顶上小叶
superior parietal lobule

中央沟
central sulcus

角回
angular gyrus

辐射冠
corona radiata

岛叶
insular lobe

横窦
transverse sinus

小脑半球
cerebellar hemisphere

中央前回
precentral gyrus

额中回
middle frontal gyrus

额下回
inferior frontal gyrus

颞上回
superior temporal gyrus

颞中回
middle temporal gyrus

251. 脑磁共振成像（矢状位1）
MRI of the brain (sagittal view 1)

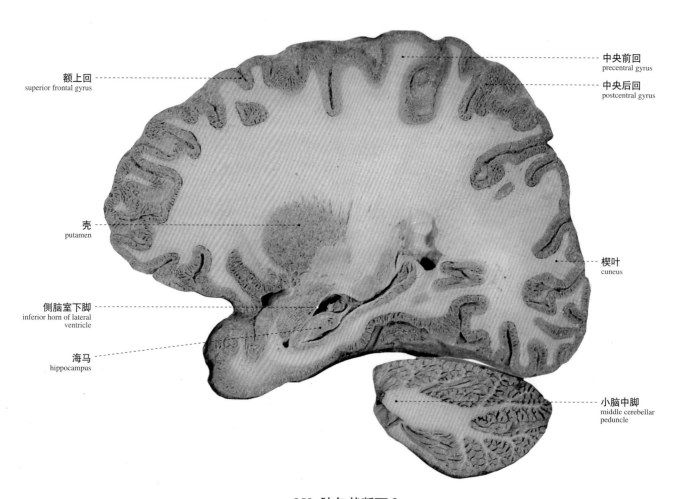

额上回
superior frontal gyrus

中央前回
precentral gyrus

中央后回
postcentral gyrus

壳
putamen

楔叶
cuneus

侧脑室下脚
inferior horn of lateral
ventricle

海马
hippocampus

小脑中脚
middle cerebellar
peduncle

252. 脑矢状断面 2

Sagittal section of the brain 2

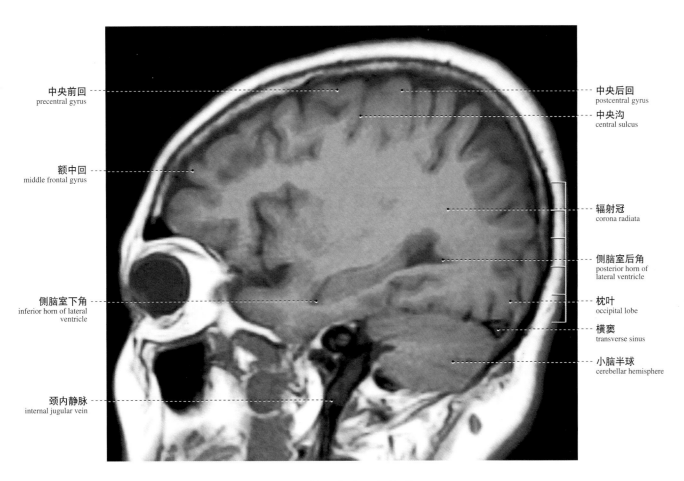

中央前回
precentral gyrus

中央后回
postcentral gyrus

中央沟
central sulcus

额中回
middle frontal gyrus

辐射冠
corona radiata

侧脑室后角
posterior horn of
lateral ventricle

枕叶
occipital lobe

侧脑室下角
inferior horn of lateral
ventricle

横窦
transverse sinus

小脑半球
cerebellar hemisphere

颈内静脉
internal jugular vein

253. 脑磁共振成像（矢状位 2）
MRI of the brain (sagittal view 2)

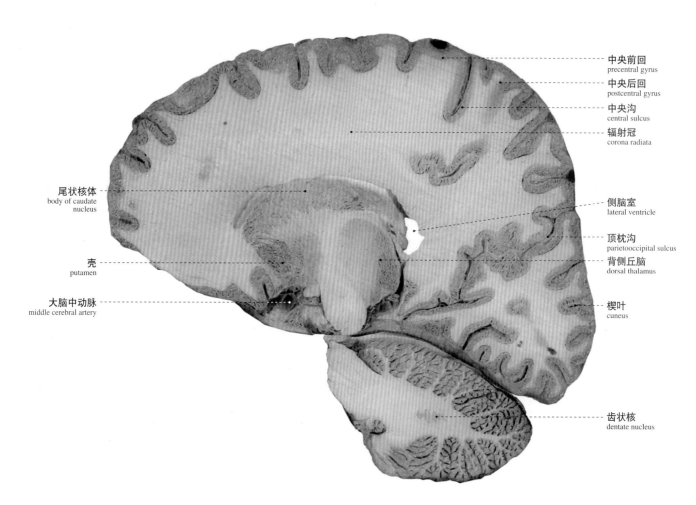

中央前回
precentral gyrus

中央后回
postcentral gyrus

中央沟
central sulcus

辐射冠
corona radiata

尾状核体
body of caudate nucleus

侧脑室
lateral ventricle

顶枕沟
parietooccipital sulcus

壳
putamen

背侧丘脑
dorsal thalamus

大脑中动脉
middle cerebral artery

楔叶
cuneus

齿状核
dentate nucleus

254. 脑矢状断面 3

Sagittal section of the brain 3

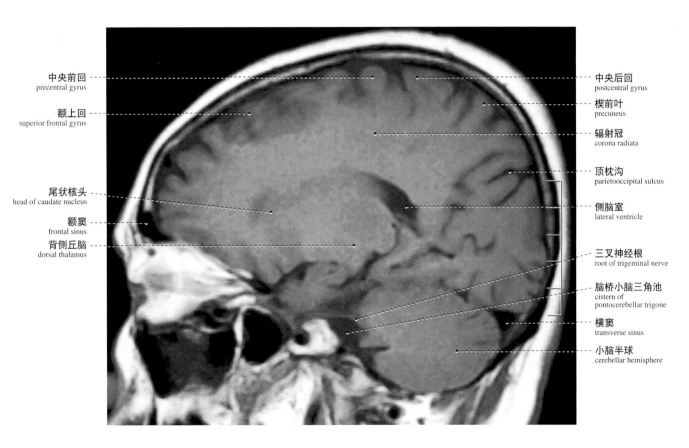

中央前回
precentral gyrus

额上回
superior frontal gyrus

尾状核头
head of caudate nucleus

额窦
frontal sinus

背侧丘脑
dorsal thalamus

中央后回
postcentral gyrus

楔前叶
precuneus

辐射冠
corona radiata

顶枕沟
parietooccipital sulcus

侧脑室
lateral ventricle

三叉神经根
root of trigeminal nerve

脑桥小脑三角池
cistern of pontocerebellar trigone

横窦
transverse sinus

小脑半球
cerebellar hemisphere

255. 脑磁共振成像（矢状位 3）
MRI of the brain (sagittal view 3)

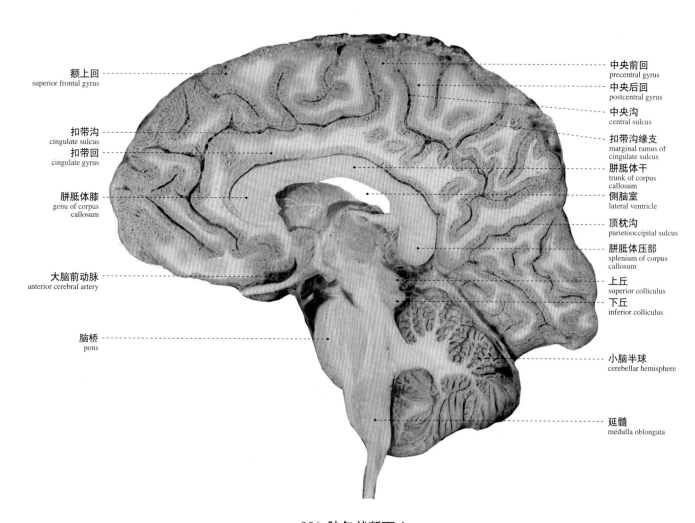

额上回
superior frontal gyrus

扣带沟
cingulate sulcus

扣带回
cingulate gyrus

胼胝体膝
genu of corpus callosum

大脑前动脉
anterior cerebral artery

脑桥
pons

中央前回
precentral gyrus

中央后回
postcentral gyrus

中央沟
central sulcus

扣带沟缘支
marginal ramus of cingulate sulcus

胼胝体干
trunk of corpus callosum

侧脑室
lateral ventricle

顶枕沟
parietooccipital sulcus

胼胝体压部
splenium of corpus callosum

上丘
superior colliculus

下丘
inferior colliculus

小脑半球
cerebellar hemisphere

延髓
medulla oblongata

256. 脑矢状断面 4

Sagittal section of the brain 4

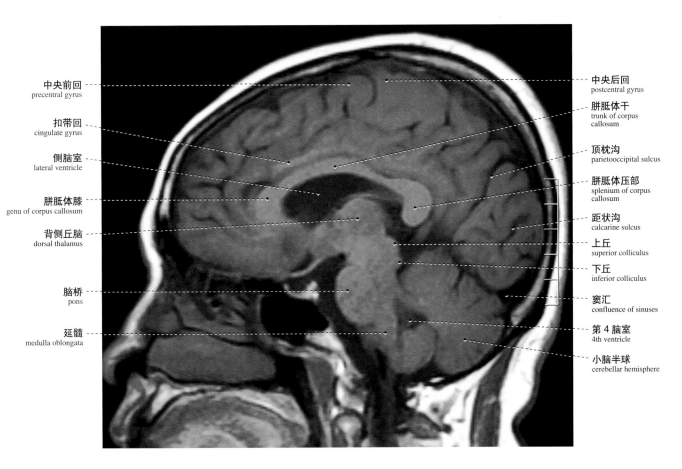

中央前回
precentral gyrus

扣带回
cingulate gyrus

侧脑室
lateral ventricle

胼胝体膝
genu of corpus callosum

背侧丘脑
dorsal thalamus

脑桥
pons

延髓
medulla oblongata

中央后回
postcentral gyrus

胼胝体干
trunk of corpus callosum

顶枕沟
parietooccipital sulcus

胼胝体压部
splenium of corpus callosum

距状沟
calcarine sulcus

上丘
superior colliculus

下丘
inferior colliculus

窦汇
confluence of sinuses

第 4 脑室
4th ventricle

小脑半球
cerebellar hemisphere

257. 脑磁共振成像（矢状位4）
MRI of the brain (sagittal view 4)

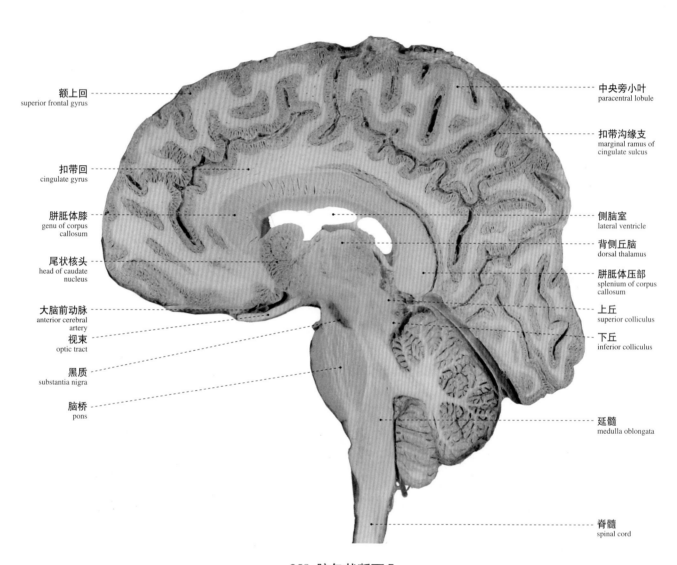

额上回
superior frontal gyrus

扣带回
cingulate gyrus

胼胝体膝
genu of corpus callosum

尾状核头
head of caudate nucleus

大脑前动脉
anterior cerebral artery

视束
optic tract

黑质
substantia nigra

脑桥
pons

中央旁小叶
paracentral lobule

扣带沟缘支
marginal ramus of cingulate sulcus

侧脑室
lateral ventricle

背侧丘脑
dorsal thalamus

胼胝体压部
splenium of corpus callosum

上丘
superior colliculus

下丘
inferior colliculus

延髓
medulla oblongata

脊髓
spinal cord

258. 脑矢状断面 5
Sagittal section of the brain 5

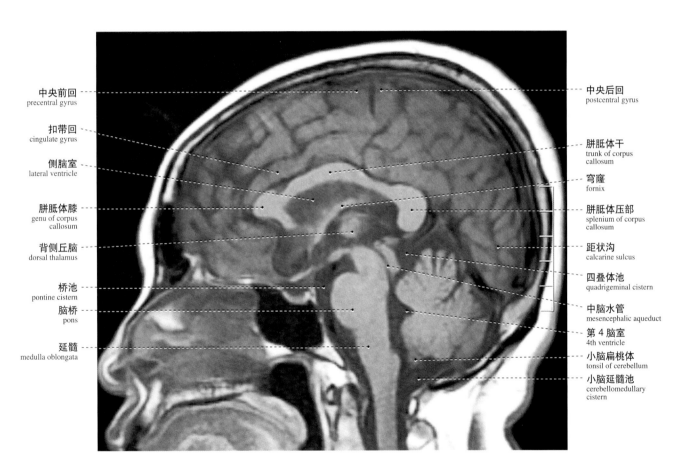

中央前回
precentral gyrus

扣带回
cingulate gyrus

侧脑室
lateral ventricle

胼胝体膝
genu of corpus
callosum

背侧丘脑
dorsal thalamus

桥池
pontine cistern

脑桥
pons

延髓
medulla oblongata

中央后回
postcentral gyrus

胼胝体干
trunk of corpus
callosum

穹窿
fornix

胼胝体压部
splenium of corpus
callosum

距状沟
calcarine sulcus

四叠体池
quadrigeminal cistern

中脑水管
mesencephalic aqueduct

第 4 脑室
4th ventricle

小脑扁桃体
tonsil of cerebellum

小脑延髓池
cerebellomedullary
cistern

259. 脑磁共振成像（矢状位 5）
MRI of the brain (sagittal view 5)

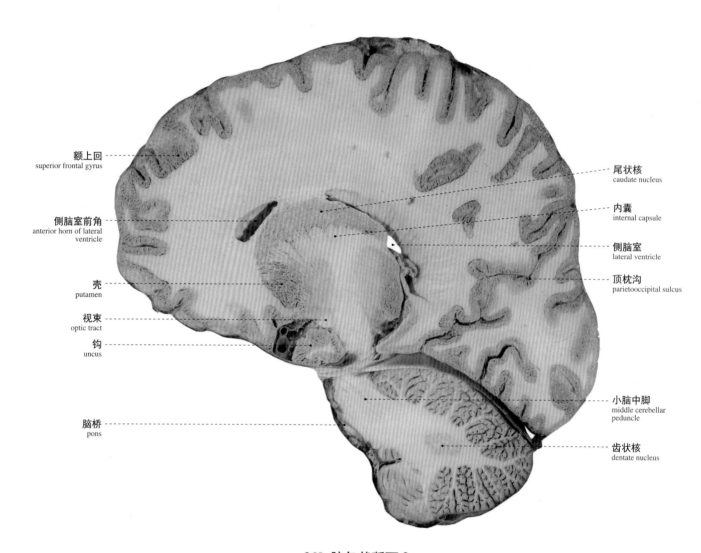

额上回
superior frontal gyrus

侧脑室前角
anterior horn of lateral
ventricle

壳
putamen

视束
optic tract

钩
uncus

脑桥
pons

尾状核
caudate nucleus

内囊
internal capsule

侧脑室
lateral ventricle

顶枕沟
parietooccipital sulcus

小脑中脚
middle cerebellar
peduncle

齿状核
dentate nucleus

260. 脑矢状断面 6
Sagittal section of the brain 6

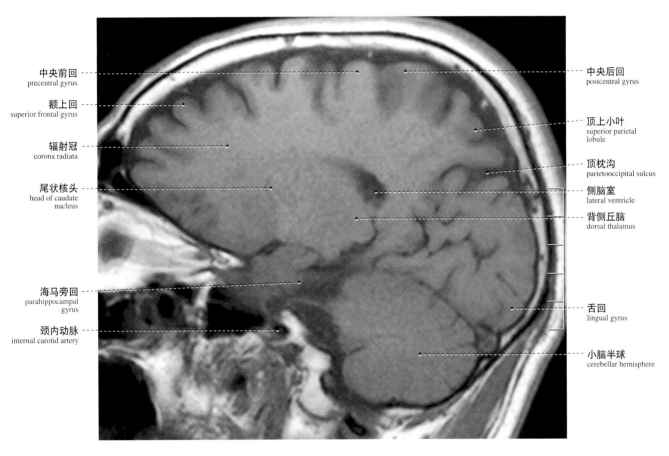

中央前回
precentral gyrus

额上回
superior frontal gyrus

辐射冠
corona radiata

尾状核头
head of caudate
nucleus

海马旁回
parahippocampal
gyrus

颈内动脉
internal carotid artery

中央后回
postcentral gyrus

顶上小叶
superior parietal
lobule

顶枕沟
parietooccipital sulcus

侧脑室
lateral ventricle

背侧丘脑
dorsal thalamus

舌回
lingual gyrus

小脑半球
cerebellar hemisphere

261. 脑磁共振成像（矢状位6）

MRI of the brain (sagittal view 6)

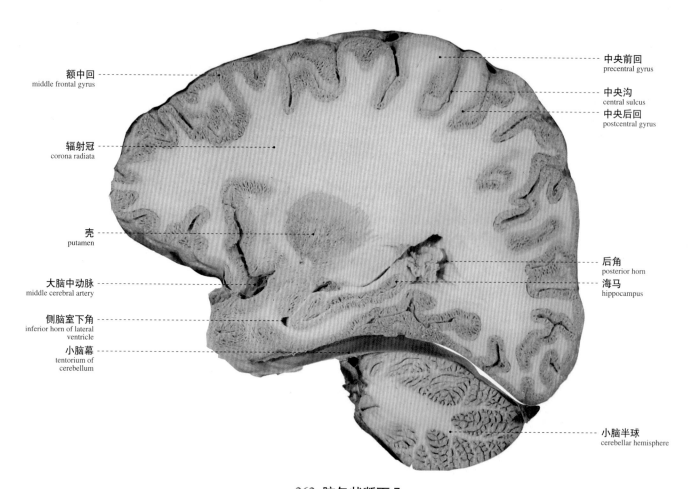

额中回
middle frontal gyrus

辐射冠
corona radiata

壳
putamen

大脑中动脉
middle cerebral artery

侧脑室下角
inferior horn of lateral
ventricle

小脑幕
tentorium of
cerebellum

中央前回
precentral gyrus

中央沟
central sulcus

中央后回
postcentral gyrus

后角
posterior horn

海马
hippocampus

小脑半球
cerebellar hemisphere

262. 脑矢状断面 7

Sagittal section of the brain 7

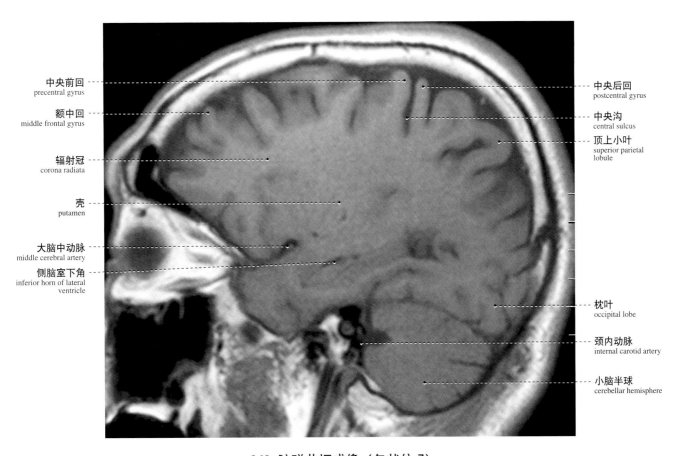

中央前回
precentral gyrus

额中回
middle frontal gyrus

辐射冠
corona radiata

壳
putamen

大脑中动脉
middle cerebral artery

侧脑室下角
inferior horn of lateral
ventricle

中央后回
postcentral gyrus

中央沟
central sulcus

顶上小叶
superior parietal
lobule

枕叶
occipital lobe

颈内动脉
internal carotid artery

小脑半球
cerebellar hemisphere

263. 脑磁共振成像（矢状位 7）
MRI of the brain (sagittal view 7)

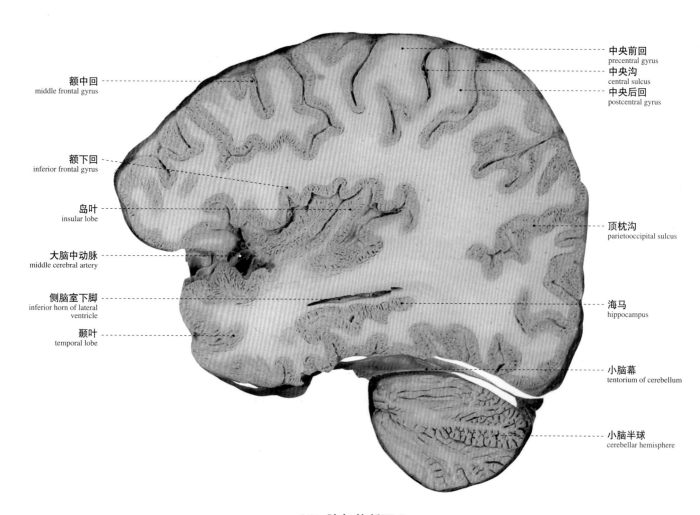

額中回
middle frontal gyrus

額下回
inferior frontal gyrus

島叶
insular lobe

大脑中动脉
middle cerebral artery

側脑室下脚
inferior horn of lateral
ventricle

颞叶
temporal lobe

中央前回
precentral gyrus

中央沟
central sulcus

中央后回
postcentral gyrus

頂枕沟
parietooccipital sulcus

海马
hippocampus

小脑幕
tentorium of cerebellum

小脑半球
cerebellar hemisphere

264. 脑矢状断面 8
Sagittal section of the brain 8

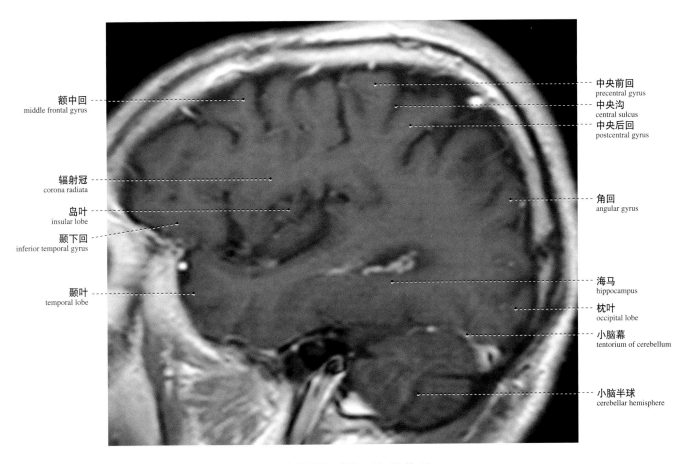

额中回
middle frontal gyrus

辐射冠
corona radiata

岛叶
insular lobe

颞下回
inferior temporal gyrus

颞叶
temporal lobe

中央前回
precentral gyrus

中央沟
central sulcus

中央后回
postcentral gyrus

角回
angular gyrus

海马
hippocampus

枕叶
occipital lobe

小脑幕
tentorium of cerebellum

小脑半球
cerebellar hemisphere

265. 脑磁共振成像（矢状位 8）
MRI of the brain (sagittal view 8)

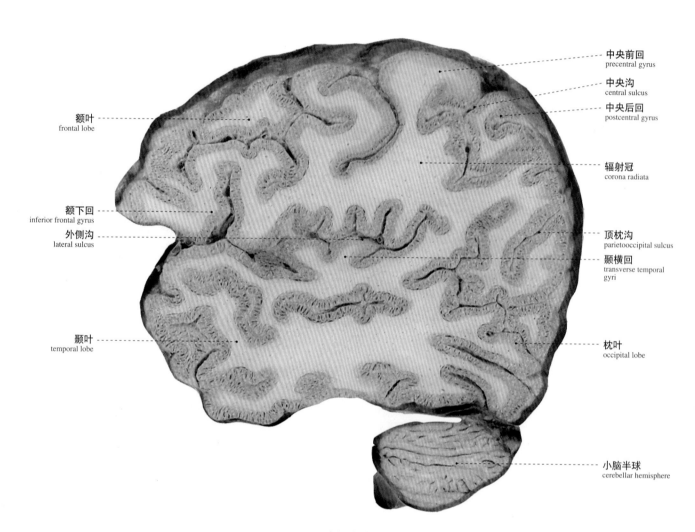

中央前回
precentral gyrus

中央沟
central sulcus

中央后回
postcentral gyrus

额叶
frontal lobe

辐射冠
corona radiata

额下回
inferior frontal gyrus

顶枕沟
parietooccipital sulcus

外侧沟
lateral sulcus

颞横回
transverse temporal gyri

颞叶
temporal lobe

枕叶
occipital lobe

小脑半球
cerebellar hemisphere

266. 脑矢状断面 9

Sagittal section of the brain 9

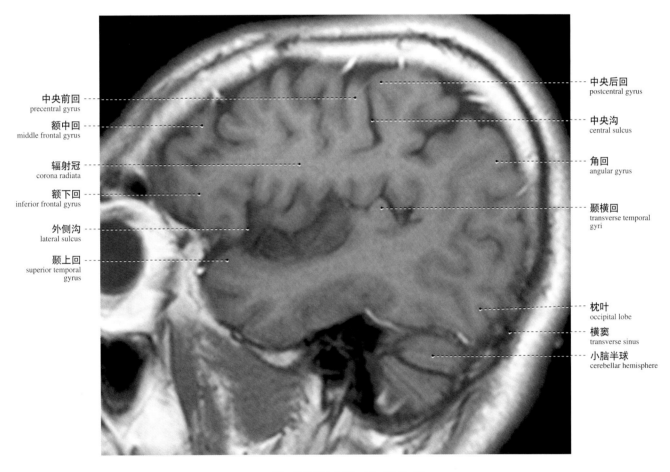

中央前回
precentral gyrus

额中回
middle frontal gyrus

辐射冠
corona radiata

额下回
inferior frontal gyrus

外侧沟
lateral sulcus

颞上回
superior temporal
gyrus

中央后回
postcentral gyrus

中央沟
central sulcus

角回
angular gyrus

颞横回
transverse temporal
gyri

枕叶
occipital lobe

横窦
transverse sinus

小脑半球
cerebellar hemisphere

267. 脑磁共振成像（矢状位 9）

MRI of the brain (sagittal view 9)

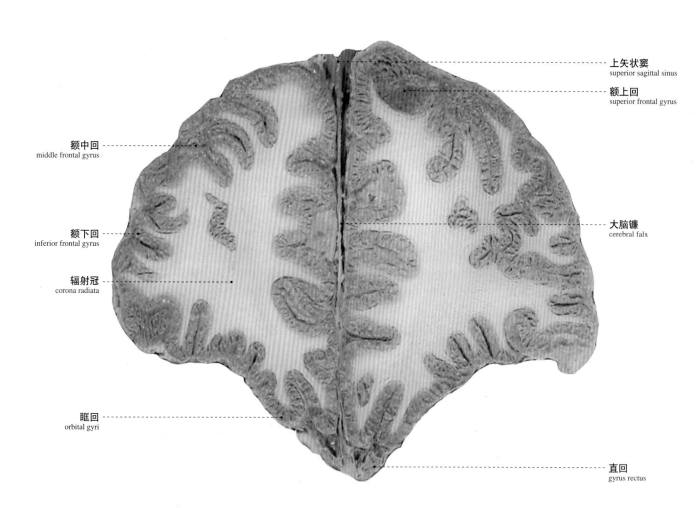

额中回
middle frontal gyrus

额下回
inferior frontal gyrus

辐射冠
corona radiata

眶回
orbital gyri

上矢状窦
superior sagittal sinus

额上回
superior frontal gyrus

大脑镰
cerebral falx

直回
gyrus rectus

268. 脑冠状断面 1
Frontal section of the brain 1

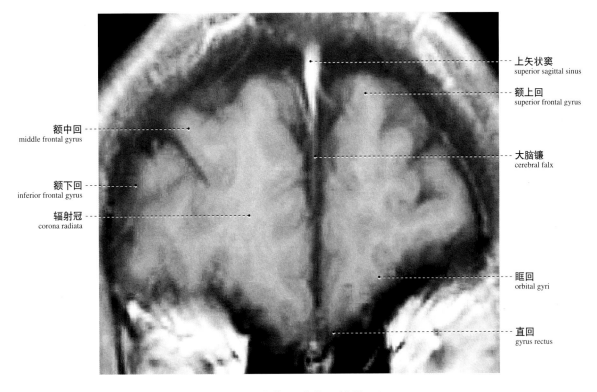

额中回
middle frontal gyrus

额下回
inferior frontal gyrus

辐射冠
corona radiata

上矢状窦
superior sagittal sinus

额上回
superior frontal gyrus

大脑镰
cerebral falx

眶回
orbital gyri

直回
gyrus rectus

269. 脑磁共振成像（轴位 1）
MRI of the brain (axial view 1)

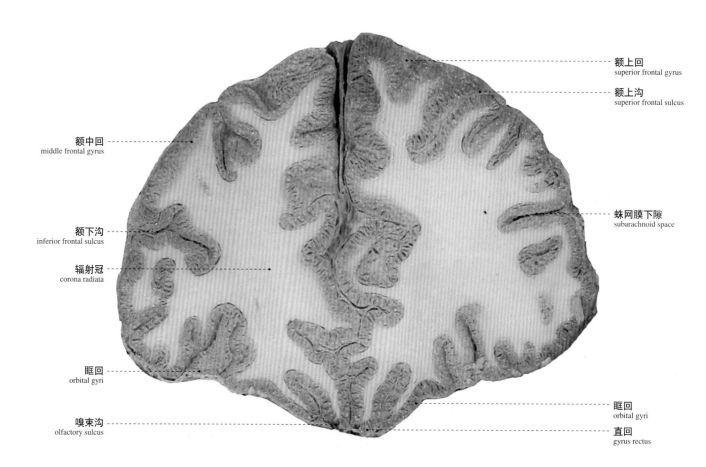

额上回
superior frontal gyrus

额上沟
superior frontal sulcus

额中回
middle frontal gyrus

蛛网膜下隙
subarachnoid space

额下沟
inferior frontal sulcus

辐射冠
corona radiata

眶回
orbital gyri

眶回
orbital gyri

嗅束沟
olfactory sulcus

直回
gyrus rectus

270. 脑冠状断面 2

Frontal section of the brain 2

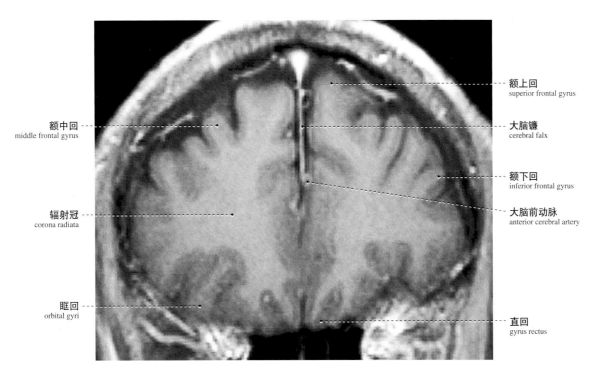

额中回
middle frontal gyrus

辐射冠
corona radiata

眶回
orbital gyri

额上回
superior frontal gyrus

大脑镰
cerebral falx

额下回
inferior frontal gyrus

大脑前动脉
anterior cerebral artery

直回
gyrus rectus

271. 脑磁共振成像（轴位 2）
MRI of the brain (axial view 2)

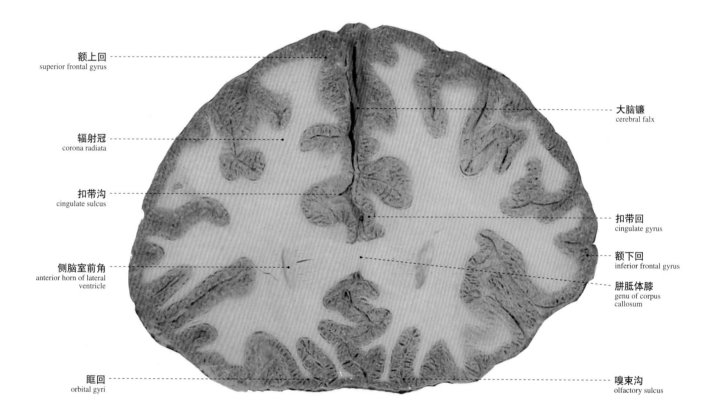

额上回
superior frontal gyrus

辐射冠
corona radiata

扣带沟
cingulate sulcus

侧脑室前角
anterior horn of lateral
ventricle

眶回
orbital gyri

大脑镰
cerebral falx

扣带回
cingulate gyrus

额下回
inferior frontal gyrus

胼胝体膝
genu of corpus
callosum

嗅束沟
olfactory sulcus

272. 脑冠状断面 3
Frontal section of the brain 3

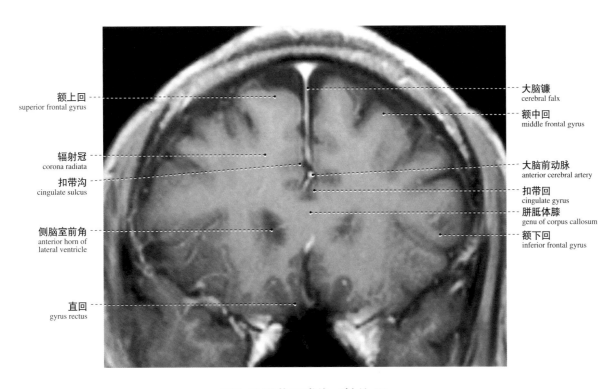

额上回
superior frontal gyrus

辐射冠
corona radiata

扣带沟
cingulate sulcus

侧脑室前角
anterior horn of
lateral ventricle

直回
gyrus rectus

大脑镰
cerebral falx

额中回
middle frontal gyrus

大脑前动脉
anterior cerebral artery

扣带回
cingulate gyrus

胼胝体膝
genu of corpus callosum

额下回
inferior frontal gyrus

273. 脑磁共振成像（轴位 3）
MRI of the brain (axial view 3)

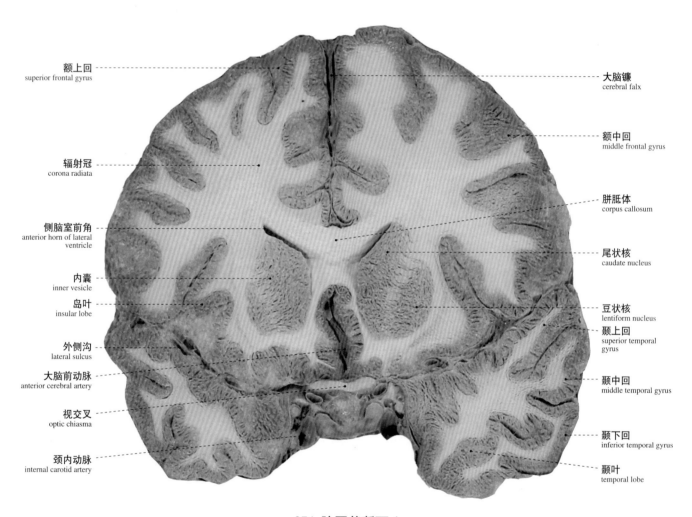

额上回
superior frontal gyrus

辐射冠
corona radiata

侧脑室前角
anterior horn of lateral ventricle

内囊
inner vesicle

岛叶
insular lobe

外侧沟
lateral sulcus

大脑前动脉
anterior cerebral artery

视交叉
optic chiasma

颈内动脉
internal carotid artery

大脑镰
cerebral falx

额中回
middle frontal gyrus

胼胝体
corpus callosum

尾状核
caudate nucleus

豆状核
lentiform nucleus

颞上回
superior temporal gyrus

颞中回
middle temporal gyrus

颞下回
inferior temporal gyrus

颞叶
temporal lobe

274. 脑冠状断面 4
Frontal section of the brain 4

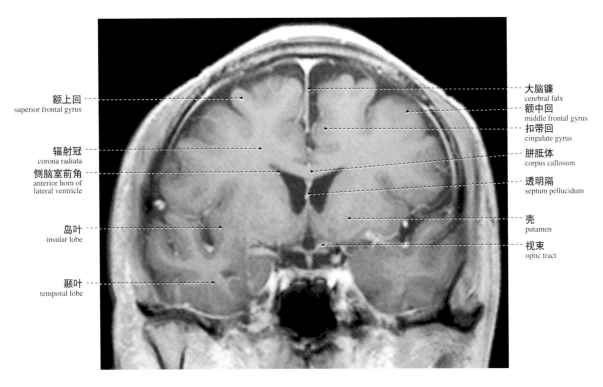

额上回
superior frontal gyrus

辐射冠
corona radiata

侧脑室前角
anterior horn of
lateral ventricle

岛叶
insular lobe

颞叶
temporal lobe

大脑镰
cerebral falx

额中回
middle frontal gyrus

扣带回
cingulate gyrus

胼胝体
corpus callosum

透明隔
septum pellucidum

壳
putamen

视束
optic tract

275. 脑磁共振成像（轴位4）
MRI of the brain (axial view 4)

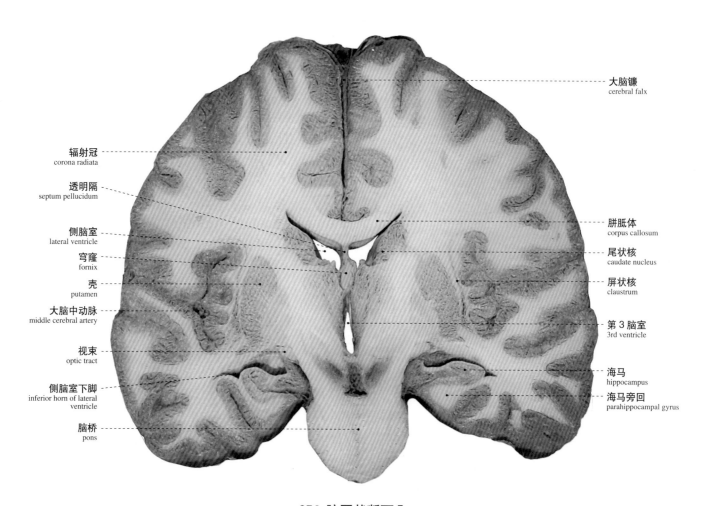

大脑镰
cerebral falx

辐射冠
corona radiata

透明隔
septum pellucidum

侧脑室
lateral ventricle

穹窿
fornix

壳
putamen

大脑中动脉
middle cerebral artery

视束
optic tract

侧脑室下脚
inferior horn of lateral ventricle

脑桥
pons

胼胝体
corpus callosum

尾状核
caudate nucleus

屏状核
claustrum

第 3 脑室
3rd ventricle

海马
hippocampus

海马旁回
parahippocampal gyrus

276. 脑冠状断面 5
Frontal section of the brain 5

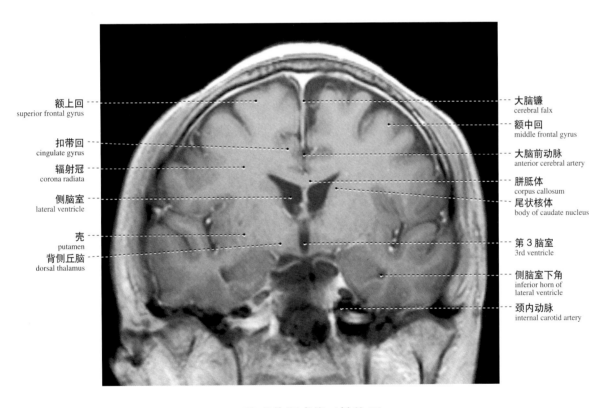

额上回
superior frontal gyrus

扣带回
cingulate gyrus

辐射冠
corona radiata

侧脑室
lateral ventricle

壳
putamen

背侧丘脑
dorsal thalamus

大脑镰
cerebral falx

额中回
middle frontal gyrus

大脑前动脉
anterior cerebral artery

胼胝体
corpus callosum

尾状核体
body of caudate nucleus

第 3 脑室
3rd ventricle

侧脑室下角
inferior horn of
lateral ventricle

颈内动脉
internal carotid artery

277. 脑磁共振成像（轴位 5）
MRI of the brain (axial view 5)

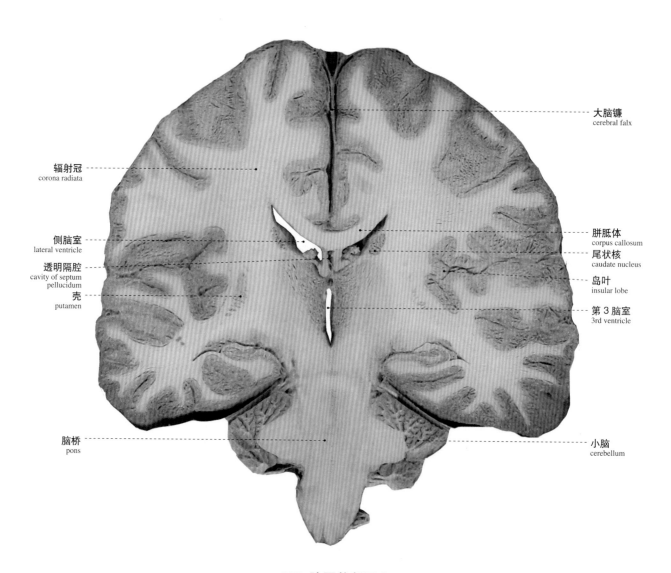

大脑镰
cerebral falx

辐射冠
corona radiata

侧脑室
lateral ventricle

透明隔腔
cavity of septum
pellucidum

壳
putamen

胼胝体
corpus callosum

尾状核
caudate nucleus

岛叶
insular lobe

第 3 脑室
3rd ventricle

脑桥
pons

小脑
cerebellum

278. 脑冠状断面 6
Frontal section of the brain 6

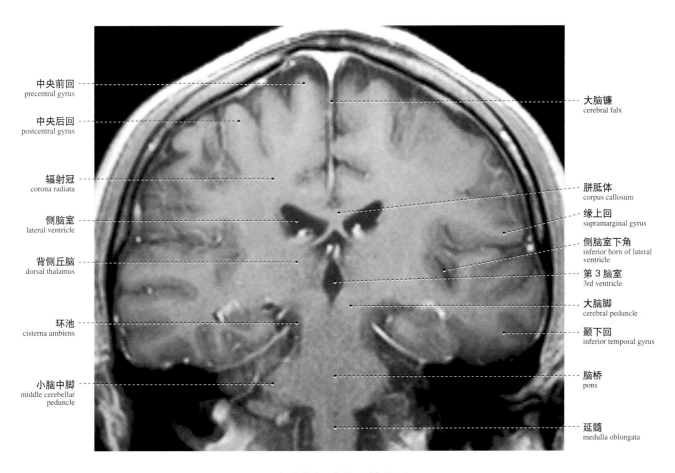

中央前回
precentral gyrus

中央后回
postcentral gyrus

辐射冠
corona radiata

侧脑室
lateral ventricle

背侧丘脑
dorsal thalamus

环池
cisterna ambiens

小脑中脚
middle cerebellar peduncle

大脑镰
cerebral falx

胼胝体
corpus callosum

缘上回
supramarginal gyrus

侧脑室下角
inferior horn of lateral ventricle

第 3 脑室
3rd ventricle

大脑脚
cerebral peduncle

颞下回
inferior temporal gyrus

脑桥
pons

延髓
medulla oblongata

279. 脑磁共振成像（轴位 6）
MRI of the brain (axial view 6)

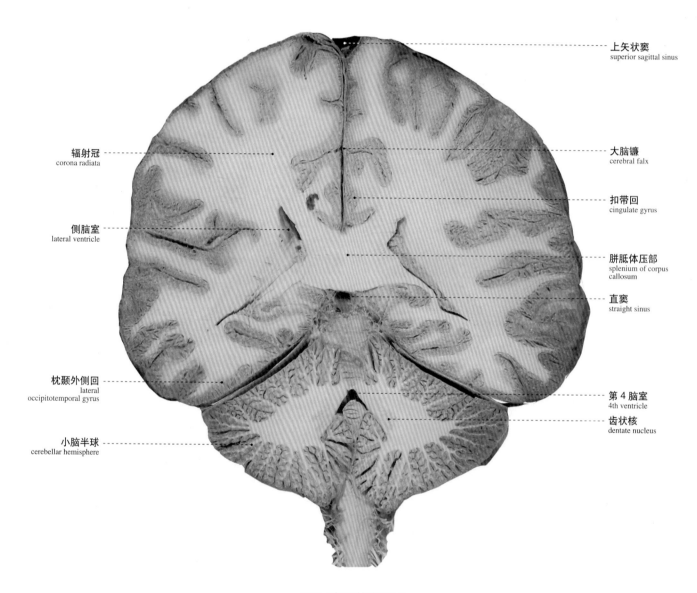

辐射冠
corona radiata

侧脑室
lateral ventricle

枕颞外侧回
lateral
occipitotemporal gyrus

小脑半球
cerebellar hemisphere

上矢状窦
superior sagittal sinus

大脑镰
cerebral falx

扣带回
cingulate gyrus

胼胝体压部
splenium of corpus
callosum

直窦
straight sinus

第 4 脑室
4th ventricle

齿状核
dentate nucleus

280. 脑冠状断面 7
Frontal section of the brain 7

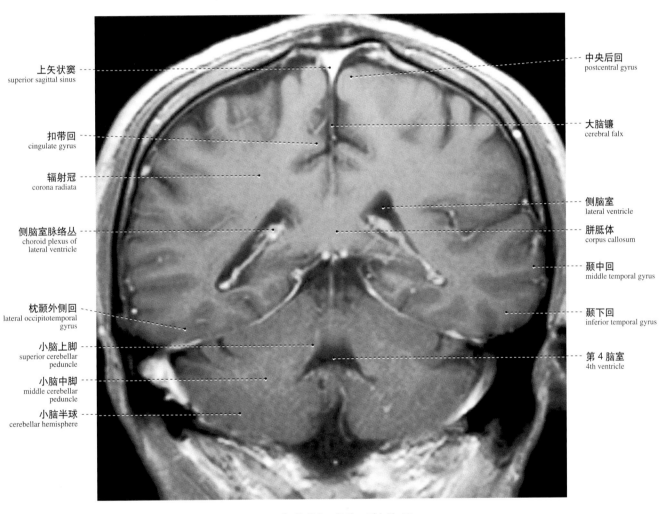

上矢状窦
superior sagittal sinus

扣带回
cingulate gyrus

辐射冠
corona radiata

侧脑室脉络丛
choroid plexus of
lateral ventricle

枕颞外侧回
lateral occipitotemporal
gyrus

小脑上脚
superior cerebellar
peduncle

小脑中脚
middle cerebellar
peduncle

小脑半球
cerebellar hemisphere

中央后回
postcentral gyrus

大脑镰
cerebral falx

侧脑室
lateral ventricle

胼胝体
corpus callosum

颞中回
middle temporal gyrus

颞下回
inferior temporal gyrus

第 4 脑室
4th ventricle

281. 脑磁共振成像（轴位 7）
MRI of the brain (axial view 7)

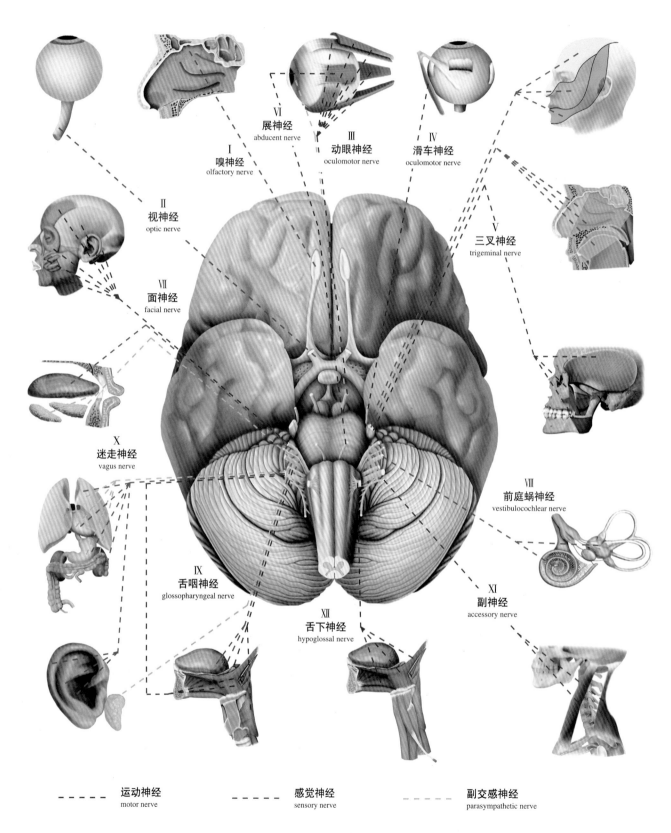

VI
展神经
abducent nerve

I
嗅神经
olfactory nerve

III
动眼神经
oculomotor nerve

IV
滑车神经
oculomotor nerve

II
视神经
optic nerve

V
三叉神经
trigeminal nerve

VII
面神经
facial nerve

X
迷走神经
vagus nerve

VIII
前庭蜗神经
vestibulocochlear nerve

IX
舌咽神经
glossopharyngeal nerve

XII
舌下神经
hypoglossal nerve

XI
副神经
accessory nerve

运动神经
motor nerve

感觉神经
sensory nerve

副交感神经
parasympathetic nerve

282. 脑神经
Cranial nerves

表3　12对脑神经

顺　序	名　称	性　质	连脑部位	进出颅腔部位
I	嗅神经	感觉性	端脑	筛孔
II	视神经	感觉性	间脑	视神经管
III	动眼神经	运动性	中脑	眶上裂
IV	滑车神经	运动性	中脑	眶上裂
V	三叉神经	混合性	脑桥	视神经经眶上裂 上颌神经经圆孔 下颌神经经卵圆孔
VI	展神经	运动性	脑桥	眶上裂
VII	面神经	混合性	脑桥	内耳门、茎乳孔
VIII	前庭蜗神经	感觉性	脑桥	内耳门
IX	舌咽神经	混合性	延髓	颈静脉孔
X	迷走神经	混合性	延髓	颈静脉孔
XI	副神经	运动性	延髓	颈静脉孔
XII	舌下神经	运动性	延髓	舌下神经管

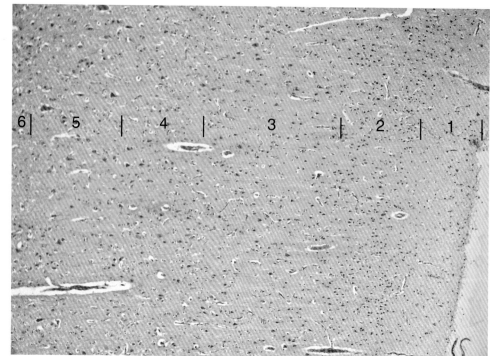

1. 分子层
   molecular layer
2. 外颗粒层
   external granular layer
3. 外锥体细胞层
   external pyramidal layer
4. 内颗粒层
   internal granular layer
5. 内锥体细胞层
   internal pyramidal layer
6. 多形细胞层
   polymorphic layer

283. 大脑皮质（人大脑，HE 染色，×40）
Cerebral cortex (human cerebrum, HE staining, ×40)

大锥体细胞
large pyramidal cell

284. 大锥体细胞（人大脑皮质中央前回运动区，HE 染色，×400）
Large pyramidal cell (motor areas of precentral gyrus of human cerebral cortex, HE staining, ×400)

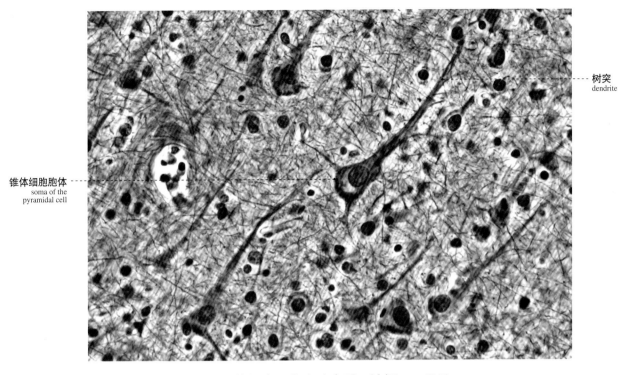

树突
dendrite

锥体细胞胞体
soma of the
pyramidal cell

285. 锥体细胞（人大脑皮质，镀银，×400）

Pyramidal cell (human cerebral cortex, silver staining, ×400)

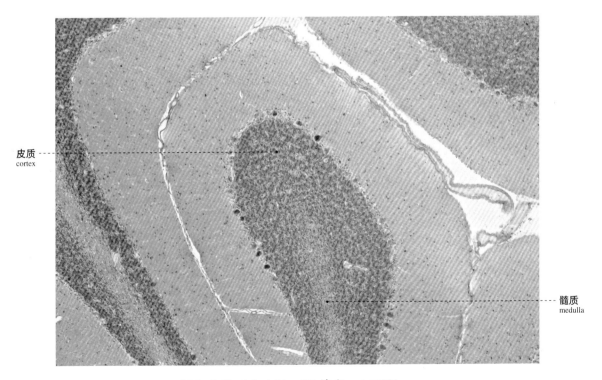

皮质
cortex

髓质
medulla

286. 小脑（人小脑，HE 染色，×100）

Cerebellum (human cerebellum, HE staining, ×100)

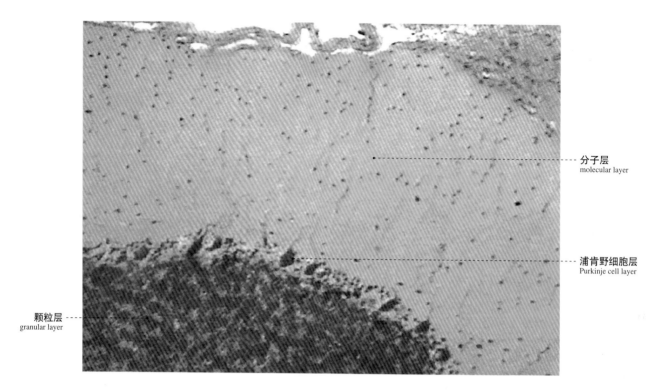

分子层
molecular layer

浦肯野细胞层
Purkinje cell layer

颗粒层
granular layer

287. 小脑皮质（人小脑，HE 染色，×400）
Cerebellar cortex (human cerebellum, HE staining, ×400)

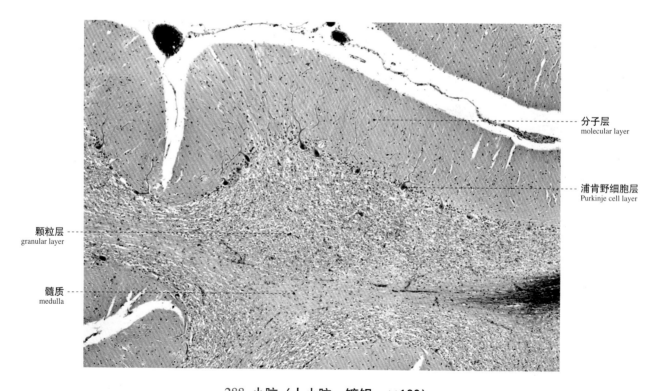

分子层
molecular layer

浦肯野细胞层
Purkinje cell layer

颗粒层
granular layer

髓质
medulla

288. 小脑（人小脑，镀银，×100）
Cerebellum (human cerebellum, silver staining, ×100)

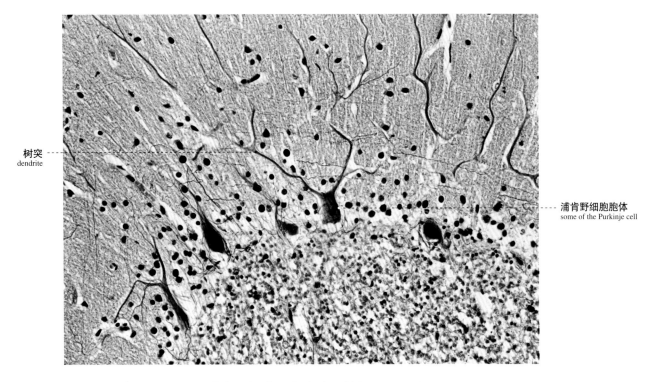

树突
dendrite

浦肯野细胞胞体
some of the Purkinje cell

289. 浦肯野细胞（人小脑，镀银，×400）
Purkinje cell (human cerebellum, silver staining, ×400)

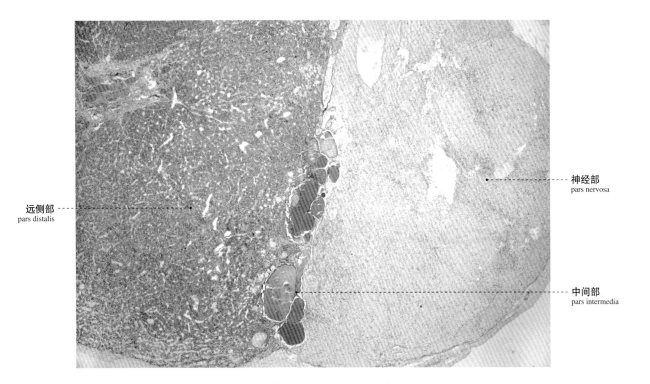

神经部
pars nervosa

远侧部
pars distalis

中间部
pars intermedia

290. 垂体（人垂体，矢状切面，HE 染色，×40）
Hypophysis (human hypophysis, sagittal section, HE staining, ×40)

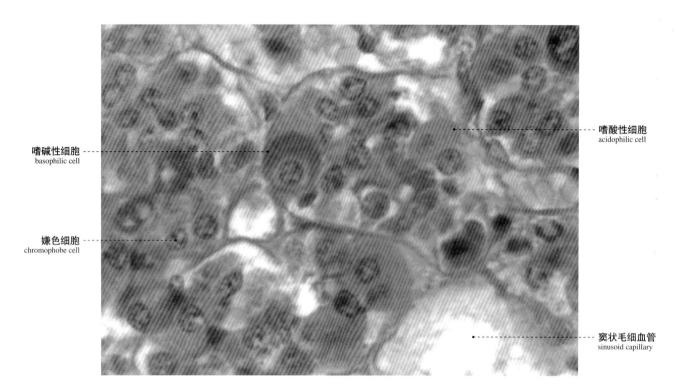

嗜碱性细胞
basophilic cell

嫌色细胞
chromophobe cell

嗜酸性细胞
acidophilic cell

窦状毛细血管
sinusoid capillary

291. 远侧部（人垂体，HE 染色，×400）
Pars distalis (human hypophysis, HE staining, ×400)

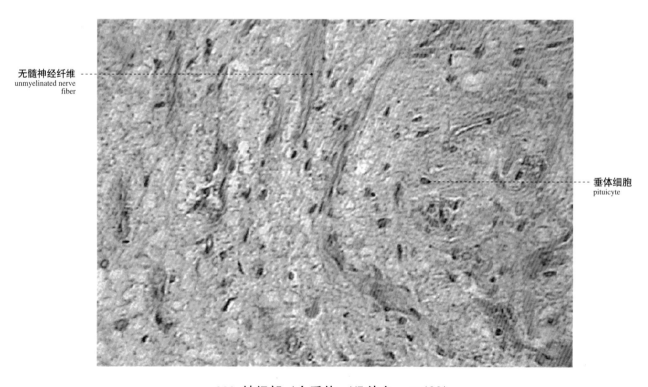

无髓神经纤维
unmyelinated nerve
fiber

垂体细胞
pituicyte

292. 神经部（人垂体，HE 染色，×400）
Pars nervosa (human hypophysis, HE staining, ×400)

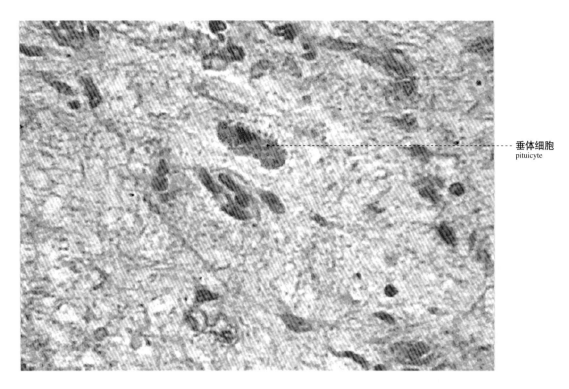

垂体细胞
pituicyte

293. 垂体细胞（人垂体，神经部，HE 染色，×400）
Pituicyte (human hypophysis, pars nervosa, HE staining, ×400)

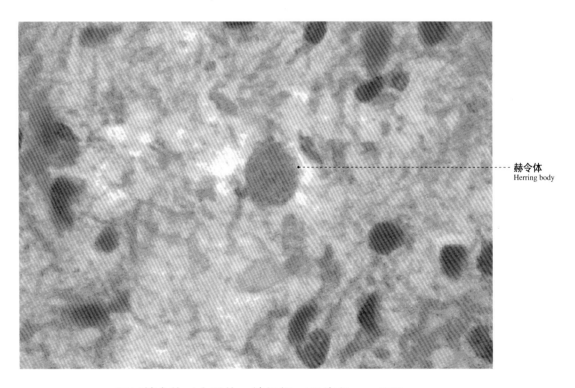

赫令体
Herring body

294. 赫令体（人垂体，神经部，HE 染色，×400）
Herring body (human hypophysis, pars nervosa, HE staining, ×400)

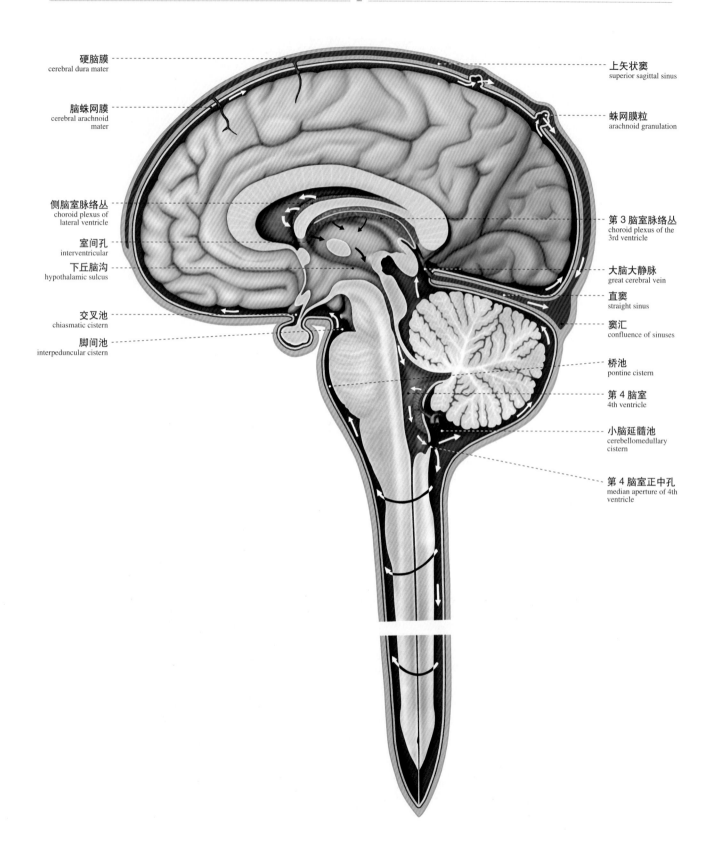

硬脑膜
cerebral dura mater

脑蛛网膜
cerebral arachnoid mater

侧脑室脉络丛
choroid plexus of lateral ventricle

室间孔
interventricular

下丘脑沟
hypothalamic sulcus

交叉池
chiasmatic cistern

脚间池
interpeduncular cistern

上矢状窦
superior sagittal sinus

蛛网膜粒
arachnoid granulation

第 3 脑室脉络丛
choroid plexus of the 3rd ventricle

大脑大静脉
great cerebral vein

直窦
straight sinus

窦汇
confluence of sinuses

桥池
pontine cistern

第 4 脑室
4th ventricle

小脑延髓池
cerebellomedullary cistern

第 4 脑室正中孔
median aperture of 4th ventricle

295. 脑脊液循环
Circulation of the cerebrospinal fluid

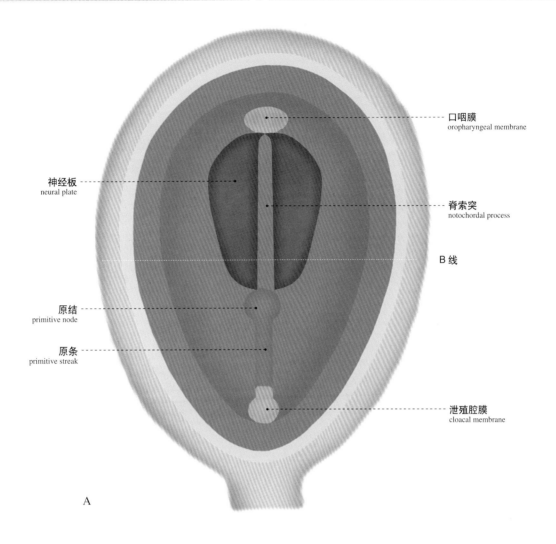

口咽膜
oropharyngeal membrane

神经板
neural plate

脊索突
notochordal process

B 线

原结
primitive node

原条
primitive streak

泄殖腔膜
cloacal membrane

A

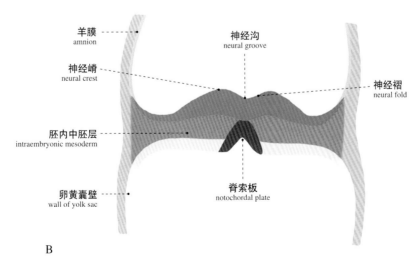

羊膜
amnion

神经沟
neural groove

神经嵴
neural crest

神经褶
neural fold

胚内中胚层
intraembryonic mesoderm

卵黄囊壁
wall of yolk sac

脊索板
notochordal plate

B

296. 神经管的形成（约 18 天）

Formation of the neural tube (about 18 days)

A. 胚背侧观；B. 为 A 图经 B 线的切面，可见早期神经沟及神经褶，也可见脊索的发生

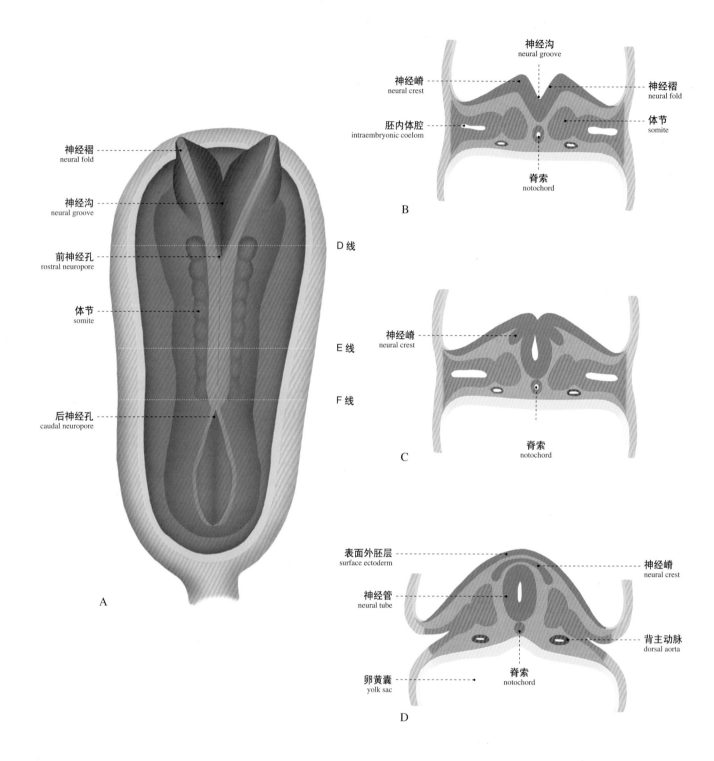

神经褶
neural fold

神经沟
neural groove

前神经孔
rostral neuropore

体节
somite

后神经孔
caudal neuropore

A

D 线

E 线

F 线

神经沟
neural groove

神经嵴
neural crest

胚内体腔
intraembryonic coelom

神经褶
neural fold

体节
somite

脊索
notochord

B

神经嵴
neural crest

脊索
notochord

C

表面外胚层
surface ectoderm

神经管
neural tube

卵黄囊
yolk sac

神经嵴
neural crest

背主动脉
dorsal aorta

脊索
notochord

D

297. 神经管的形成（约 22 天）

Formation of the neural tube (about 22 days)

A. 胚背侧观（约 22 天），两边神经褶按对应体节处融合，分别向头尾侧扩展，留有未融合的前、后神经孔；

B~D. 为 C 之横切面，示神经管、神经嵴的形成

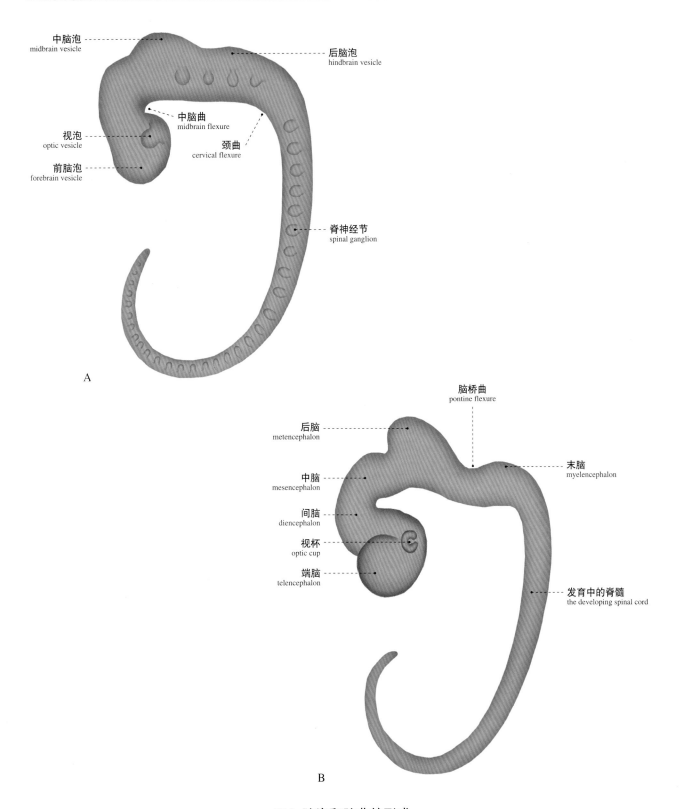

中脑泡
midbrain vesicle

后脑泡
hindbrain vesicle

中脑曲
midbrain flexure

视泡
optic vesicle

颈曲
cervical flexure

前脑泡
forebrain vesicle

脊神经节
spinal ganglion

A

脑桥曲
pontine flexure

后脑
metencephalon

末脑
myelencephalon

中脑
mesencephalon

间脑
diencephalon

视杯
optic cup

发育中的脊髓
the developing spinal cord

端脑
telencephalon

B

298. 脑泡和脑曲的形成
Formation of the brain vesicle and the brain flexure

A. 约 28 天胚脑的外侧观；B. 6 周胚脑的外侧观

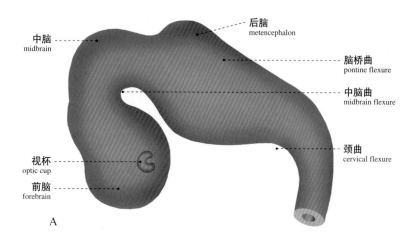

中脑 midbrain
后脑 metencephalon
脑桥曲 pontine flexure
中脑曲 midbrain flexure
颈曲 cervical flexure
视杯 optic cup
前脑 forebrain

A

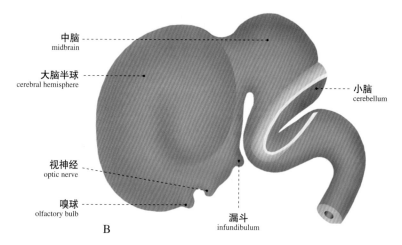

中脑 midbrain
大脑半球 cerebral hemisphere
小脑 cerebellum
视神经 optic nerve
嗅球 olfactory bulb
漏斗 infundibulum

B

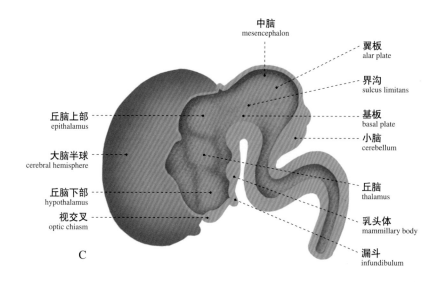

中脑 mesencephalon
翼板 alar plate
界沟 sulcus limitans
基板 basal plate
小脑 cerebellum
丘脑上部 epithalamus
大脑半球 cerebral hemisphere
丘脑 thalamus
丘脑下部 hypothalamus
乳头体 mammillary body
视交叉 optic chiasm
漏斗 infundibulum

C

299. 脑的发生（5 周，7 周）
Development of the brain (5 weeks, 7 weeks)

A. 5 周末脑的外侧观；B. 7 周脑的外侧观；C. 脑的矢状面观，示前、中脑泡的内表面

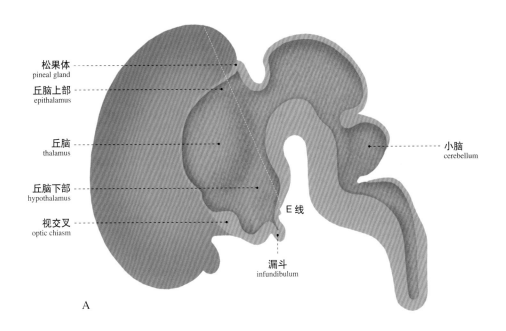

松果体
pineal gland

丘脑上部
epithalamus

丘脑
thalamus

丘脑下部
hypothalamus

视交叉
optic chiasm

小脑
cerebellum

E 线

漏斗
infundibulum

A

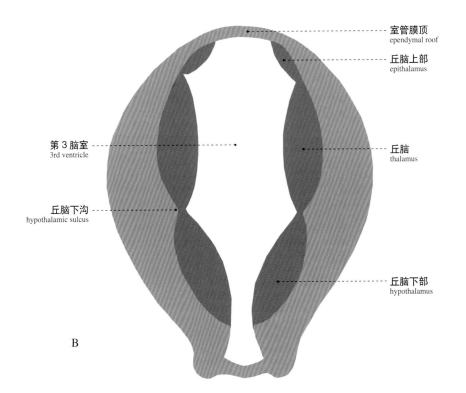

室管膜顶
ependymal roof

丘脑上部
epithalamus

第 3 脑室
3rd ventricle

丘脑
thalamus

丘脑下沟
hypothalamic sulcus

丘脑下部
hypothalamus

B

300. 脑的发生（8 周）
Development of the brain (8 weeks)

A. 8 周脑矢状切面观，示内表面；B. 经间脑（经 E 线）横切面，示背侧丘脑上部，两侧丘脑和腹侧丘脑下部

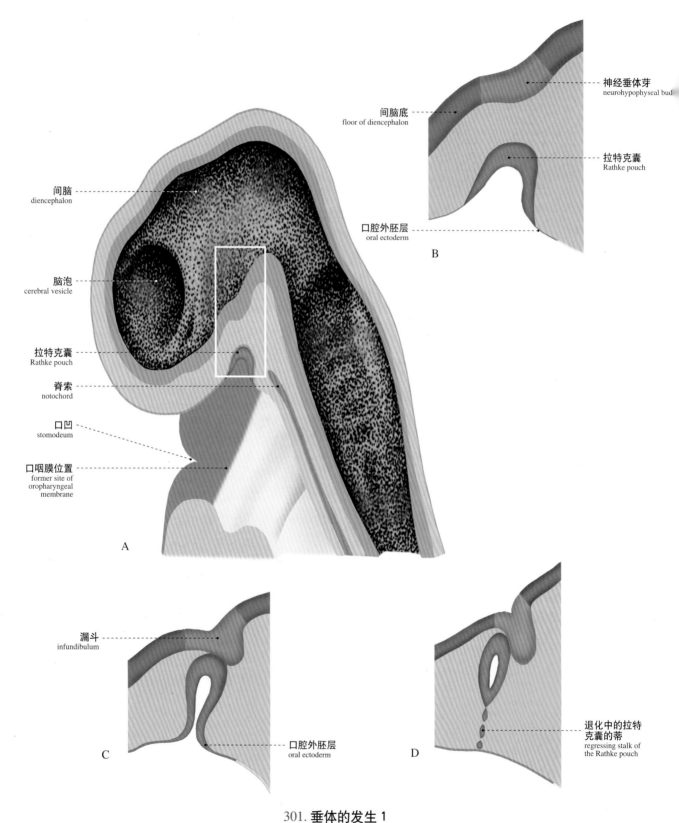

间脑
diencephalon

脑泡
cerebral vesicle

拉特克囊
Rathke pouch

脊索
notochord

口凹
stomodeum

口咽膜位置
former site of
oropharyngeal
membrane

A

神经垂体芽
neurohypophyseal bud

间脑底
floor of diencephalon

拉特克囊
Rathke pouch

口腔外胚层
oral ectoderm

B

漏斗
infundibulum

口腔外胚层
oral ectoderm

C

退化中的拉特
克囊的蒂
regressing stalk of
the Rathke pouch

D

301. 垂体的发生 1
Development of the hypophysis 1

A. 胚（约 36 天）脑末端矢状切面，示拉特克囊 (Rathke pouch) 从原始口腔顶往上生长以及前脑泡神经垂体芽往下生长；B、C、D. 示垂体发生的各个时期，约 8 周，拉特克囊失去与口腔的连接而与漏斗紧密相贴

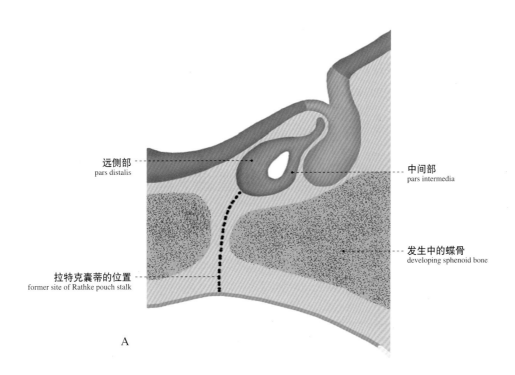

远侧部
pars distalis

中间部
pars intermedia

发生中的蝶骨
developing sphenoid bone

拉特克囊蒂的位置
former site of Rathke pouch stalk

A

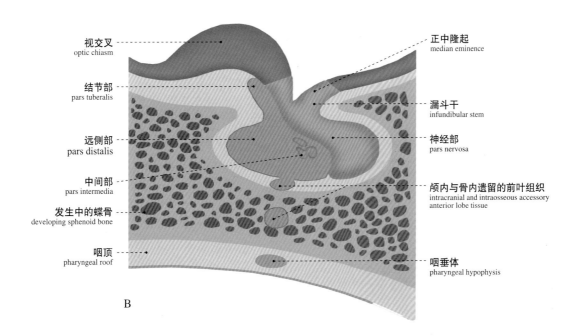

视交叉
optic chiasm

正中隆起
median eminence

结节部
pars tuberalis

漏斗干
infundibular stem

远侧部
pars distalis

神经部
pars nervosa

中间部
pars intermedia

颅内与骨内遗留的前叶组织
intracranial and intraosseous accessory
anterior lobe tissue

发生中的蝶骨
developing sphenoid bone

咽顶
pharyngeal roof

咽垂体
pharyngeal hypophysis

B

302. 垂体的发生 2
Development of the hypophysis 2

A、B. 为垂体发生的后期，示拉特克囊的前壁增殖形成腺垂体的远侧部（前叶）；拉特克囊的后壁形成腺垂体的中间部

眼

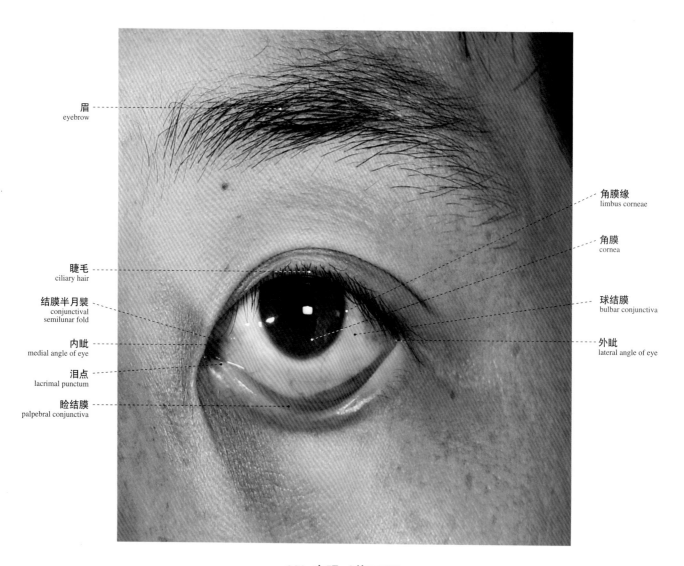

眉
eyebrow

睫毛
ciliary hair

结膜半月襞
conjunctival
semilunar fold

内眦
medial angle of eye

泪点
lacrimal punctum

睑结膜
palpebral conjunctiva

角膜缘
limbus corneae

角膜
cornea

球结膜
bulbar conjunctiva

外眦
lateral angle of eye

303. 左眼（前面观）
Left eye (anterior aspect)

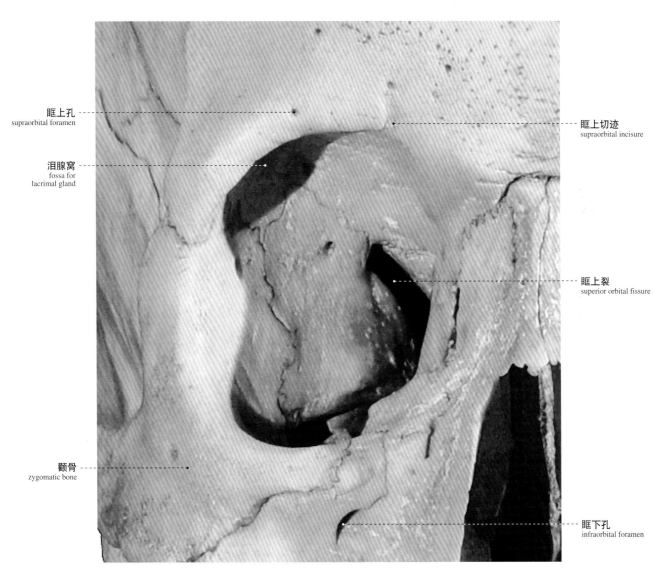

眶上孔
supraorbital foramen

泪腺窝
fossa for
lacrimal gland

颧骨
zygomatic bone

眶上切迹
supraorbital incisure

眶上裂
superior orbital fissure

眶下孔
infraorbital foramen

304. 眼眶（前面观）
Orbit (anterior aspect)

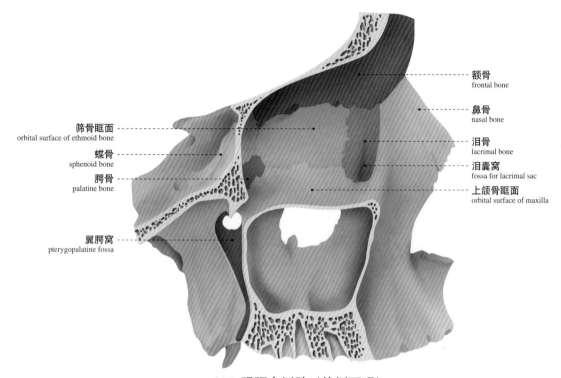

筛骨眶面
orbital surface of ethmoid bone

蝶骨
sphenoid bone

腭骨
palatine bone

翼腭窝
pterygopalatine fossa

额骨
frontal bone

鼻骨
nasal bone

泪骨
lacrimal bone

泪囊窝
fossa for lacrimal sac

上颌骨眶面
orbital surface of maxilla

305. 眼眶内侧壁（外侧面观）
Medial wall of the orbit (lateral aspect)

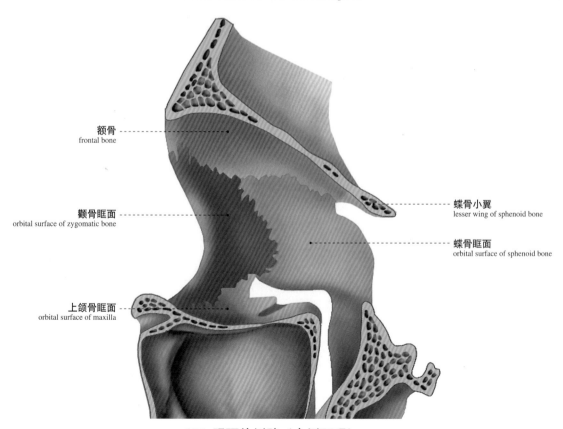

额骨
frontal bone

颧骨眶面
orbital surface of zygomatic bone

上颌骨眶面
orbital surface of maxilla

蝶骨小翼
lesser wing of sphenoid bone

蝶骨眶面
orbital surface of sphenoid bone

306. 眼眶外侧壁（内侧面观）
Lateral wall of the orbit (medial aspect)

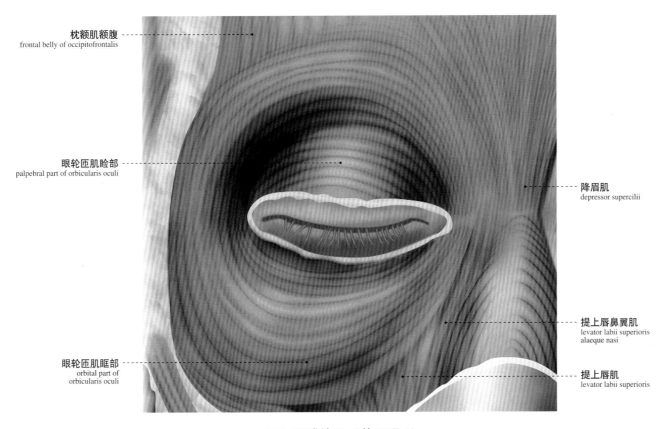

枕额肌额腹
frontal belly of occipitofrontalis

眼轮匝肌睑部
palpebral part of orbicularis oculi

降眉肌
depressor supercilii

提上唇鼻翼肌
levator labii superioris alaeque nasi

眼轮匝肌眶部
orbital part of orbicularis oculi

提上唇肌
levator labii superioris

307. 眼球外肌（前面观 1）
Ocular muscles (anterior aspect 1)

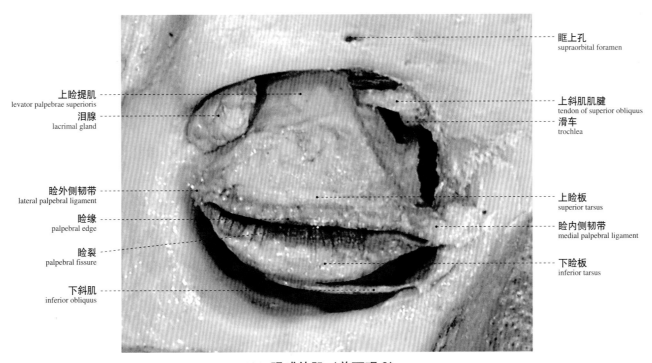

眶上孔
supraorbital foramen

上睑提肌
levator palpebrae superioris

泪腺
lacrimal gland

上斜肌肌腱
tendon of superior obliquus

滑车
trochlea

睑外侧韧带
lateral palpebral ligament

上睑板
superior tarsus

睑缘
palpebral edge

睑内侧韧带
medial palpebral ligament

睑裂
palpebral fissure

下睑板
inferior tarsus

下斜肌
inferior obliquus

308. 眼球外肌（前面观 2）
Ocular muscles (anterior aspect 2)

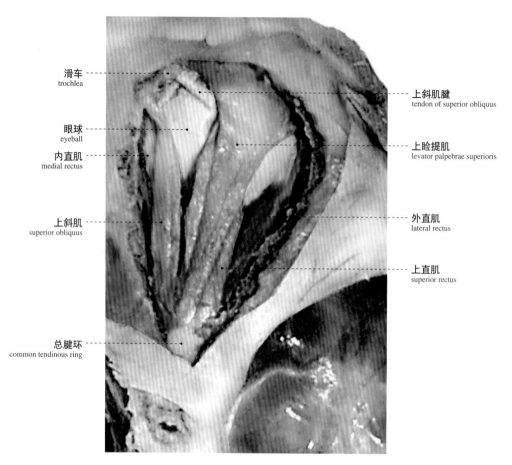

309. 眼球外肌（上面观 1）

Ocular muscles (superior aspect 1)

滑车
trochlea

眼球
eyeball

内直肌
medial rectus

上斜肌
superior obliquus

总腱环
common tendinous ring

上斜肌腱
tendon of superior obliquus

上睑提肌
levator palpebrae superioris

外直肌
lateral rectus

上直肌
superior rectus

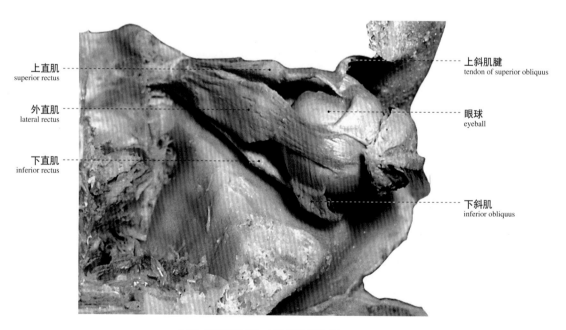

310. 眼球外肌（外侧面观 1）

Ocular muscles (lateral aspect 1)

上直肌
superior rectus

外直肌
lateral rectus

下直肌
inferior rectus

上斜肌腱
tendon of superior obliquus

眼球
eyeball

下斜肌
inferior obliquus

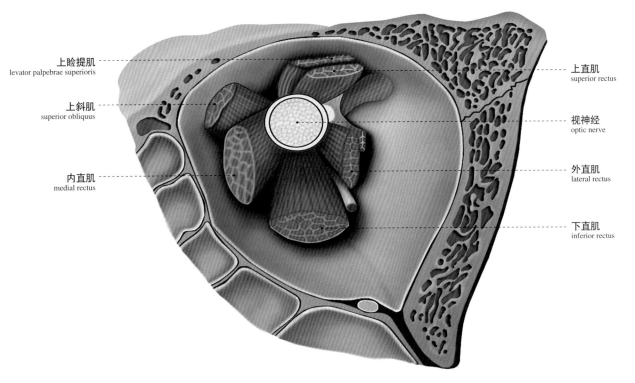

上睑提肌
levator palpebrae superioris

上斜肌
superior obliquus

内直肌
medial rectus

上直肌
superior rectus

视神经
optic nerve

外直肌
lateral rectus

下直肌
inferior rectus

311. 眼球外肌（前面观 3）
Ocular muscles (anterior aspect 3)

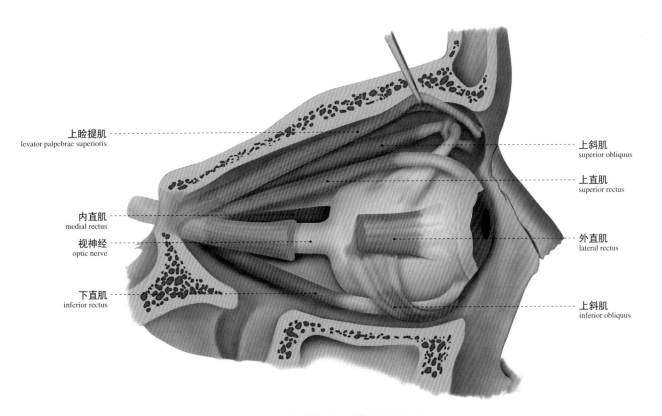

上睑提肌
levator palpebrae superioris

内直肌
medial rectus

视神经
optic nerve

下直肌
inferior rectus

上斜肌
superior obliquus

上直肌
superior rectus

外直肌
lateral rectus

上斜肌
inferior obliquus

312. 眼球外肌（外侧面观 2）
Ocular muscles (lateral aspect 2)

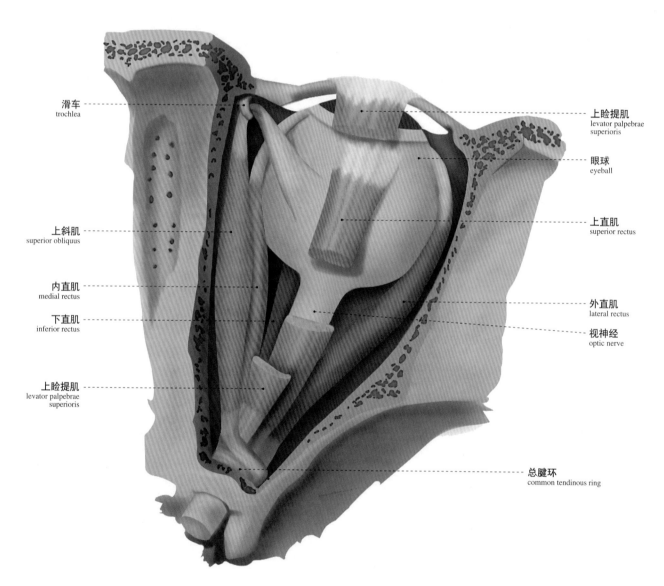

滑车
trochlea

上斜肌
superior obliquus

内直肌
medial rectus

下直肌
inferior rectus

上睑提肌
levator palpebrae
superioris

上睑提肌
levator palpebrae
superioris

眼球
eyeball

上直肌
superior rectus

外直肌
lateral rectus

视神经
optic nerve

总腱环
common tendinous ring

313. 眼球外肌（上面观 2）
Ocular muscles (superior aspect 2)

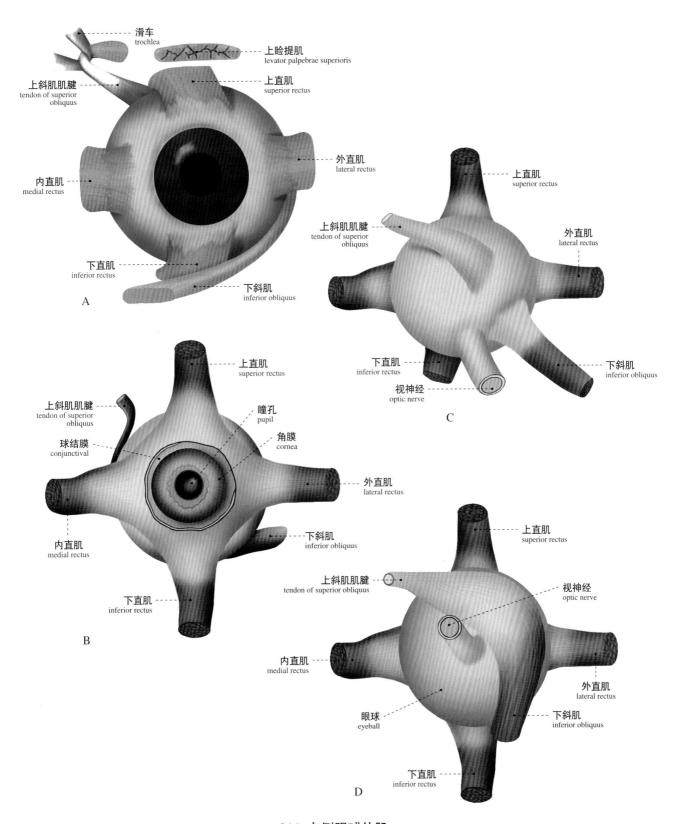

滑车
trochlea

上睑提肌
levator palpebrae superioris

上斜肌肌腱
tendon of superior obliquus

上直肌
superior rectus

外直肌
lateral rectus

内直肌
medial rectus

下直肌
inferior rectus

下斜肌
inferior obliquus

A

上直肌
superior rectus

上斜肌肌腱
tendon of superior obliquus

外直肌
lateral rectus

下直肌
inferior rectus

下斜肌
inferior obliquus

视神经
optic nerve

C

上直肌
superior rectus

上斜肌肌腱
tendon of superior obliquus

球结膜
conjunctival

瞳孔
pupil

角膜
cornea

外直肌
lateral rectus

内直肌
medial rectus

下斜肌
inferior obliquus

下直肌
inferior rectus

B

上直肌
superior rectus

上斜肌肌腱
tendon of superior obliquus

视神经
optic nerve

内直肌
medial rectus

外直肌
lateral rectus

眼球
eyeball

下斜肌
inferior obliquus

下直肌
inferior rectus

D

314. 右侧眼球外肌
Right ocular muscles
A. 前面观 1；B. 前面观 2；C. 后上面观；D. 后面观

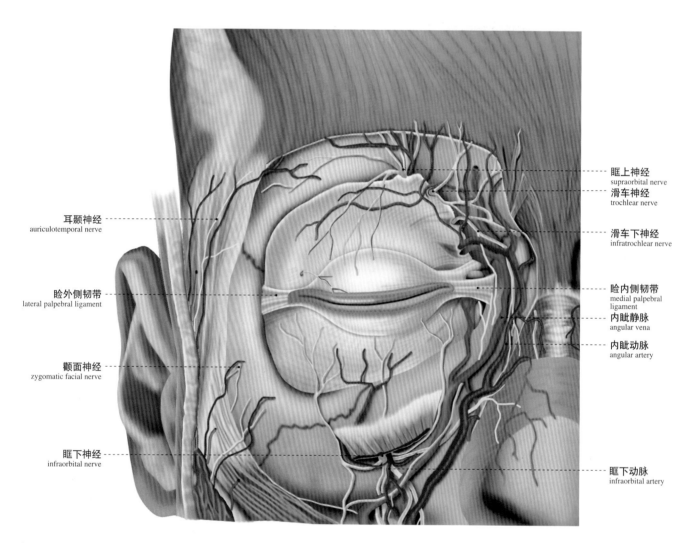

耳颞神经
auriculotemporal nerve

睑外侧韧带
lateral palpebral ligament

颧面神经
zygomatic facial nerve

眶下神经
infraorbital nerve

眶上神经
supraorbital nerve

滑车神经
trochlear nerve

滑车下神经
infratrochlear nerve

睑内侧韧带
medial palpebral ligament

内眦静脉
angular vena

内眦动脉
angular artery

眶下动脉
infraorbital artery

315. 眼眶神经血管（前面观 1）
Orbital nerves and blood vessels (anterior aspect 1)

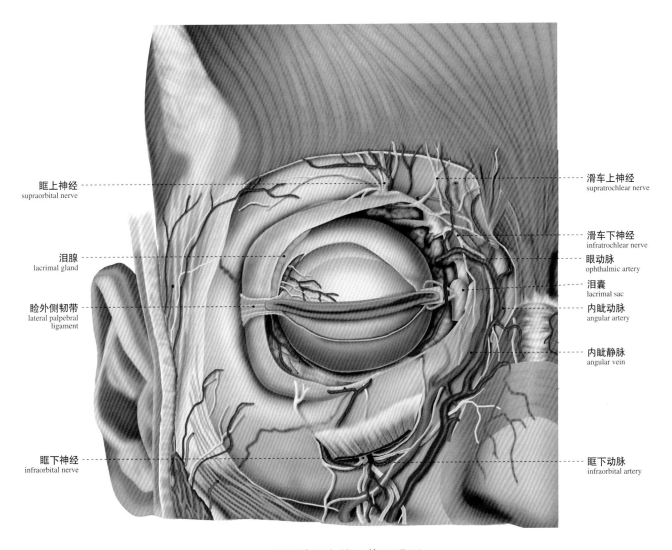

眶上神经
supraorbital nerve

泪腺
lacrimal gland

睑外侧韧带
lateral palpebral
ligament

眶下神经
infraorbital nerve

滑车上神经
supratrochlear nerve

滑车下神经
infratrochlear nerve

眼动脉
ophthalmic artery

泪囊
lacrimal sac

内眦动脉
angular artery

内眦静脉
angular vein

眶下动脉
infraorbital artery

316. 眼眶神经血管（前面观2）
Orbital nerves and blood vessels (anterior aspect 2)

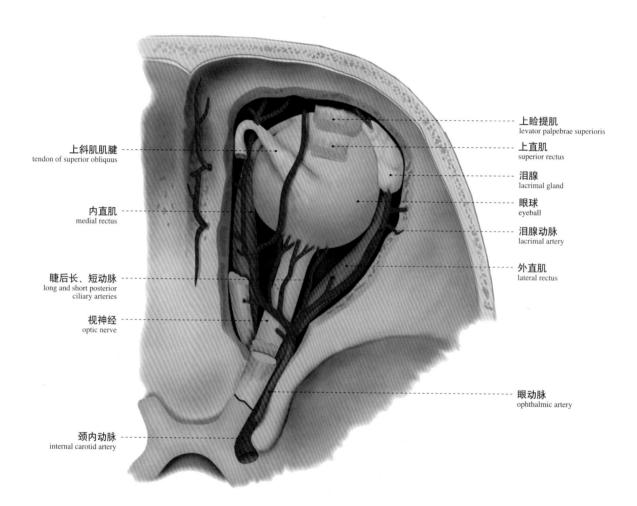

上斜肌肌腱
tendon of superior obliquus

内直肌
medial rectus

睫后长、短动脉
long and short posterior
ciliary arteries

视神经
optic nerve

颈内动脉
internal carotid artery

上睑提肌
levator palpebrae superioris

上直肌
superior rectus

泪腺
lacrimal gland

眼球
eyeball

泪腺动脉
lacrimal artery

外直肌
lateral rectus

眼动脉
ophthalmic artery

317. 右侧眶动脉（上面观）
Right orbital arteries (superior aspect)

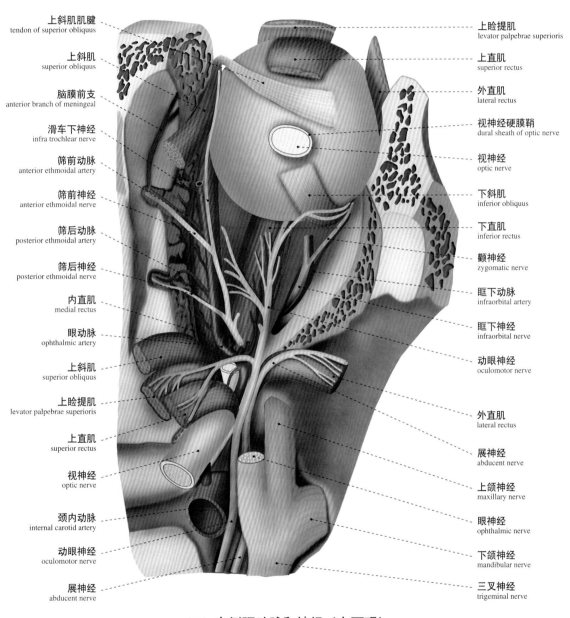

上斜肌肌腱
tendon of superior obliquus

上斜肌
superior obliquus

脑膜前支
anterior branch of meningeal

滑车下神经
infra trochlear nerve

筛前动脉
anterior ethmoidal artery

筛前神经
anterior ethmoidal nerve

筛后动脉
posterior ethmoidal artery

筛后神经
posterior ethmoidal nerve

内直肌
medial rectus

眼动脉
ophthalmic artery

上斜肌
superior obliquus

上睑提肌
levator palpebrae superioris

上直肌
superior rectus

视神经
optic nerve

颈内动脉
internal carotid artery

动眼神经
oculomotor nerve

展神经
abducent nerve

上睑提肌
levator palpebrae superioris

上直肌
superior rectus

外直肌
lateral rectus

视神经硬膜鞘
dural sheath of optic nerve

视神经
optic nerve

下斜肌
inferior obliquus

下直肌
inferior rectus

颧神经
zygomatic nerve

眶下动脉
infraorbital artery

眶下神经
infraorbital nerve

动眼神经
oculomotor nerve

外直肌
lateral rectus

展神经
abducent nerve

上颌神经
maxillary nerve

眼神经
ophthalmic nerve

下颌神经
mandibular nerve

三叉神经
trigeminal nerve

318. 右侧眶动脉和神经（上面观）
Right orbital arteries and nerves (superior aspect)

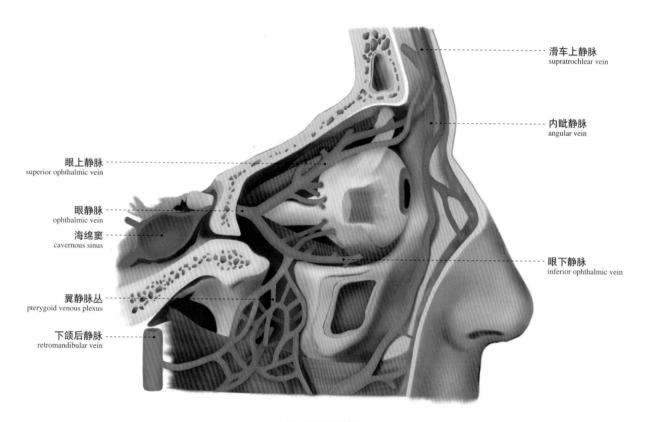

滑车上静脉
supratrochlear vein

内眦静脉
angular vein

眼上静脉
superior ophthalmic vein

眼静脉
ophthalmic vein

海绵窦
cavernous sinus

眼下静脉
inferior ophthalmic vein

翼静脉丛
pterygoid venous plexus

下颌后静脉
retromandibular vein

319. 眼周围静脉
Veins around the eye

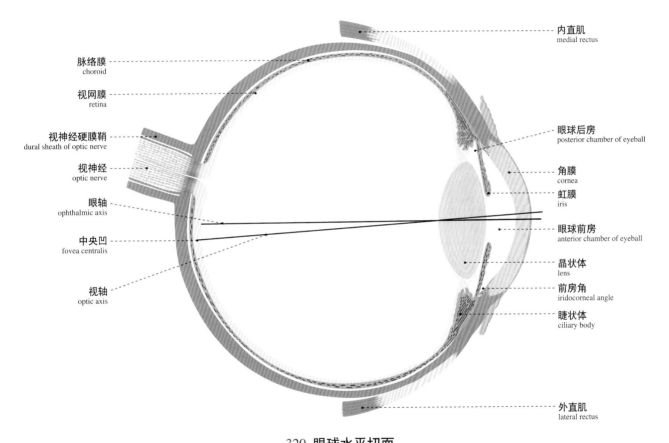

脉络膜
choroid

视网膜
retina

视神经硬膜鞘
dural sheath of optic nerve

视神经
optic nerve

眼轴
ophthalmic axis

中央凹
fovea centralis

视轴
optic axis

内直肌
medial rectus

眼球后房
posterior chamber of eyeball

角膜
cornea

虹膜
iris

眼球前房
anterior chamber of eyeball

晶状体
lens

前房角
iridocorneal angle

睫状体
ciliary body

外直肌
lateral rectus

320. 眼球水平切面
Horizontal section through the eyeball

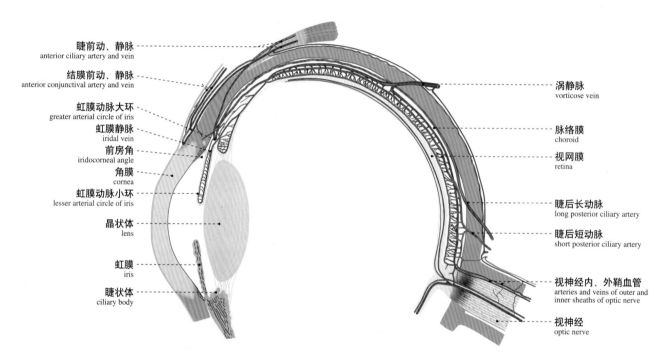

睫前动、静脉
anterior ciliary artery and vein

结膜前动、静脉
anterior conjunctival artery and vein

虹膜动脉大环
greater arterial circle of iris

虹膜静脉
iridal vein

前房角
iridocorneal angle

角膜
cornea

虹膜动脉小环
lesser arterial circle of iris

晶状体
lens

虹膜
iris

睫状体
ciliary body

涡静脉
vorticose vein

脉络膜
choroid

视网膜
retina

睫后长动脉
long posterior ciliary artery

睫后短动脉
short posterior ciliary artery

视神经内、外鞘血管
arteries and veins of outer and inner sheaths of optic nerve

视神经
optic nerve

321. 眼球的血管
Blood vessels of the eyeball

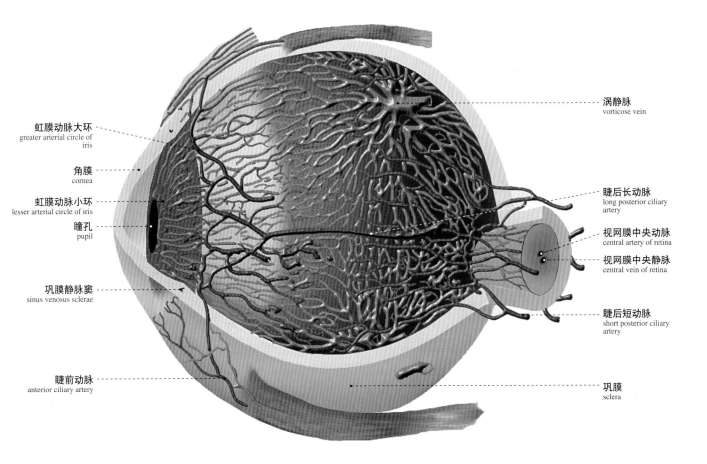

虹膜动脉大环
greater arterial circle of iris

角膜
cornea

虹膜动脉小环
lesser arterial circle of iris

瞳孔
pupil

巩膜静脉窦
sinus venosus sclerae

睫前动脉
anterior ciliary artery

涡静脉
vorticose vein

睫后长动脉
long posterior ciliary artery

视网膜中央动脉
central artery of retina

视网膜中央静脉
central vein of retina

睫后短动脉
short posterior ciliary artery

巩膜
sclera

322. 眼球血管分布
Distribution of the blood vessels of the eyeball

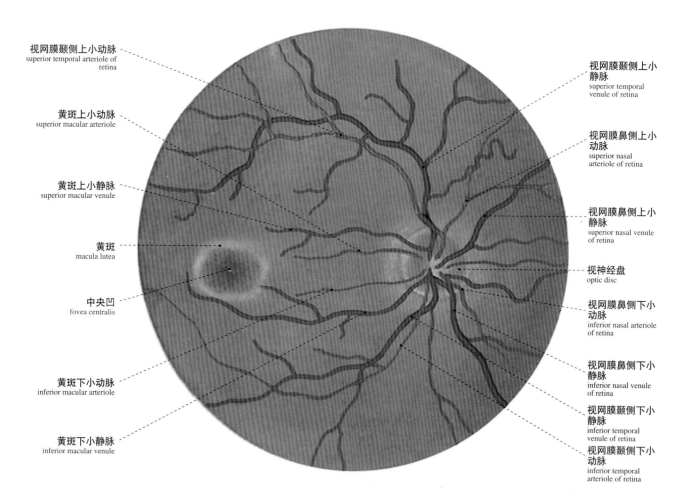

视网膜颞侧上小动脉
superior temporal arteriole of retina

黄斑上小动脉
superior macular arteriole

黄斑上小静脉
superior macular venule

黄斑
macula lutea

中央凹
fovea centralis

黄斑下小动脉
inferior macular arteriole

黄斑下小静脉
inferior macular venule

视网膜颞侧上小静脉
superior temporal venule of retina

视网膜鼻侧上小动脉
superior nasal arteriole of retina

视网膜鼻侧上小静脉
superior nasal venule of retina

视神经盘
optic disc

视网膜鼻侧下小动脉
inferior nasal arteriole of retina

视网膜鼻侧下小静脉
inferior nasal venule of retina

视网膜颞侧下小静脉
inferior temporal venule of retina

视网膜颞侧下小动脉
inferior temporal arteriole of retina

323. 右侧眼底镜图

Right ophthalmoscopic image of the fundus of the eyeball

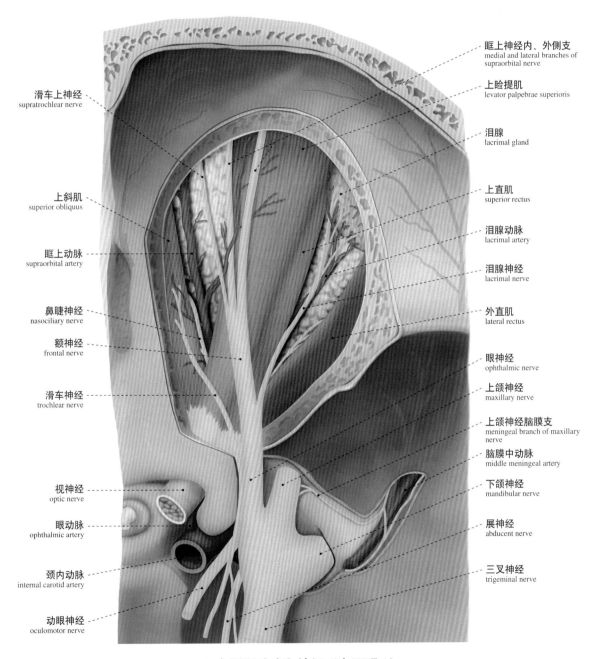

滑车上神经
supratrochlear nerve

上斜肌
superior obliquus

眶上动脉
supraorbital artery

鼻睫神经
nasociliary nerve

额神经
frontal nerve

滑车神经
trochlear nerve

视神经
optic nerve

眼动脉
ophthalmic artery

颈内动脉
internal carotid artery

动眼神经
oculomotor nerve

眶上神经内、外侧支
medial and lateral branches of supraorbital nerve

上睑提肌
levator palpebrae superioris

泪腺
lacrimal gland

上直肌
superior rectus

泪腺动脉
lacrimal artery

泪腺神经
lacrimal nerve

外直肌
lateral rectus

眼神经
ophthalmic nerve

上颌神经
maxillary nerve

上颌神经脑膜支
meningeal branch of maxillary nerve

脑膜中动脉
middle meningeal artery

下颌神经
mandibular nerve

展神经
abducent nerve

三叉神经
trigeminal nerve

324. 右侧眶动脉和神经（上面观 1）
Right orbital arteries and nerves (superior aspect 1)

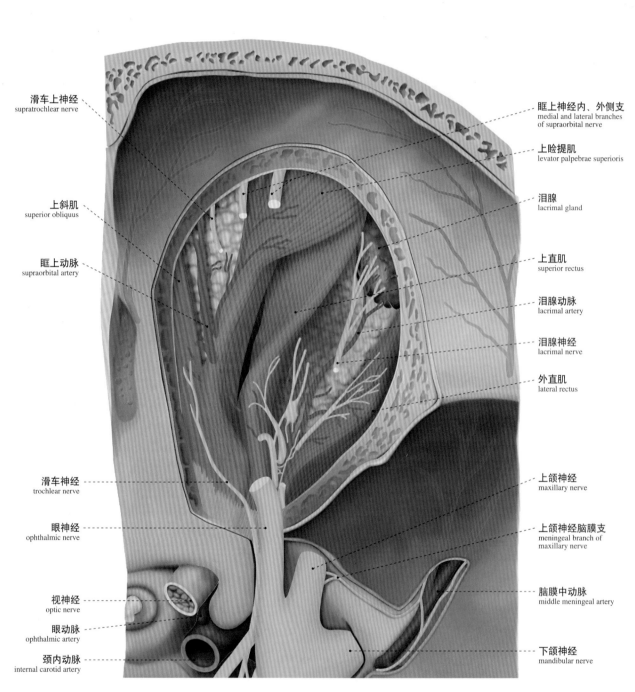

滑车上神经
supratrochlear nerve

上斜肌
superior obliquus

眶上动脉
supraorbital artery

滑车神经
trochlear nerve

眼神经
ophthalmic nerve

视神经
optic nerve

眼动脉
ophthalmic artery

颈内动脉
internal carotid artery

眶上神经内、外侧支
medial and lateral branches of supraorbital nerve

上睑提肌
levator palpebrae superioris

泪腺
lacrimal gland

上直肌
superior rectus

泪腺动脉
lacrimal artery

泪腺神经
lacrimal nerve

外直肌
lateral rectus

上颌神经
maxillary nerve

上颌神经脑膜支
meningeal branch of maxillary nerve

脑膜中动脉
middle meningeal artery

下颌神经
mandibular nerve

325. 右侧眶动脉和神经（上面观 2）

Right orbital arteries and nerves (superior aspect 2)

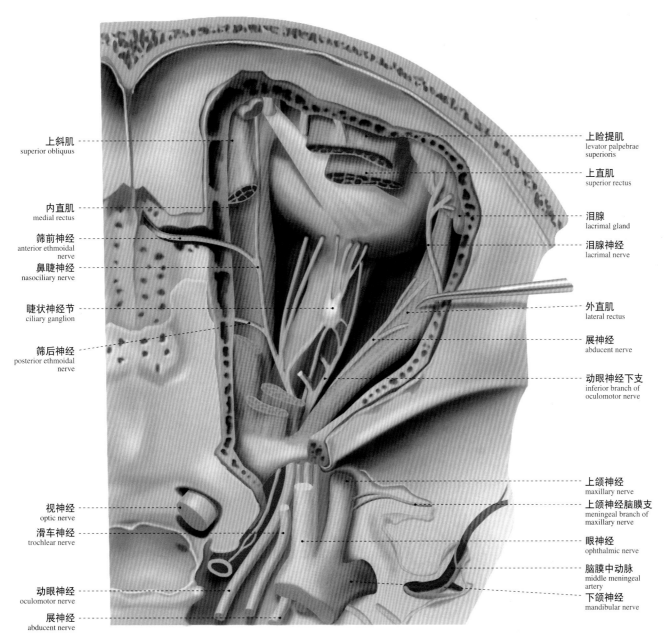

上斜肌
superior obliquus

内直肌
medial rectus

筛前神经
anterior ethmoidal nerve

鼻睫神经
nasociliary nerve

睫状神经节
ciliary ganglion

筛后神经
posterior ethmoidal nerve

视神经
optic nerve

滑车神经
trochlear nerve

动眼神经
oculomotor nerve

展神经
abducent nerve

上睑提肌
levator palpebrae superioris

上直肌
superior rectus

泪腺
lacrimal gland

泪腺神经
lacrimal nerve

外直肌
lateral rectus

展神经
abducent nerve

动眼神经下支
inferior branch of oculomotor nerve

上颌神经
maxillary nerve

上颌神经脑膜支
meningeal branch of maxillary nerve

眼神经
ophthalmic nerve

脑膜中动脉
middle meningeal artery

下颌神经
mandibular nerve

326. 右侧眶动脉和神经（上面观 3）
Right orbital arteries and nerves (superior aspect 3)

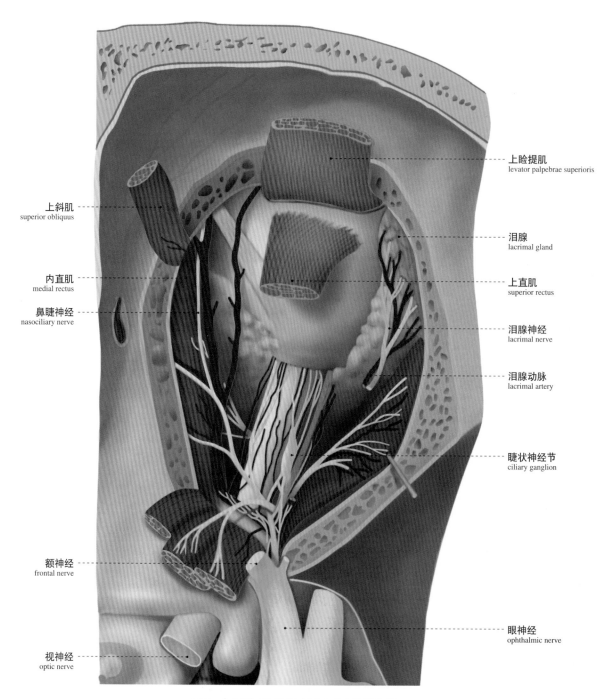

上睑提肌
levator palpebrae superioris

上斜肌
superior obliquus

泪腺
lacrimal gland

内直肌
medial rectus

上直肌
superior rectus

鼻睫神经
nasociliary nerve

泪腺神经
lacrimal nerve

泪腺动脉
lacrimal artery

睫状神经节
ciliary ganglion

额神经
frontal nerve

眼神经
ophthalmic nerve

视神经
optic nerve

327. 右侧眶动脉和神经（上面观 4）

Right orbital arteries and nerves (superior aspect 4)

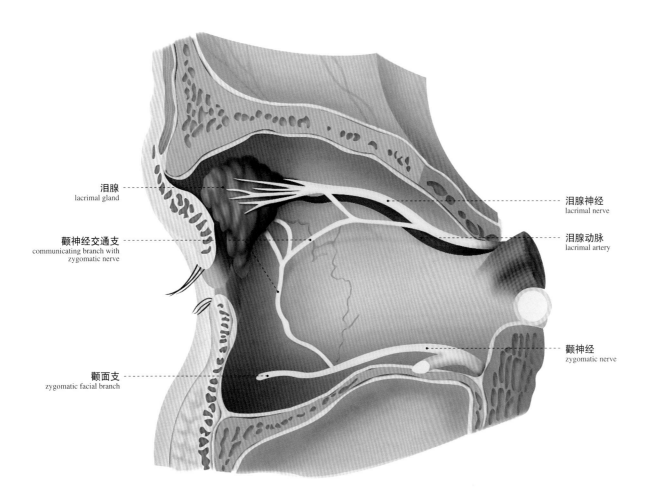

泪腺
lacrimal gland

颧神经交通支
communicating branch with
zygomatic nerve

颧面支
zygomatic facial branch

泪腺神经
lacrimal nerve

泪腺动脉
lacrimal artery

颧神经
zygomatic nerve

328. 泪腺的神经分布
Innervation of the lacrimal gland

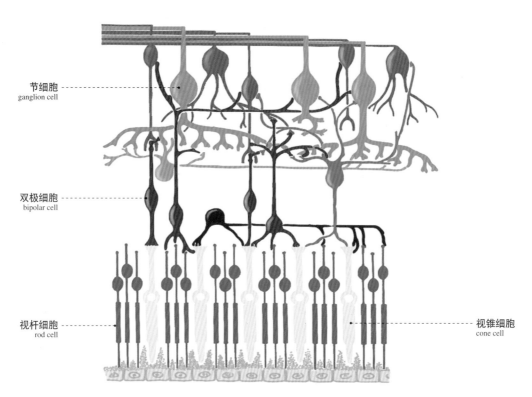

节细胞
ganglion cell

双极细胞
bipolar cell

视杆细胞
rod cell

视锥细胞
cone cell

329. 视网膜的神经细胞
Nerve cells of the retina

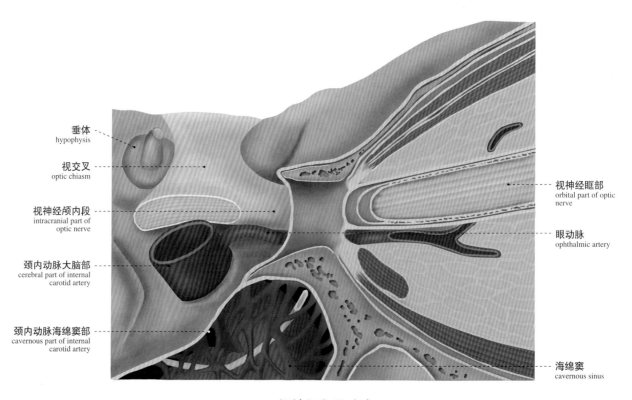

垂体
hypophysis

视交叉
optic chiasm

视神经颅内段
intracranial part of
optic nerve

颈内动脉大脑部
cerebral part of internal
carotid artery

颈内动脉海绵窦部
cavernous part of internal
carotid artery

视神经眶部
orbital part of optic
nerve

眼动脉
ophthalmic artery

海绵窦
cavernous sinus

330. 视神经和眼动脉
Optic nerve and ophthalmic artery

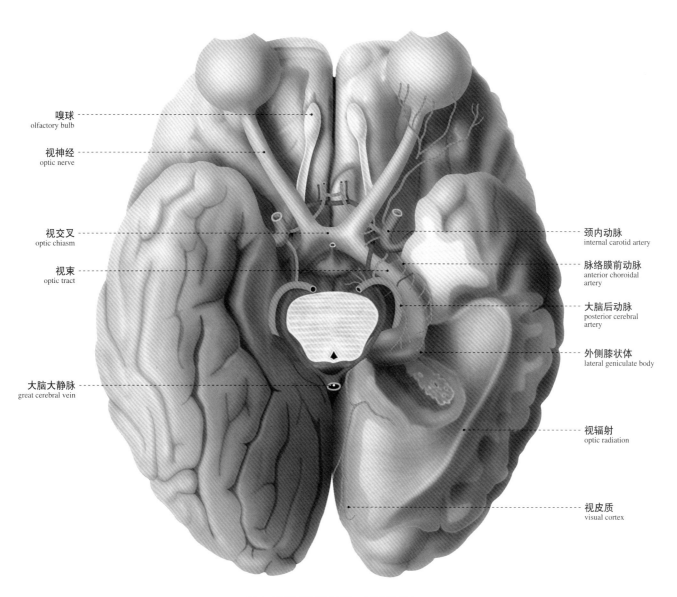

嗅球
olfactory bulb

视神经
optic nerve

视交叉
optic chiasm

视束
optic tract

大脑大静脉
great cerebral vein

颈内动脉
internal carotid artery

脉络膜前动脉
anterior choroidal artery

大脑后动脉
posterior cerebral artery

外侧膝状体
lateral geniculate body

视辐射
optic radiation

视皮质
visual cortex

331. 脑和视觉通路（下面观）
Brain and visual pathway (inferior aspect)

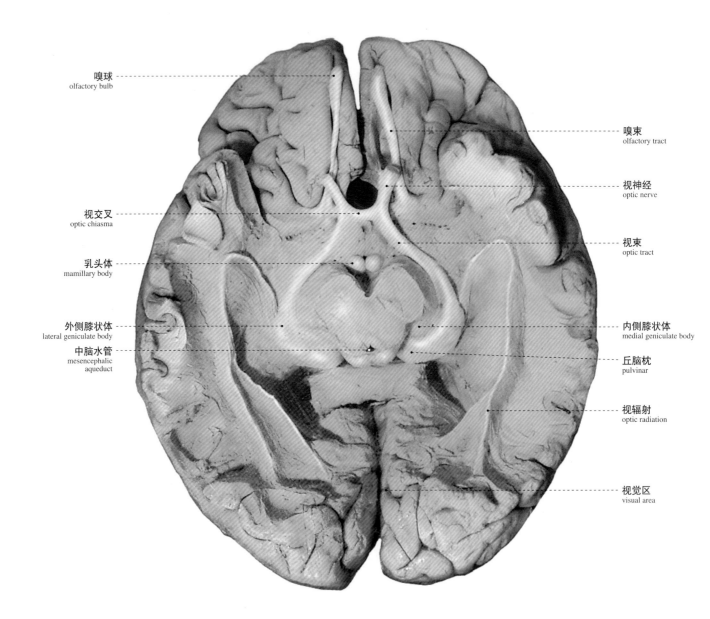

嗅球
olfactory bulb

嗅束
olfactory tract

视神经
optic nerve

视交叉
optic chiasma

视束
optic tract

乳头体
mamillary body

外侧膝状体
lateral geniculate body

内侧膝状体
medial geniculate body

中脑水管
mesencephalic
aqueduct

丘脑枕
pulvinar

视辐射
optic radiation

视觉区
visual area

332. 视觉传导通路 1
Visual pathway 1

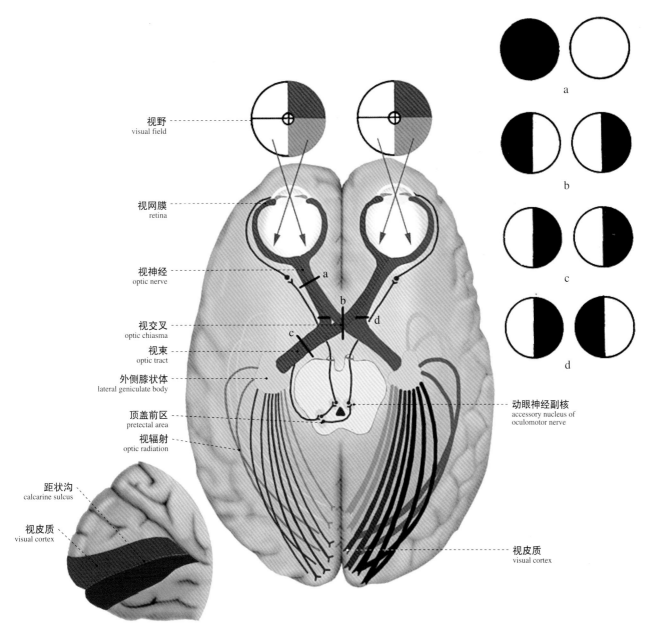

视野
visual field

视网膜
retina

视神经
optic nerve

视交叉
optic chiasma

视束
optic tract

外侧膝状体
lateral geniculate body

顶盖前区
pretectal area

视辐射
optic radiation

距状沟
calcarine sulcus

视皮质
visual cortex

动眼神经副核
accessory nucleus of
oculomotor nerve

视皮质
visual cortex

333. 视觉传导通路 2
Visual pathway 2

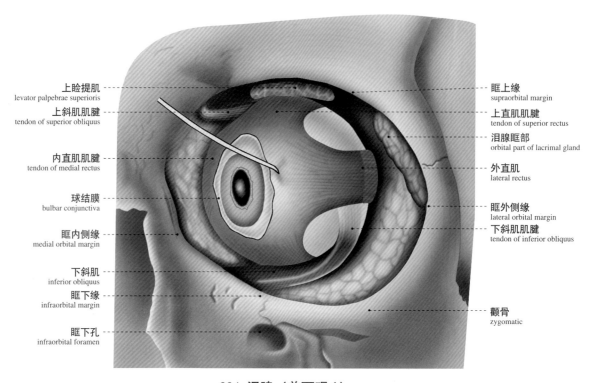

上睑提肌
levator palpebrae superioris

上斜肌肌腱
tendon of superior obliquus

内直肌肌腱
tendon of medial rectus

球结膜
bulbar conjunctiva

眶内侧缘
medial orbital margin

下斜肌
inferior obliquus

眶下缘
infraorbital margin

眶下孔
infraorbital foramen

眶上缘
supraorbital margin

上直肌肌腱
tendon of superior rectus

泪腺眶部
orbital part of lacrimal gland

外直肌
lateral rectus

眶外侧缘
lateral orbital margin

下斜肌肌腱
tendon of inferior obliquus

颧骨
zygomatic

334. 泪腺（前面观 1）
Lacrimal gland (anterior aspect 1)

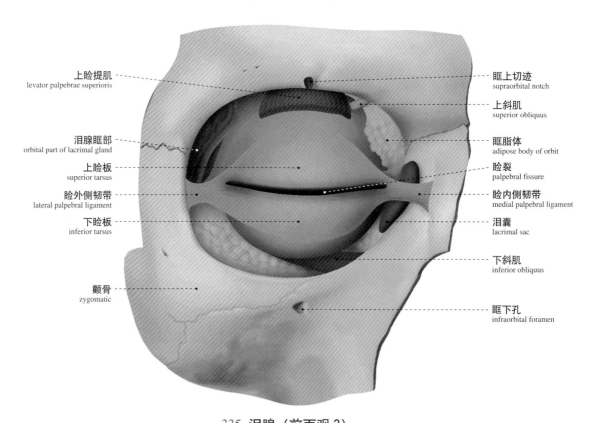

上睑提肌
levator palpebrae superioris

泪腺眶部
orbital part of lacrimal gland

上睑板
superior tarsus

睑外侧韧带
lateral palpebral ligament

下睑板
inferior tarsus

颧骨
zygomatic

眶上切迹
supraorbital notch

上斜肌
superior obliquus

眶脂体
adipose body of orbit

睑裂
palpebral fissure

睑内侧韧带
medial palpebral ligament

泪囊
lacrimal sac

下斜肌
inferior obliquus

眶下孔
infraorbital foramen

335. 泪腺（前面观 2）
Lacrimal gland (anterior aspect 2)

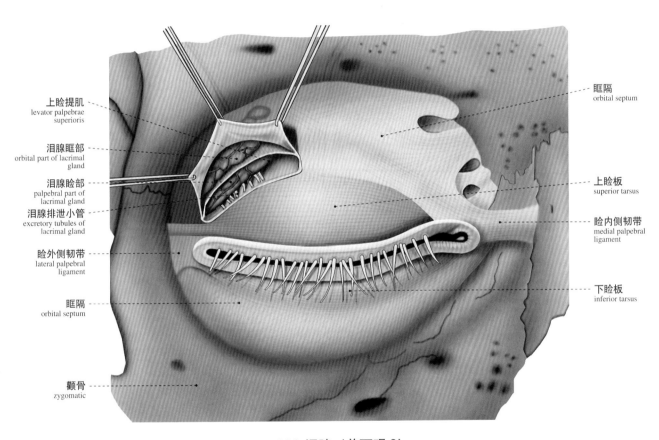

上睑提肌
levator palpebrae
superioris

泪腺眶部
orbital part of lacrimal
gland

泪腺睑部
palpebral part of
lacrimal gland

泪腺排泄小管
excretory tubules of
lacrimal gland

睑外侧韧带
lateral palpebral
ligament

眶隔
orbital septum

颧骨
zygomatic

眶隔
orbital septum

上睑板
superior tarsus

睑内侧韧带
medial palpebral
ligament

下睑板
inferior tarsus

336. 泪腺（前面观 3）
Lacrimal gland (anterior aspect 3)

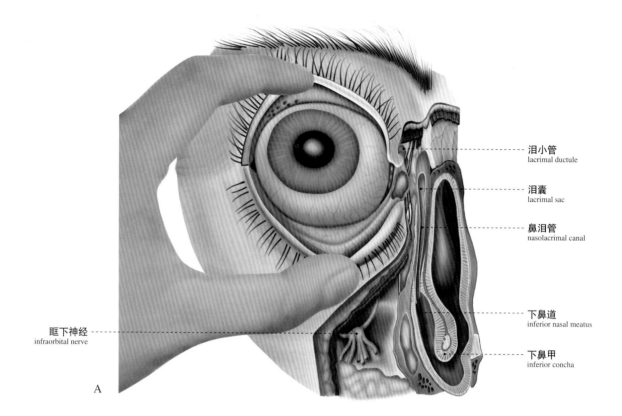

泪小管
lacrimal ductule

泪囊
lacrimal sac

鼻泪管
nasolacrimal canal

下鼻道
inferior nasal meatus

下鼻甲
inferior concha

眶下神经
infraorbital nerve

A

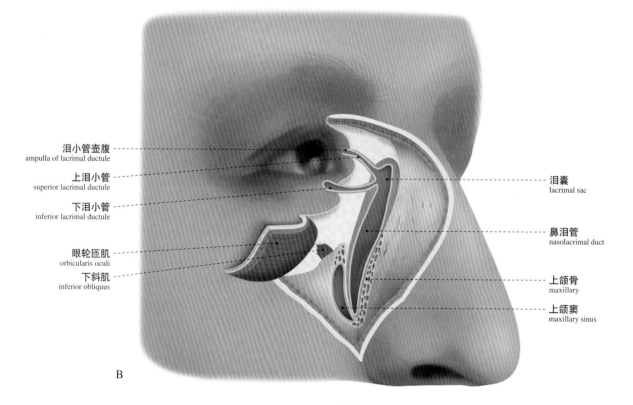

泪小管壶腹
ampulla of lacrimal ductule

上泪小管
superior lacrimal ductule

下泪小管
inferior lacrimal ductule

眼轮匝肌
orbicularis oculi

下斜肌
inferior obliquus

泪囊
lacrimal sac

鼻泪管
nasolacrimal duct

上颌骨
maxillary

上颌窦
maxillary sinus

B

337. 泪器
Lacrimal apparatus

A. 前面观；B. 前外侧面观

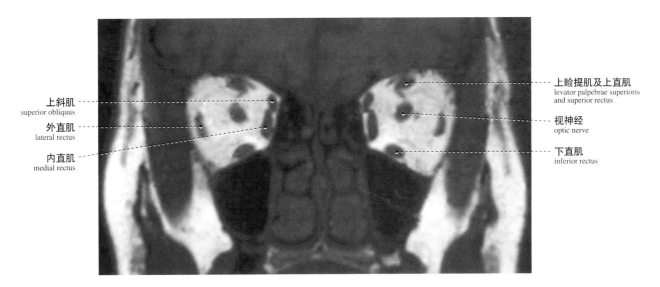

上睑提肌及上直肌
levator palpebrae superioris
and superior rectus

视神经
optic nerve

下直肌
inferior rectus

上斜肌
superior obliquus

外直肌
lateral rectus

内直肌
medial rectus

338. 眼磁共振成像 1

MRI of the eye 1

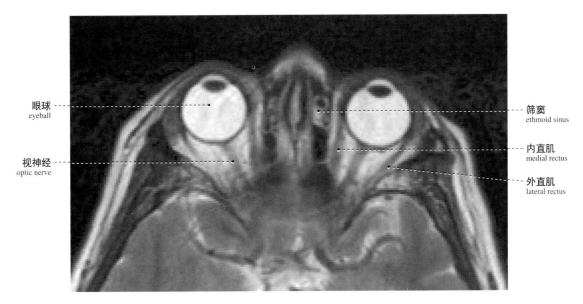

眼球
eyeball

视神经
optic nerve

筛窦
ethmoid sinus

内直肌
medial rectus

外直肌
lateral rectus

339. 眼磁共振成像 2

MRI of the eye 2

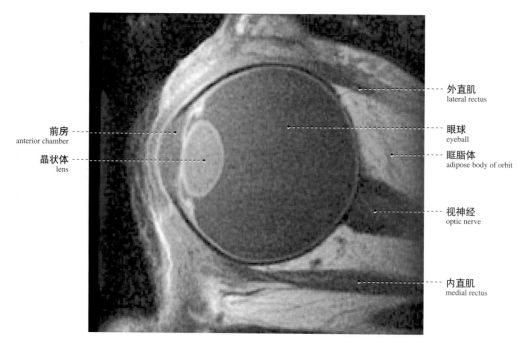

前房
anterior chamber

晶状体
lens

外直肌
lateral rectus

眼球
eyeball

眶脂体
adipose body of orbit

视神经
optic nerve

内直肌
medial rectus

340. 眼磁共振成像 3
MRI of the eye 3

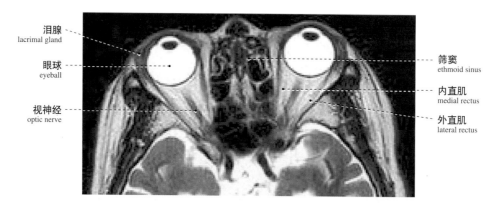

泪腺
lacrimal gland

眼球
eyeball

视神经
optic nerve

筛窦
ethmoid sinus

内直肌
medial rectus

外直肌
lateral rectus

341. 眼磁共振成像 4
MRI of the eye 4

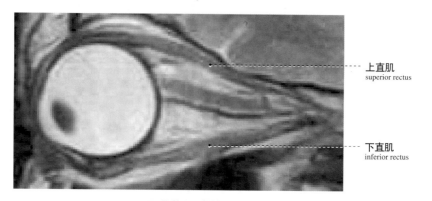

上直肌
superior rectus

下直肌
inferior rectus

342. 眼磁共振成像 5
MRI of the eye 5

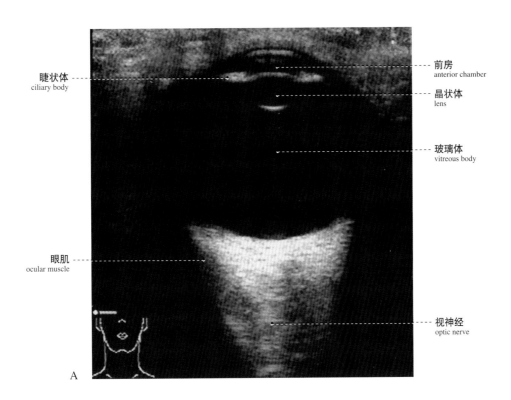

睫状体
ciliary body

前房
anterior chamber

晶状体
lens

玻璃体
vitreous body

眼肌
ocular muscle

视神经
optic nerve

A

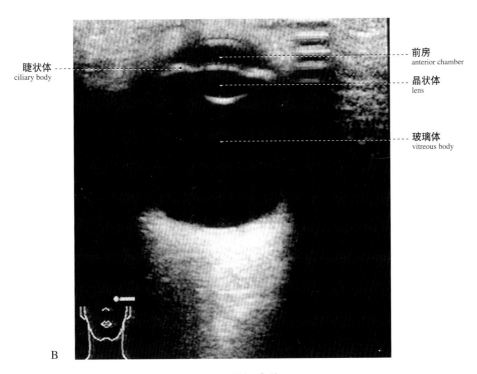

睫状体
ciliary body

前房
anterior chamber

晶状体
lens

玻璃体
vitreous body

B

343. 眼超声像

Ultrasound image of the eye

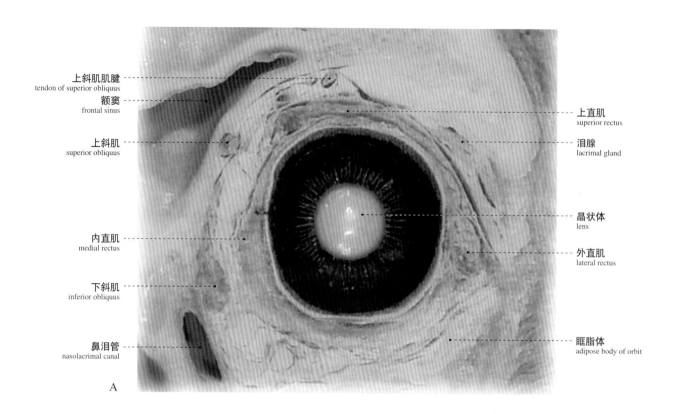

上斜肌肌腱
tendon of superior obliquus

额窦
frontal sinus

上斜肌
superior obliquus

内直肌
medial rectus

下斜肌
inferior obliquus

鼻泪管
nasolacrimal canal

上直肌
superior rectus

泪腺
lacrimal gland

晶状体
lens

外直肌
lateral rectus

眶脂体
adipose body of orbit

A

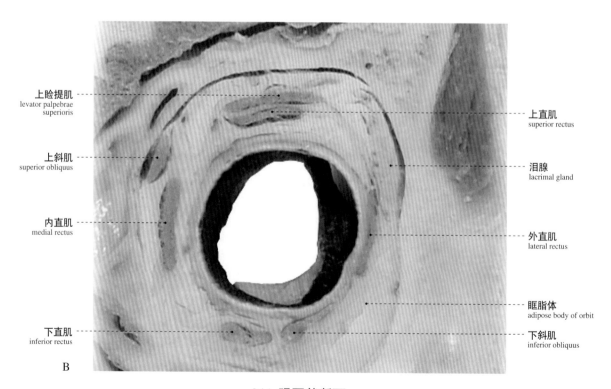

上睑提肌
levator palpebrae
superioris

上斜肌
superior obliquus

内直肌
medial rectus

下直肌
inferior rectus

上直肌
superior rectus

泪腺
lacrimal gland

外直肌
lateral rectus

眶脂体
adipose body of orbit

下斜肌
inferior obliquus

B

344. 眼冠状断面
Frontal section of the eye

角膜
cornea

眼球
eyeball

内直肌
medial rectus

视神经
optic nerve

眶脂体
adipose body of orbit

晶状体
lens

泪腺
lacrimal gland

巩膜
sclera

外直肌
lateral rectus

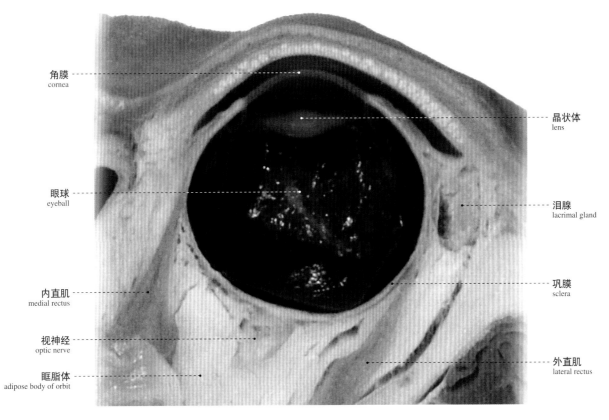

345. 眼水平断面
Horizontal section of the eye

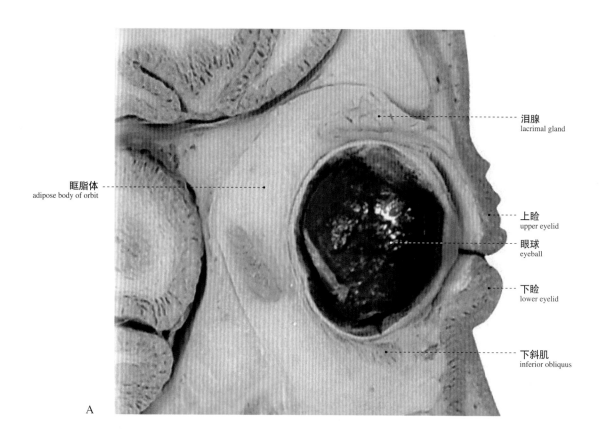

泪腺
lacrimal gland

眶脂体
adipose body of orbit

上睑
upper eyelid

眼球
eyeball

下睑
lower eyelid

下斜肌
inferior obliquus

A

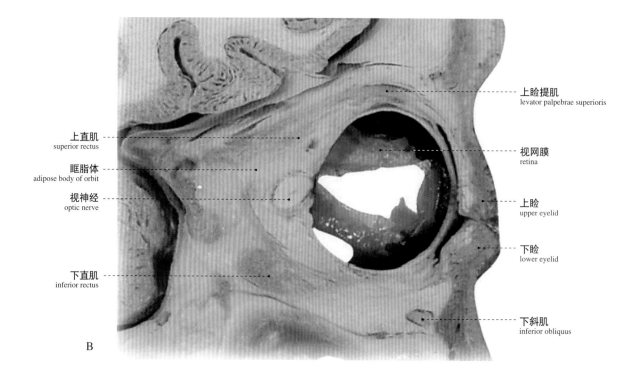

上睑提肌
levator palpebrae superioris

上直肌
superior rectus

眶脂体
adipose body of orbit

视神经
optic nerve

下直肌
inferior rectus

视网膜
retina

上睑
upper eyelid

下睑
lower eyelid

下斜肌
inferior obliquus

B

346. 眼矢状断面
Sagittal section of the eye

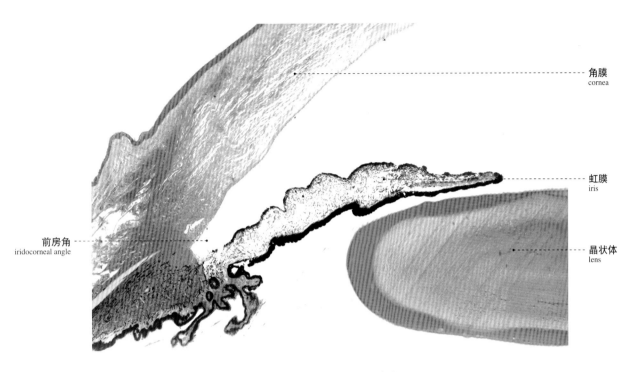

角膜
cornea

虹膜
iris

前房角
iridocorneal angle

晶状体
lens

347. 眼球前部（人眼球，HE 染色，×40）

Anterior portion of the eyeball (human eyeball, HE staining, ×40)

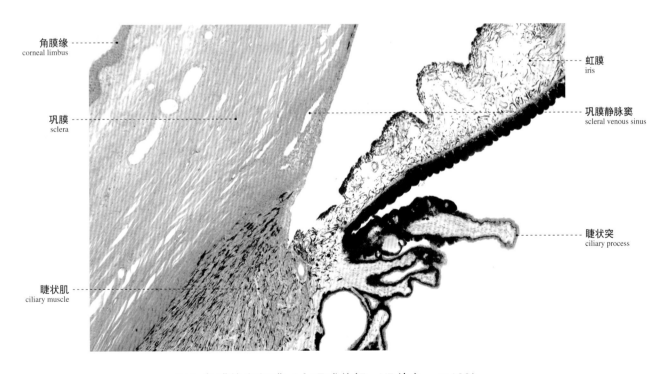

角膜缘
corneal limbus

虹膜
iris

巩膜
sclera

巩膜静脉窦
scleral venous sinus

睫状突
ciliary process

睫状肌
ciliary muscle

348. 角膜缘和虹膜（人眼球前部，HE 染色，×100）

Corneal limbus and iris (anterior portion of human eyeball, HE staining, ×100)

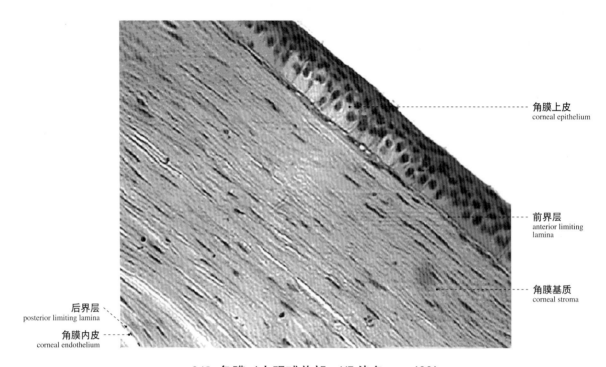

角膜上皮
corneal epithelium

前界层
anterior limiting lamina

角膜基质
corneal stroma

后界层
posterior limiting lamina

角膜内皮
corneal endothelium

349. 角膜（人眼球前部，HE 染色，×400）
Cornea (anterior portion of human eyeball, HE staining, ×400)

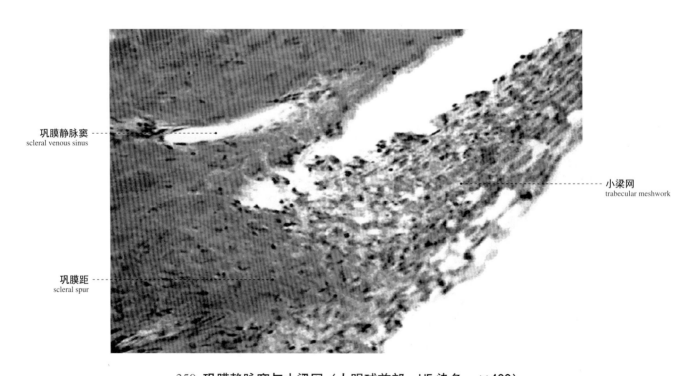

巩膜静脉窦
scleral venous sinus

小梁网
trabecular meshwork

巩膜距
scleral spur

350. 巩膜静脉窦与小梁网（人眼球前部，HE 染色，×400）
Scleral venous sinus and trabecular meshwork (anterior portion of human eyeball, HE staining, ×400)

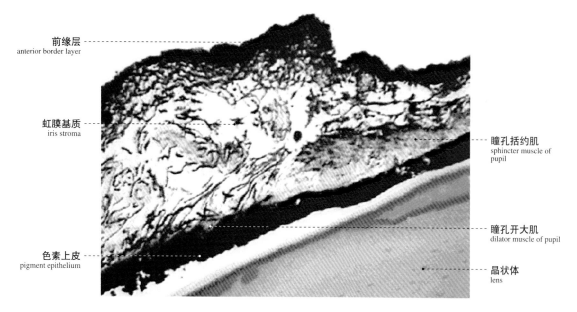

前缘层
anterior border layer

虹膜基质
iris stroma

瞳孔括约肌
sphincter muscle of pupil

瞳孔开大肌
dilator muscle of pupil

色素上皮
pigment epithelium

晶状体
lens

351. 虹膜（人眼球前部，HE 染色，×400）
Iris (anterior portion of human eyeball, HE staining, ×400)

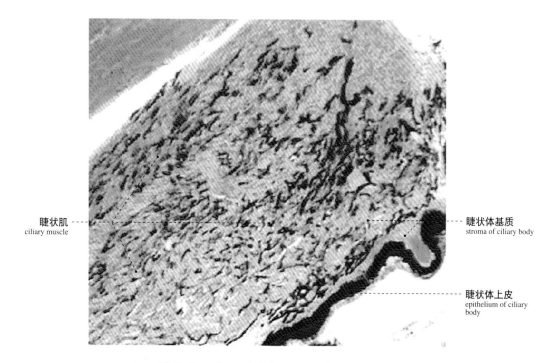

睫状肌
ciliary muscle

睫状体基质
stroma of ciliary body

睫状体上皮
epithelium of ciliary body

352. 睫状体（人眼球前部 1，HE 染色，×100）
Ciliary body (anterior portion of human eyeball 1, HE staining, ×100)

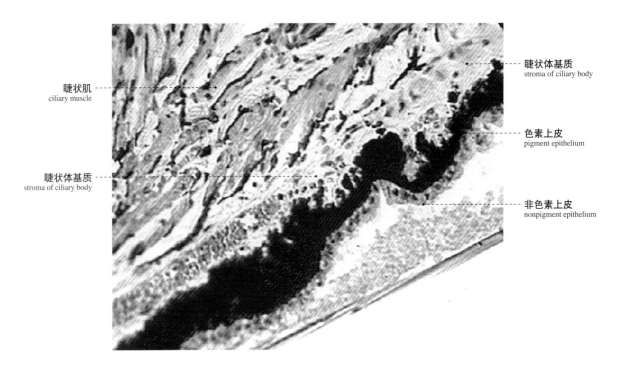

睫状肌
ciliary muscle

睫状体基质
stroma of ciliary body

睫状体基质
stroma of ciliary body

色素上皮
pigment epithelium

非色素上皮
nonpigment epithelium

353. 睫状体（人眼球前部 2，HE 染色，×400）
Ciliary body (anterior portion of human eyeball 2, HE staining, ×400)

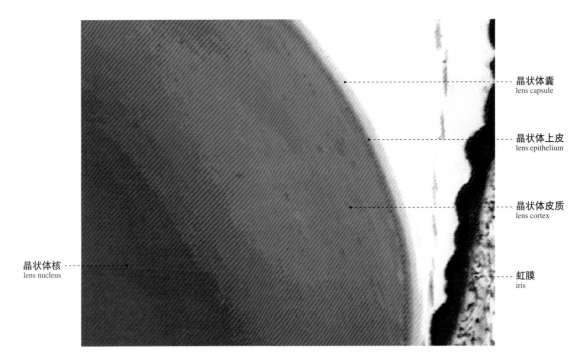

晶状体囊
lens capsule

晶状体上皮
lens epithelium

晶状体皮质
lens cortex

晶状体核
lens nucleus

虹膜
iris

354. 晶状体（人眼球前部，HE 染色，×400）
Lens (anterior portion of human eyeball, HE staining, ×400)

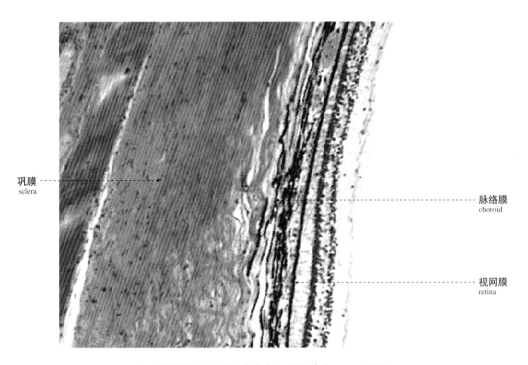

巩膜
sclera

脉络膜
choroid

视网膜
retina

355. 脉络膜（人眼球前部，HE 染色，×100）
Choroid (anterior portion of human eyeball, HE staining, ×100)

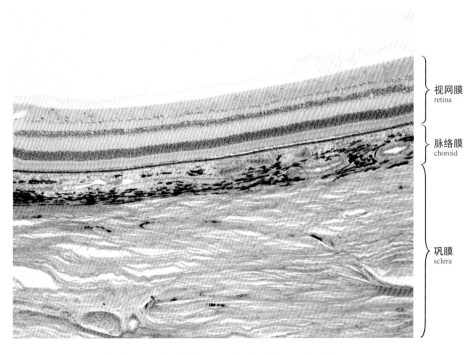

视网膜
retina

脉络膜
choroid

巩膜
sclera

356. 眼球后部（人眼球，HE 染色，×100）
Posterior portion of the eyeball (human eyeball, HE staining, ×100)

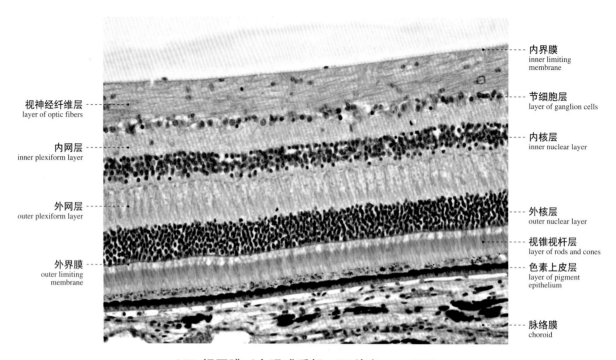

视神经纤维层
layer of optic fibers

内网层
inner plexiform layer

外网层
outer plexiform layer

外界膜
outer limiting
membrane

内界膜
inner limiting
membrane

节细胞层
layer of ganglion cells

内核层
inner nuclear layer

外核层
outer nuclear layer

视锥视杆层
layer of rods and cones

色素上皮层
layer of pigment
epithelium

脉络膜
choroid

357. 视网膜（人眼球后部，HE 染色，×400）
Retina (posterior portion of human eyeball, HE staining, ×400)

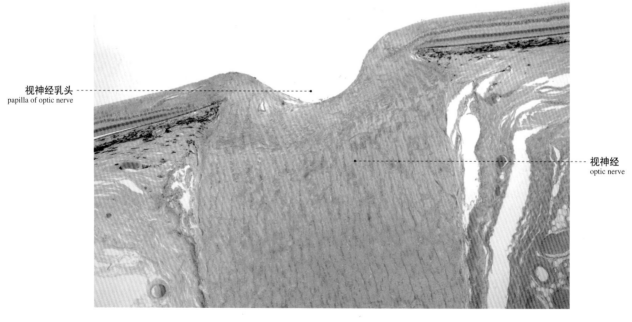

视神经乳头
papilla of optic nerve

视神经
optic nerve

358. 视神经乳头（人眼球后部，HE 染色，×40）
Papilla of optic nerve (posterior portion of human eyeball, HE staining, ×40)

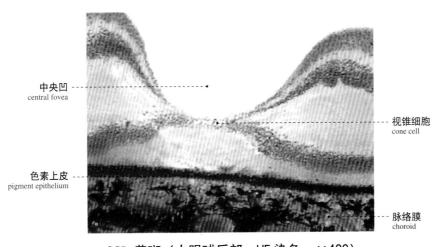

中央凹
central fovea

视锥细胞
cone cell

色素上皮
pigment epithelium

脉络膜
choroid

359. 黄斑（人眼球后部，HE 染色，×400）
Macula lutea (posterior portion of human eyeball, HE staining, ×400)

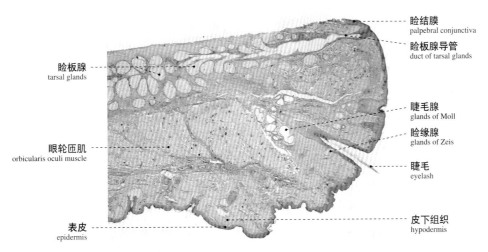

睑结膜
palpebral conjunctiva

睑板腺导管
duct of tarsal glands

睑板腺
tarsal glands

睫毛腺
glands of Moll

睑缘腺
glands of Zeis

眼轮匝肌
orbicularis oculi muscle

睫毛
eyelash

表皮
epidermis

皮下组织
hypodermis

360. 眼睑（人眼睑，HE 染色，×40）
Eyelid (human eyelids, HE staining, ×40)

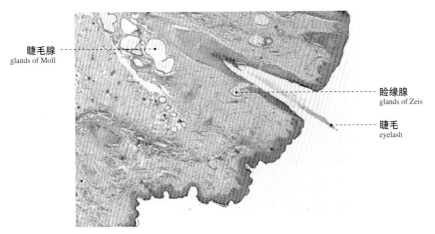

睫毛腺
glands of Moll

睑缘腺
glands of Zeis

睫毛
eyelash

361. 睑缘腺（Zeis 腺）与睫毛腺（Moll 腺）（人眼睑，HE 染色，×100）
Glands of Zeis and glands of Moll (human eyelids, HE staining, ×100)

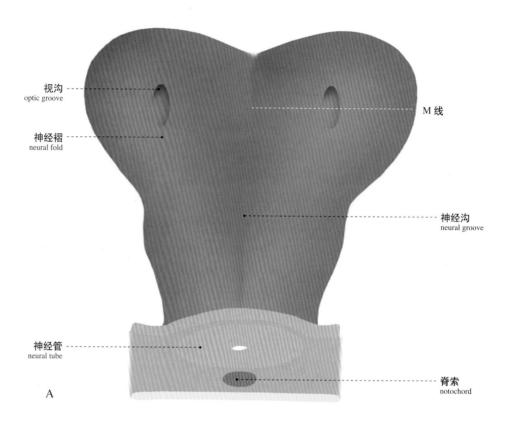

视沟
optic groove

M 线

神经褶
neural fold

神经沟
neural groove

神经管
neural tube

脊索
notochord

A

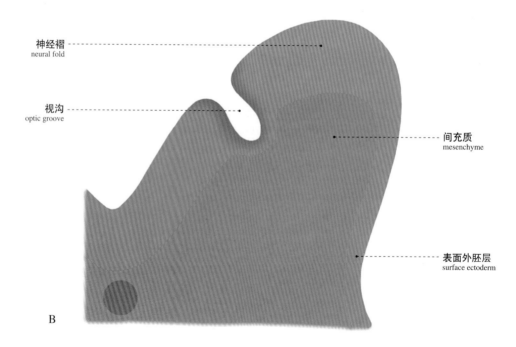

神经褶
neural fold

视沟
optic groove

间充质
mesenchyme

表面外胚层
surface ectoderm

B

362. 眼的发生（约 22 天）
Development of eyes (about 22 days)

A. 胚脑末端的背侧观，首先显示眼（视沟）的发生，此时神经褶没有融合形成前脑泡；B. 经视沟横切面（M 线）

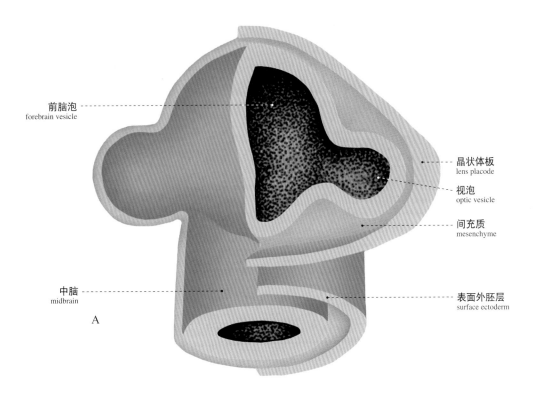

前脑泡
forebrain vesicle

晶状体板
lens placode

视泡
optic vesicle

间充质
mesenchyme

中脑
midbrain

表面外胚层
surface ectoderm

A

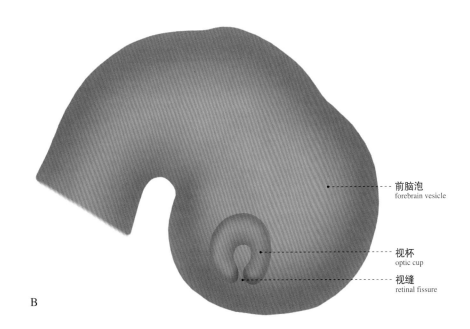

前脑泡
forebrain vesicle

视杯
optic cup

视缝
retinal fissure

B

363. 眼的发生（约 28 天、32 天）

Development of the eye (about 28 days, 32days)

A.示前脑泡（约 28 天）已形成，其表面外胚层下覆盖有一层间充质；B.胚（约 32 天）脑侧面观，示视杯的外部轮廓

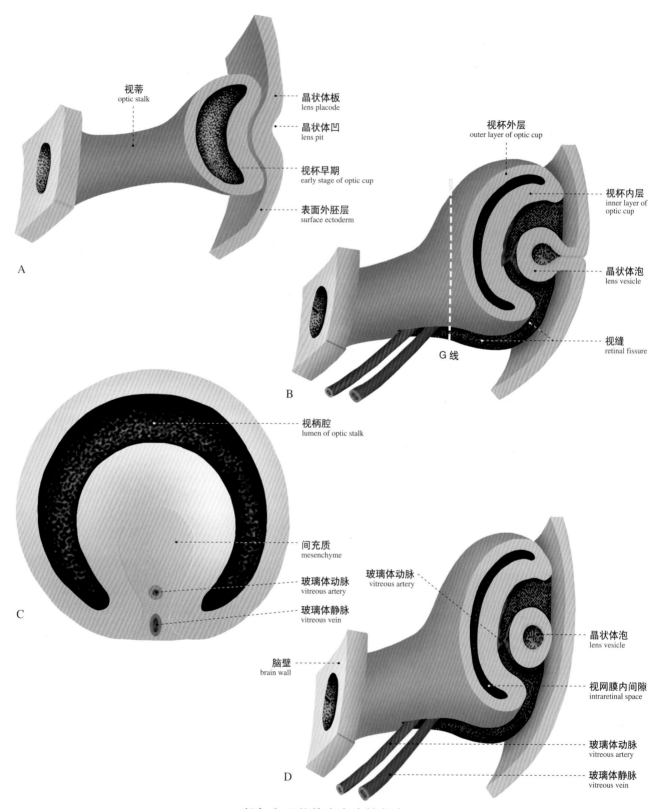

视蒂
optic stalk

晶状体板
lens placode

晶状体凹
lens pit

视杯早期
early stage of optic cup

表面外胚层
surface ectoderm

A

视杯外层
outer layer of optic cup

视杯内层
inner layer of optic cup

晶状体泡
lens vesicle

视缝
retinal fissure

G 线

B

视柄腔
lumen of optic stalk

间充质
mesenchyme

玻璃体动脉
vitreous artery

玻璃体静脉
vitreous vein

C

玻璃体动脉
vitreous artery

晶状体泡
lens vesicle

视网膜内间隙
intraretinal space

玻璃体动脉
vitreous artery

玻璃体静脉
vitreous vein

脑壁
brain wall

D

364. 视杯和晶状体泡发生的各个时期

Successive stages in the development of the optic cup and lens vesicle

A、B、D. 示视杯和晶状体泡发生各个时期, 眼发生的图解切面; C. 经过视柄的横切面 (G 线), 示视缝及其内容物, 视缝向边缘生长并融合,
最后生长成完整的视杯, 在视杯内包有视神经、视网膜中央动脉和静脉

第七章

耳

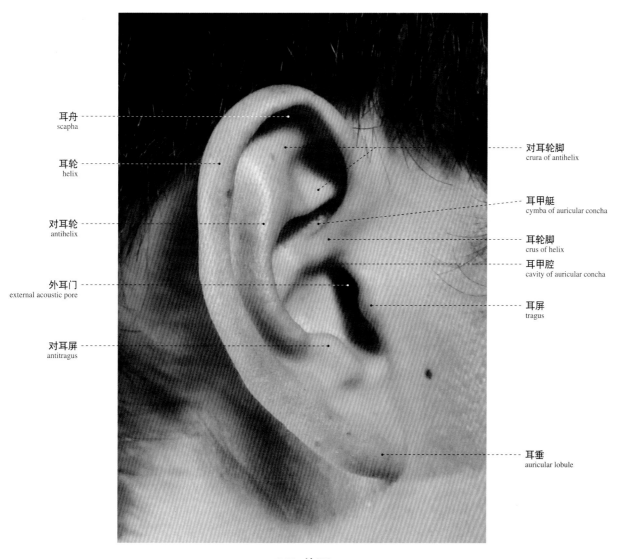

耳舟
scapha

耳轮
helix

对耳轮
antihelix

外耳门
external acoustic pore

对耳屏
antitragus

对耳轮脚
crura of antihelix

耳甲艇
cymba of auricular concha

耳轮脚
crus of helix

耳甲腔
cavity of auricular concha

耳屏
tragus

耳垂
auricular lobule

365. 外耳
External ear

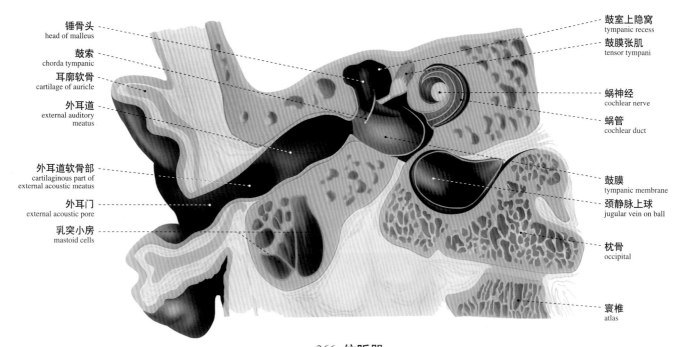

锤骨头
head of malleus

鼓索
chorda tympanic

耳廓软骨
cartilage of auricle

外耳道
external auditory
meatus

外耳道软骨部
cartilaginous part of
external acoustic meatus

外耳门
external acoustic pore

乳突小房
mastoid cells

鼓室上隐窝
tympanic recess

鼓膜张肌
tensor tympani

蜗神经
cochlear nerve

蜗管
cochlear duct

鼓膜
tympanic membrane

颈静脉上球
jugular vein on ball

枕骨
occipital

寰椎
atlas

366. 位听器
Organum vestibulocochleare

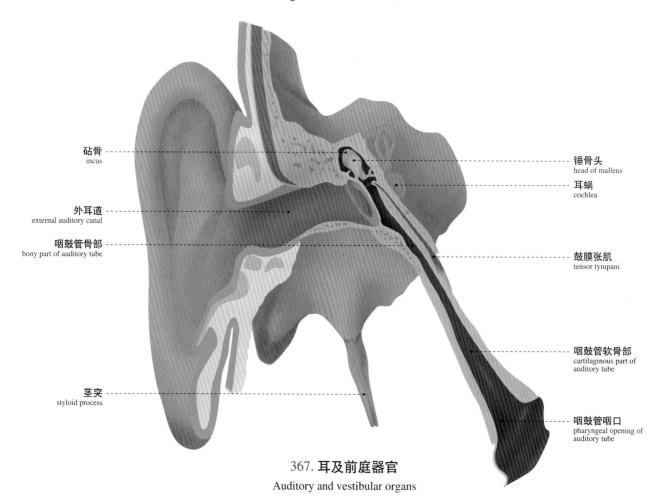

砧骨
incus

外耳道
external auditory canal

咽鼓管骨部
bony part of auditory tube

茎突
styloid process

锤骨头
head of malleus

耳蜗
cochlea

鼓膜张肌
tensor tympani

咽鼓管软骨部
cartilaginous part of
auditory tube

咽鼓管咽口
pharyngeal opening of
auditory tube

367. 耳及前庭器官
Auditory and vestibular organs

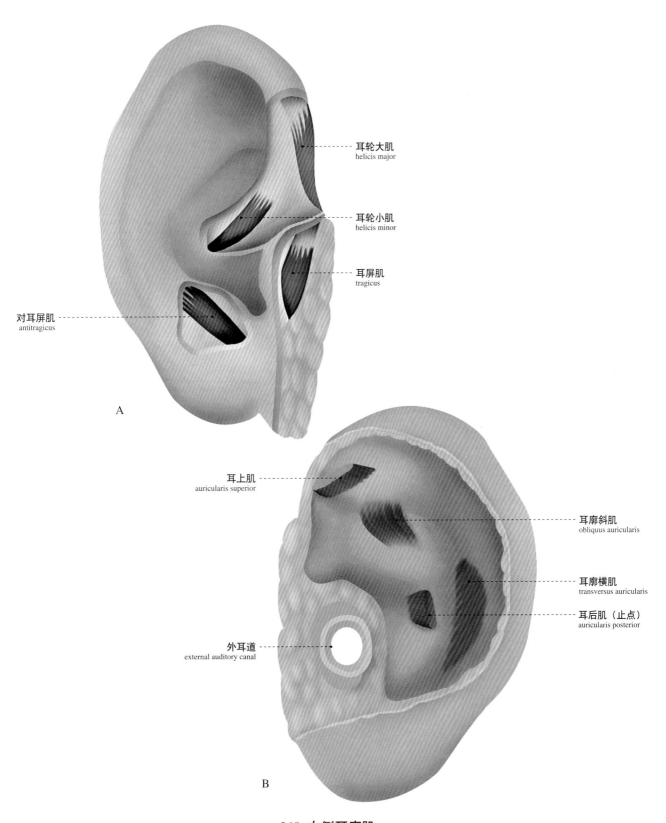

耳轮大肌
helicis major

耳轮小肌
helicis minor

耳屏肌
tragicus

对耳屏肌
antitragicus

A

耳上肌
auricularis superior

耳廓斜肌
obliquus auricularis

耳廓横肌
transversus auricularis

耳后肌（止点）
auricularis posterior

外耳道
external auditory canal

B

368. 右侧耳廓肌

Muscles of the right auricle

A. 前面观；B. 后面观

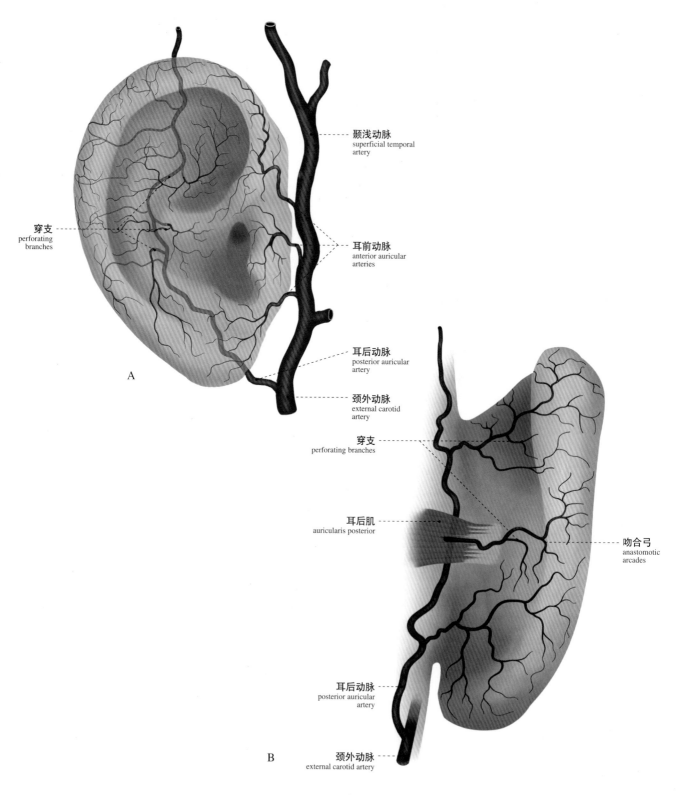

颞浅动脉
superficial temporal artery

穿支
perforating branches

耳前动脉
anterior auricular arteries

耳后动脉
posterior auricular artery

颈外动脉
external carotid artery

A

穿支
perforating branches

耳后肌
auricularis posterior

吻合弓
anastomotic arcades

耳后动脉
posterior auricular artery

颈外动脉
external carotid artery

B

369. 耳廓动脉

Arteries of the auricle

A. 外侧面观；B. 后面观

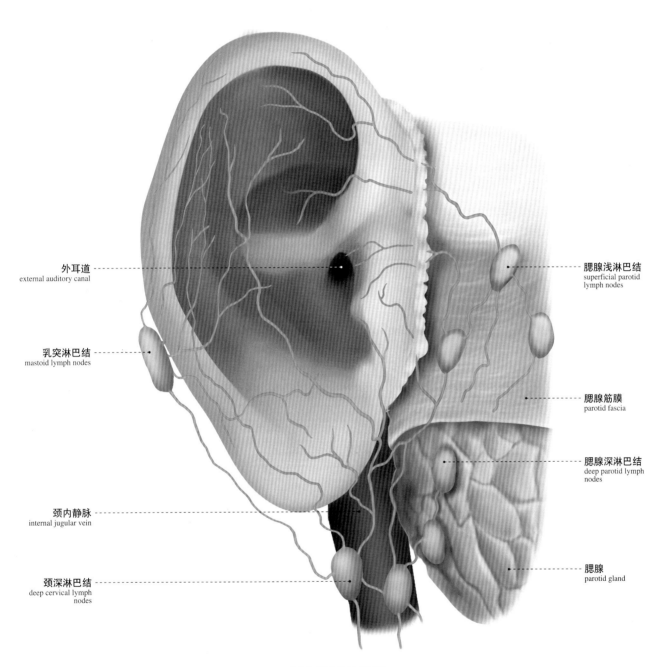

外耳道
external auditory canal

乳突淋巴结
mastoid lymph nodes

颈内静脉
internal jugular vein

颈深淋巴结
deep cervical lymph nodes

腮腺浅淋巴结
superficial parotid lymph nodes

腮腺筋膜
parotid fascia

腮腺深淋巴结
deep parotid lymph nodes

腮腺
parotid gland

370. 耳廓的淋巴
Lymph of the auricle

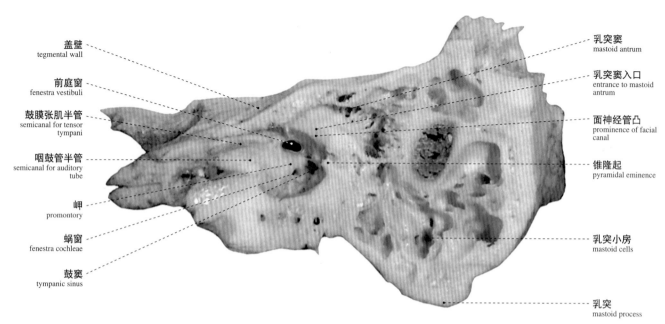

盖壁
tegmental wall

前庭窗
fenestra vestibuli

鼓膜张肌半管
semicanal for tensor tympani

咽鼓管半管
semicanal for auditory tube

岬
promontory

蜗窗
fenestra cochleae

鼓窦
tympanic sinus

乳突窦
mastoid antrum

乳突窦入口
entrance to mastoid antrum

面神经管凸
prominence of facial canal

锥隆起
pyramidal eminence

乳突小房
mastoid cells

乳突
mastoid process

371. 鼓室内侧壁
Medial wall of the tympanic cavity

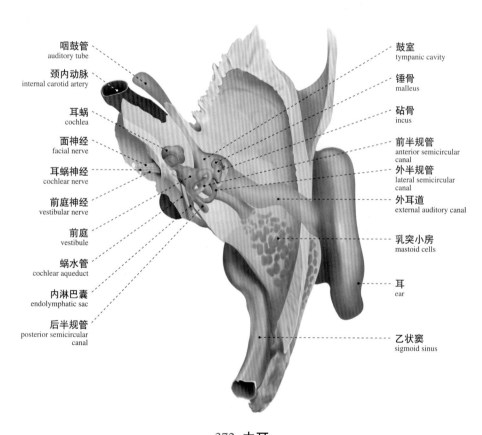

咽鼓管
auditory tube

颈内动脉
internal carotid artery

耳蜗
cochlea

面神经
facial nerve

耳蜗神经
cochlear nerve

前庭神经
vestibular nerve

前庭
vestibule

蜗水管
cochlear aqueduct

内淋巴囊
endolymphatic sac

后半规管
posterior semicircular canal

鼓室
tympanic cavity

锤骨
malleus

砧骨
incus

前半规管
anterior semicircular canal

外半规管
lateral semicircular canal

外耳道
external auditory canal

乳突小房
mastoid cells

耳
ear

乙状窦
sigmoid sinus

372. 中耳
Middle ear

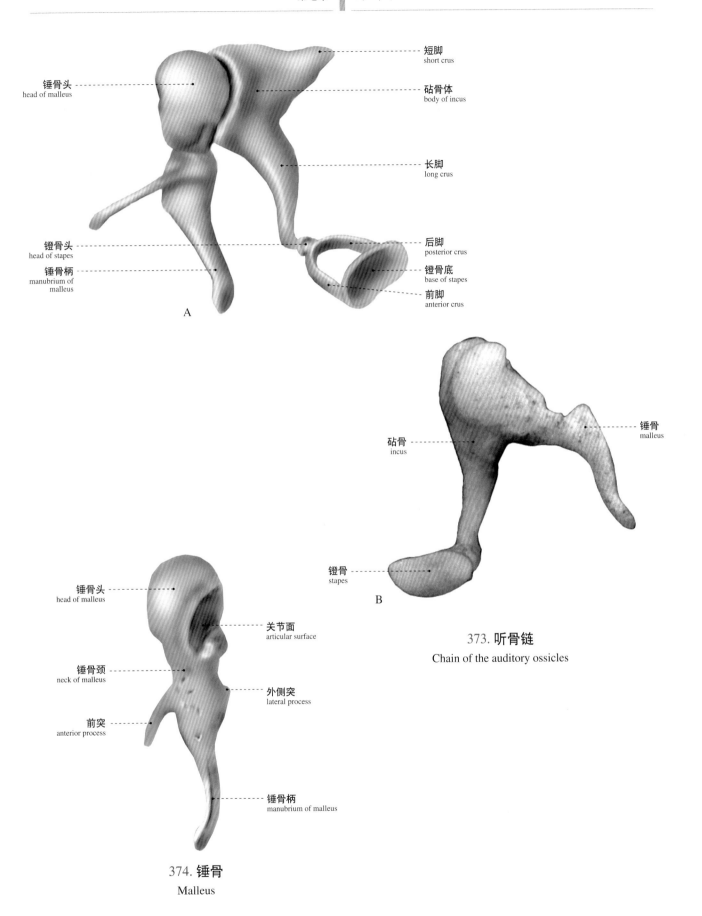

短脚
short crus

砧骨体
body of incus

锤骨头
head of malleus

长脚
long crus

镫骨头
head of stapes

后脚
posterior crus

镫骨底
base of stapes

锤骨柄
manubrium of malleus

前脚
anterior crus

A

砧骨
incus

锤骨
malleus

镫骨
stapes

B

373. 听骨链
Chain of the auditory ossicles

锤骨头
head of malleus

关节面
articular surface

锤骨颈
neck of malleus

外侧突
lateral process

前突
anterior process

锤骨柄
manubrium of malleus

374. 锤骨
Malleus

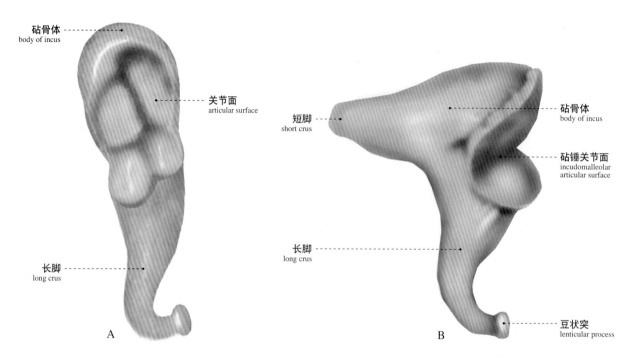

砧骨体
body of incus

关节面
articular surface

长脚
long crus

A

短脚
short crus

砧骨体
body of incus

砧锤关节面
incudomalleolar
articular surface

长脚
long crus

豆状突
lenticular process

B

375. 砧骨
Incus

A. 前面观；B. 内侧面观

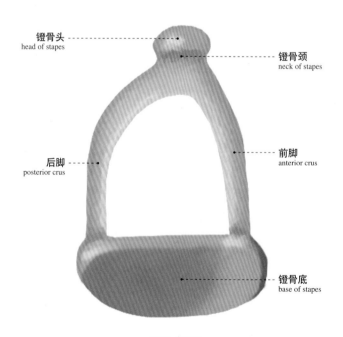

镫骨头
head of stapes

镫骨颈
neck of stapes

后脚
posterior crus

前脚
anterior crus

镫骨底
base of stapes

376. 镫骨
Stapes

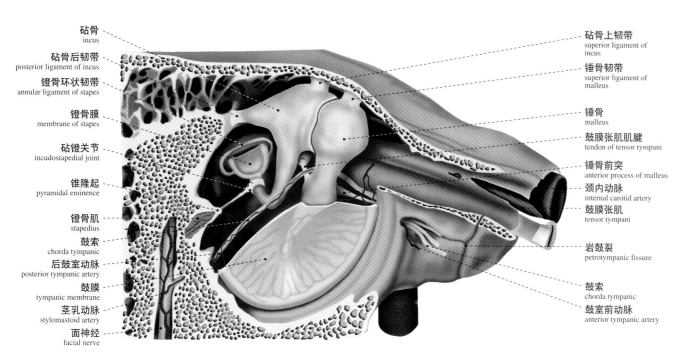

砧骨
incus

砧骨后韧带
posterior ligament of incus

镫骨环状韧带
annular ligament of stapes

镫骨膜
membrane of stapes

砧镫关节
incudostapedial joint

锥隆起
pyramidal eminence

镫骨肌
stapedius

鼓索
chorda tympanic

后鼓室动脉
posterior tympanic artery

鼓膜
tympanic membrane

茎乳动脉
stylomastoid artery

面神经
facial nerve

砧骨上韧带
superior ligament of incus

锤骨韧带
superior ligament of malleus

锤骨
malleus

鼓膜张肌肌腱
tendon of tensor tympani

锤骨前突
anterior process of malleus

颈内动脉
internal carotid artery

鼓膜张肌
tensor tympani

岩鼓裂
petrotympanic fissure

鼓索
chorda tympanic

鼓室前动脉
anterior tympanic artery

377. 鼓室听小骨链
Ossicular chain in the tympanic cavity

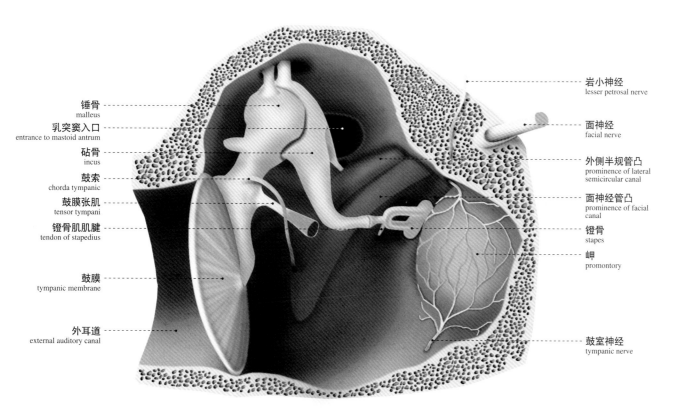

锤骨
malleus

乳突窦入口
entrance to mastoid antrum

砧骨
incus

鼓索
chorda tympanic

鼓膜张肌
tensor tympani

镫骨肌肌腱
tendon of stapedius

鼓膜
tympanic membrane

外耳道
external auditory canal

岩小神经
lesser petrosal nerve

面神经
facial nerve

外侧半规管凸
prominence of lateral semicircular canal

面神经管凸
prominence of facial canal

镫骨
stapes

岬
promontory

鼓室神经
tympanic nerve

378. 鼓室壁
Walls of the tympanic cavity

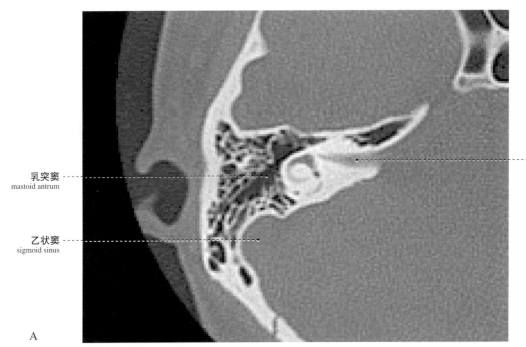

乳突窦
mastoid antrum

乙状窦
sigmoid sinus

内耳道
internal acoustic meatus

A

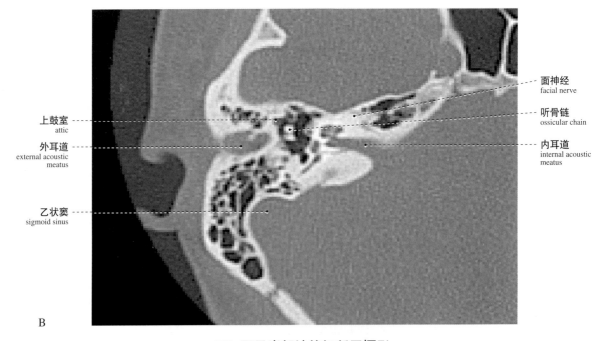

上鼓室
attic

外耳道
external acoustic meatus

乙状窦
sigmoid sinus

面神经
facial nerve

听骨链
ossicular chain

内耳道
internal acoustic meatus

B

379. 颞骨岩部计算机断层摄影
CT of the petrous
A. 冠状位；B. 轴位

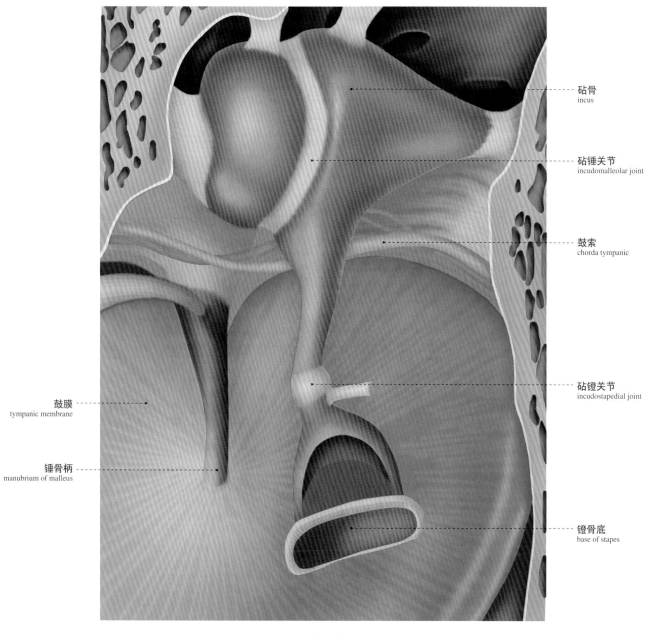

砧骨
incus

砧锤关节
incudomalleolar joint

鼓索
chorda tympanic

砧镫关节
incudostapedial joint

鼓膜
tympanic membrane

锤骨柄
manubrium of malleus

镫骨底
base of stapes

380. 右侧听小骨的关节和韧带（上内侧面观）
Joints and ligaments of the right ossicular (superior medial aspect)

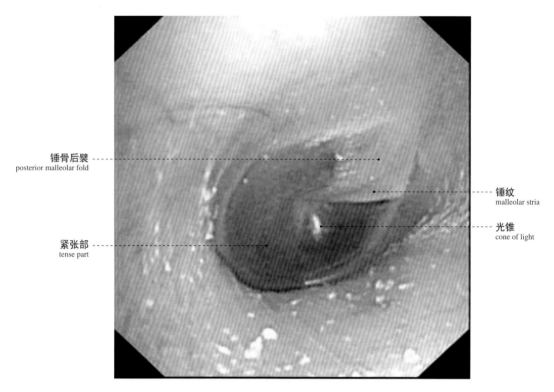

锤骨后襞
posterior malleolar fold

紧张部
tense part

锤纹
malleolar stria

光锥
cone of light

381. 右侧鼓膜
Right tympanic membrane

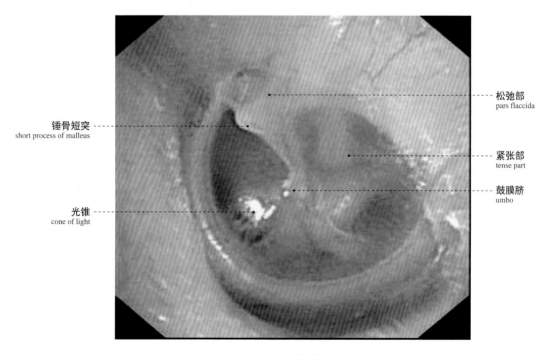

锤骨短突
short process of malleus

光锥
cone of light

松弛部
pars flaccida

紧张部
tense part

鼓膜脐
umbo

382. 左侧鼓膜
Left tympanic membrane

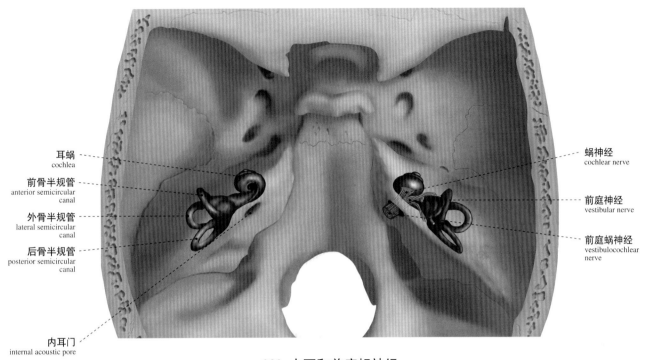

耳蜗
cochlea

前骨半规管
anterior semicircular
canal

外骨半规管
lateral semicircular
canal

后骨半规管
posterior semicircular
canal

内耳门
internal acoustic pore

蜗神经
cochlear nerve

前庭神经
vestibular nerve

前庭蜗神经
vestibulocochlear
nerve

383. 内耳和前庭蜗神经
Internal ear and the vestibulocochlear nerve

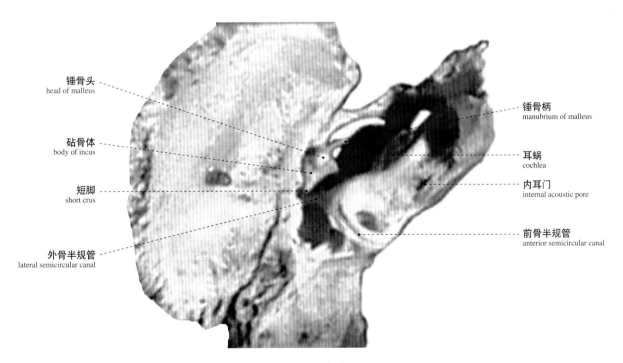

锤骨头
head of malleus

砧骨体
body of incus

短脚
short crus

外骨半规管
lateral semicircular canal

锤骨柄
manubrium of malleus

耳蜗
cochlea

内耳门
internal acoustic pore

前骨半规管
anterior semicircular canal

384. 骨迷路
Bony labyrinth

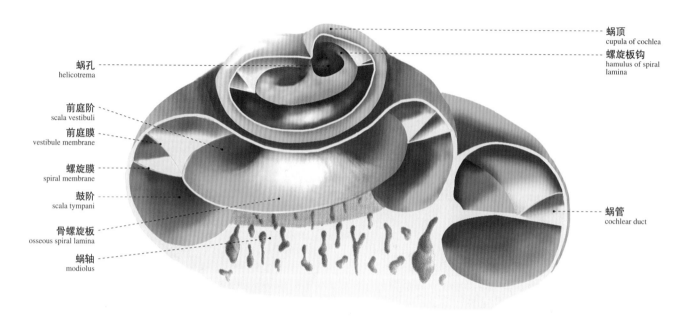

蜗顶
cupula of cochlea

螺旋板钩
hamulus of spiral lamina

蜗孔
helicotrema

前庭阶
scala vestibuli

前庭膜
vestibule membrane

螺旋膜
spiral membrane

鼓阶
scala tympani

骨螺旋板
osseous spiral lamina

蜗轴
modiolus

蜗管
cochlear duct

385. 耳蜗切面
Section of the cochlea

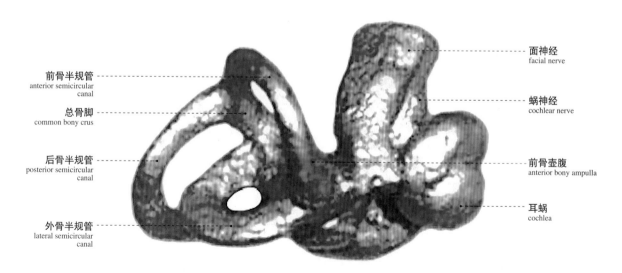

前骨半规管
anterior semicircular canal

总骨脚
common bony crus

后骨半规管
posterior semicircular canal

外骨半规管
lateral semicircular canal

面神经
facial nerve

蜗神经
cochlear nerve

前骨壶腹
anterior bony ampulla

耳蜗
cochlea

386. 骨迷路铸型
Cast of the bony labyrinth

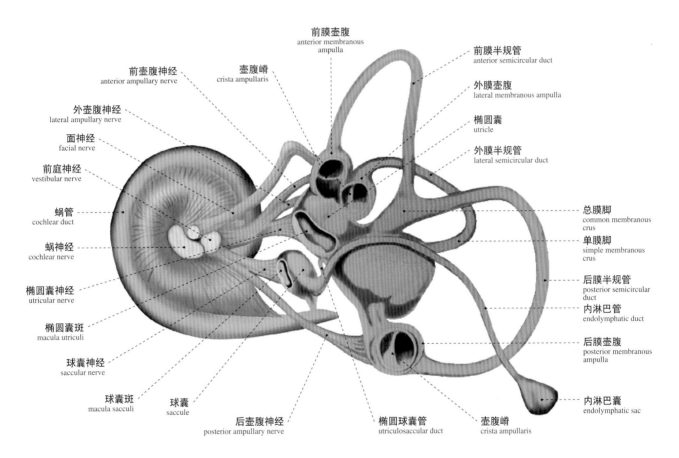

前膜壶腹
anterior membranous ampulla

前壶腹神经
anterior ampullary nerve

壶腹嵴
crista ampullaris

外壶腹神经
lateral ampullary nerve

面神经
facial nerve

前庭神经
vestibular nerve

蜗管
cochlear duct

蜗神经
cochlear nerve

椭圆囊神经
utricular nerve

椭圆囊斑
macula utriculi

球囊神经
saccular nerve

球囊斑
macula sacculi

球囊
saccule

后壶腹神经
posterior ampullary nerve

椭圆球囊管
utriculosaccular duct

壶腹嵴
crista ampullaris

前膜半规管
anterior semicircular duct

外膜壶腹
lateral membranous ampulla

椭圆囊
utricle

外膜半规管
lateral semicircular duct

总膜脚
common membranous crus

单膜脚
simple membranous crus

后膜半规管
posterior semicircular duct

内淋巴管
endolymphatic duct

后膜壶腹
posterior membranous ampulla

内淋巴囊
endolymphatic sac

387. 膜迷路
Membranous labyrinth

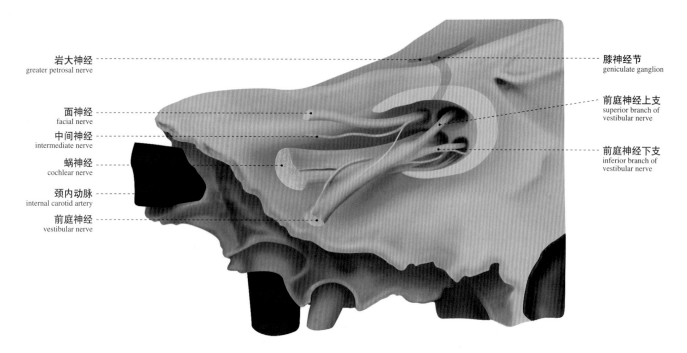

岩大神经
greater petrosal nerve

面神经
facial nerve

中间神经
intermediate nerve

蜗神经
cochlear nerve

颈内动脉
internal carotid artery

前庭神经
vestibular nerve

膝神经节
geniculate ganglion

前庭神经上支
superior branch of vestibular nerve

前庭神经下支
inferior branch of vestibular nerve

388. 通过内耳道的脑神经
Cranial nerves through the internal acoustic meatus

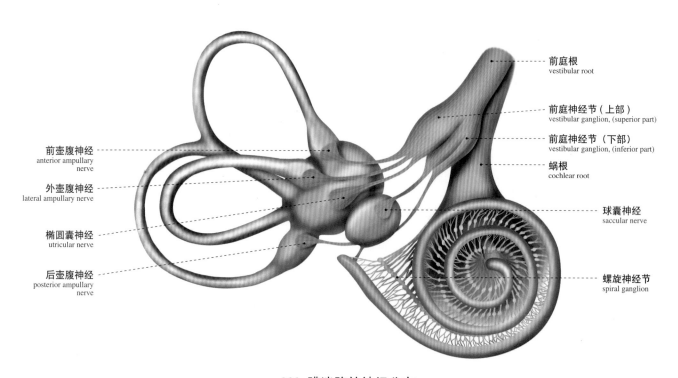

前壶腹神经
anterior ampullary nerve

外壶腹神经
lateral ampullary nerve

椭圆囊神经
utricular nerve

后壶腹神经
posterior ampullary nerve

前庭根
vestibular root

前庭神经节（上部）
vestibular ganglion, (superior part)

前庭神经节（下部）
vestibular ganglion, (inferior part)

蜗根
cochlear root

球囊神经
saccular nerve

螺旋神经节
spiral ganglion

389. 膜迷路的神经分布
Innervation of the membranous labyrinth

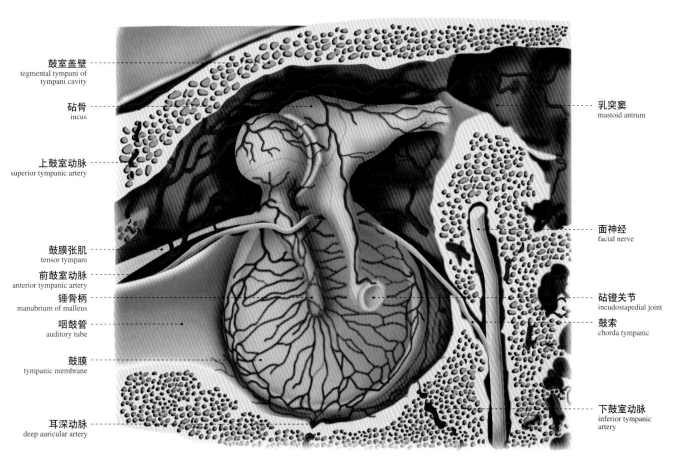

鼓室盖壁
tegmental tympani of
tympani cavity

砧骨
incus

上鼓室动脉
superior tympanic artery

鼓膜张肌
tensor tympani

前鼓室动脉
anterior tympanic artery

锤骨柄
manubrium of malleus

咽鼓管
auditory tube

鼓膜
tympanic membrane

耳深动脉
deep auricular artery

乳突窦
mastoid antrum

面神经
facial nerve

砧镫关节
incudostapedial joint

鼓索
chorda tympanic

下鼓室动脉
inferior tympanic
artery

390. 听小骨及鼓膜的动脉
Arteries of the auditory ossicles and the tympanic membrane

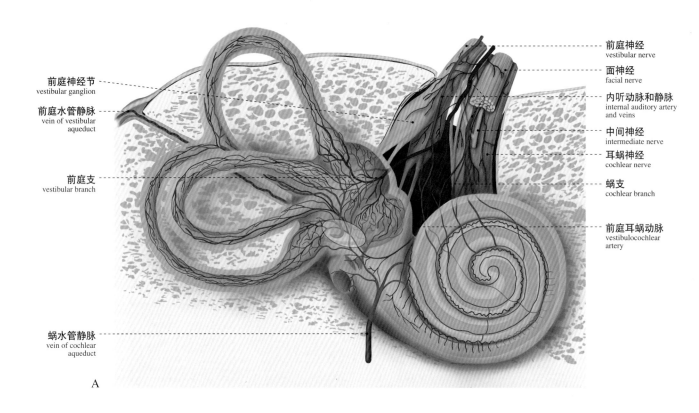

前庭神经节
vestibular ganglion

前庭水管静脉
vein of vestibular
aqueduct

前庭支
vestibular branch

蜗水管静脉
vein of cochlear
aqueduct

前庭神经
vestibular nerve

面神经
facial nerve

内听动脉和静脉
internal auditory artery
and veins

中间神经
intermediate nerve

耳蜗神经
cochlear nerve

蜗支
cochlear branch

前庭耳蜗动脉
vestibulocochlear
artery

A

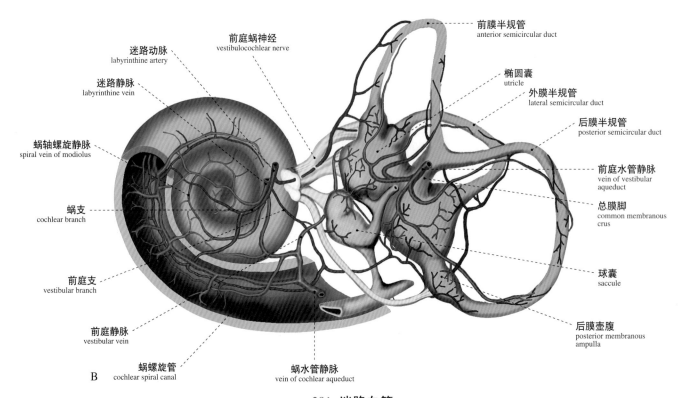

迷路动脉
labyrinthine artery

迷路静脉
labyrinthine vein

蜗轴螺旋静脉
spiral vein of modiolus

蜗支
cochlear branch

前庭支
vestibular branch

前庭静脉
vestibular vein

蜗螺旋管
cochlear spiral canal

前庭蜗神经
vestibulocochlear nerve

蜗水管静脉
vein of cochlear aqueduct

前膜半规管
anterior semicircular duct

椭圆囊
utricle

外膜半规管
lateral semicircular duct

后膜半规管
posterior semicircular duct

前庭水管静脉
vein of vestibular
aqueduct

总膜脚
common membranous
crus

球囊
saccule

后膜壶腹
posterior membranous
ampulla

B

391. 迷路血管
Blood vessels of the labyrinth

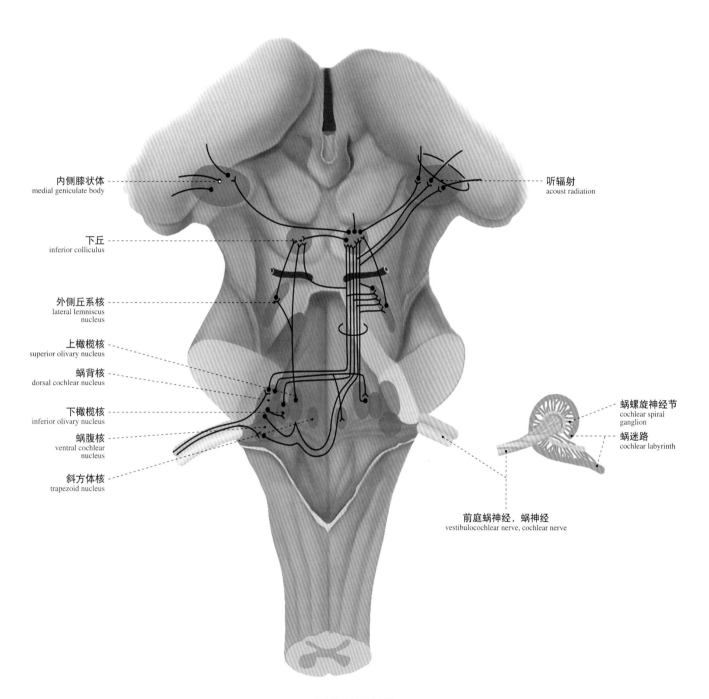

内侧膝状体
medial geniculate body

听辐射
acoust radiation

下丘
inferior colliculus

外侧丘系核
lateral lemniscus
nucleus

上橄榄核
superior olivary nucleus

蜗背核
dorsal cochlear nucleus

下橄榄核
inferior olivary nucleus

蜗腹核
ventral cochlear
nucleus

斜方体核
trapezoid nucleus

蜗螺旋神经节
cochlear spiral
ganglion

蜗迷路
cochlear labyrinth

前庭蜗神经，蜗神经
vestibulocochlear nerve, cochlear nerve

392. 听觉传导通路 1
Auditory pathway 1

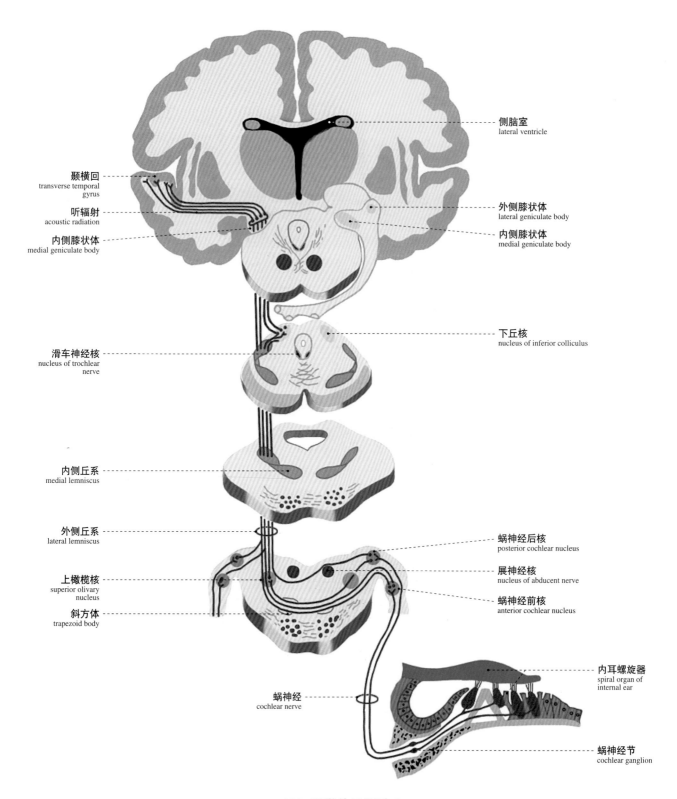

颞横回
transverse temporal gyrus

听辐射
acoustic radiation

内侧膝状体
medial geniculate body

滑车神经核
nucleus of trochlear nerve

内侧丘系
medial lemniscus

外侧丘系
lateral lemniscus

上橄榄核
superior olivary nucleus

斜方体
trapezoid body

蜗神经
cochlear nerve

侧脑室
lateral ventricle

外侧膝状体
lateral geniculate body

内侧膝状体
medial geniculate body

下丘核
nucleus of inferior colliculus

蜗神经后核
posterior cochlear nucleus

展神经核
nucleus of abducent nerve

蜗神经前核
anterior cochlear nucleus

内耳螺旋器
spiral organ of internal ear

蜗神经节
cochlear ganglion

393. 听觉传导通路 2
Auditory pathway 2

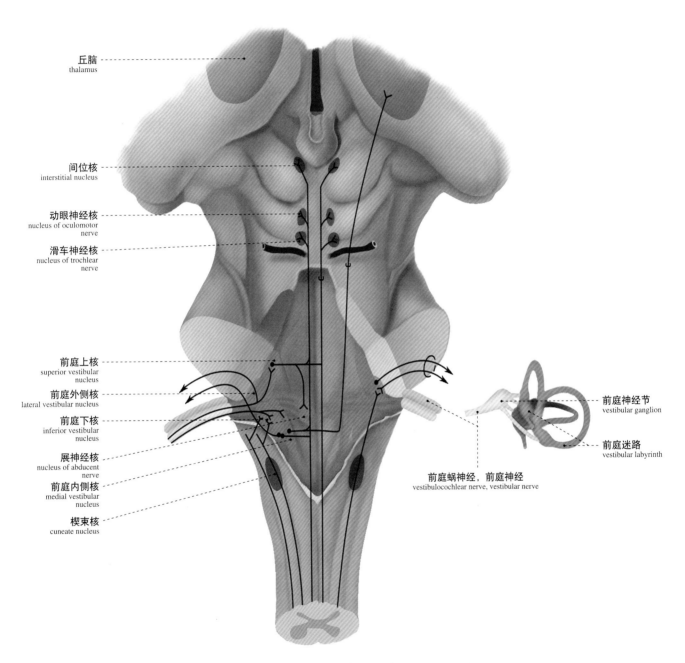

丘脑
thalamus

间位核
interstitial nucleus

动眼神经核
nucleus of oculomotor
nerve

滑车神经核
nucleus of trochlear
nerve

前庭上核
superior vestibular
nucleus

前庭外侧核
lateral vestibular nucleus

前庭下核
inferior vestibular
nucleus

展神经核
nucleus of abducent
nerve

前庭内侧核
medial vestibular
nucleus

楔束核
cuneate nucleus

前庭神经节
vestibular ganglion

前庭迷路
vestibular labyrinth

前庭蜗神经，前庭神经
vestibulocochlear nerve, vestibular nerve

394. 平衡觉传导通路
Pathway of equilibrium sense

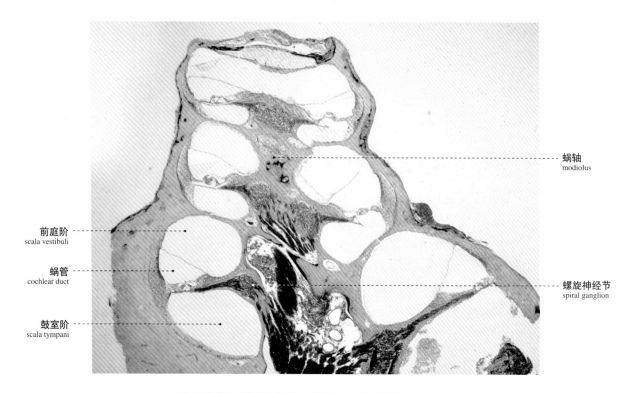

前庭阶
scala vestibuli

蜗管
cochlear duct

鼓室阶
scala tympani

蜗轴
modiolus

螺旋神经节
spiral ganglion

395. 耳蜗（豚鼠内耳，垂直切面，镀银，×40）
Cochlea (inner ear of the guinea pig, midmodiolar section, silver staining, ×40)

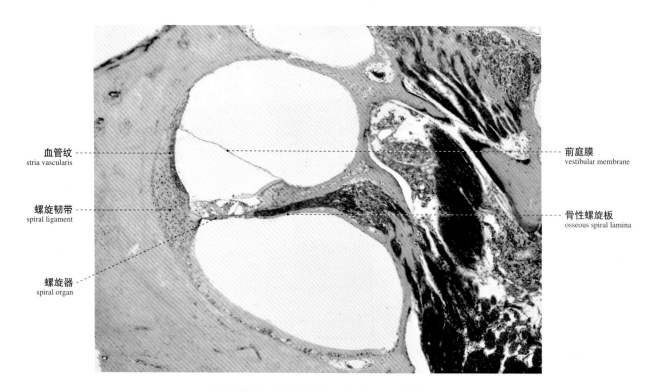

血管纹
stria vascularis

螺旋韧带
spiral ligament

螺旋器
spiral organ

前庭膜
vestibular membrane

骨性螺旋板
osseous spiral lamina

396. 蜗管（豚鼠内耳，镀银，×100）
Cochlear duct (inner ear of the guinea pig, silver staining, ×100)

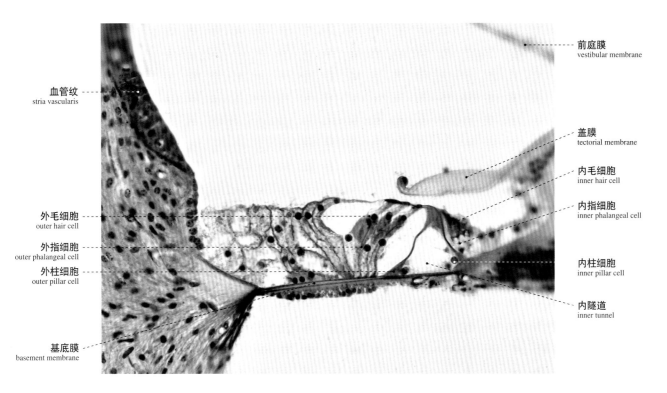

血管纹
stria vascularis

外毛细胞
outer hair cell

外指细胞
outer phalangeal cell

外柱细胞
outer pillar cell

基底膜
basement membrane

前庭膜
vestibular membrane

盖膜
tectorial membrane

内毛细胞
inner hair cell

内指细胞
inner phalangeal cell

内柱细胞
inner pillar cell

内隧道
inner tunnel

397. 螺旋器（豚鼠内耳，镀银，×400）

Spiral organ (inner ear of the guinea pig, silver staining, ×400)

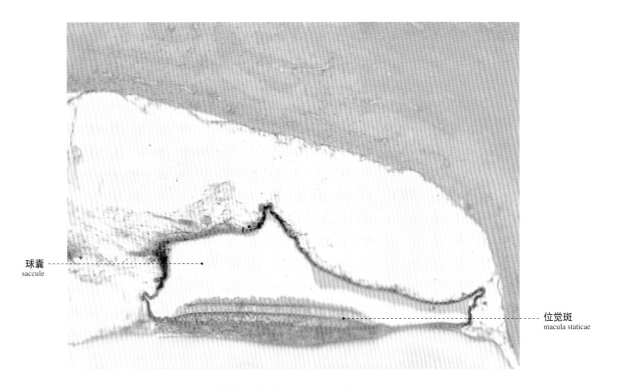

球囊
saccule

位觉斑
macula staticae

398. 位觉斑（豚鼠内耳，HE 染色，×40）

Macula staticae (inner ear of the guinea pig, HE staining, ×40)

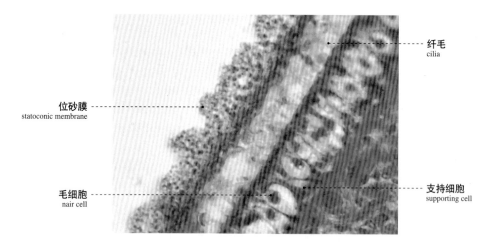

纤毛
cilia

位砂膜
statoconic membrane

毛细胞
nair cell

支持细胞
supporting cell

399. 位觉斑（豚鼠内耳，HE 染色，×400）
Macula staticae (inner ear of the guinea pig, HE staining, ×400)

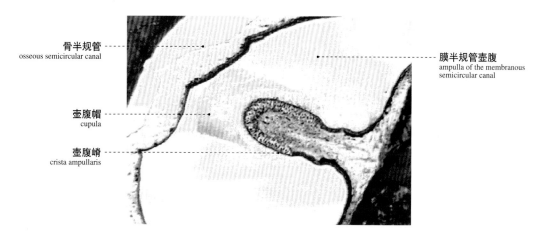

骨半规管
osseous semicircular canal

膜半规管壶腹
ampulla of the membranous
semicircular canal

壶腹帽
cupula

壶腹嵴
crista ampullaris

400. 壶腹嵴（豚鼠内耳，HE 染色，×40）
Crista ampullaris (inner ear of the guinea pig, HE staining, ×40)

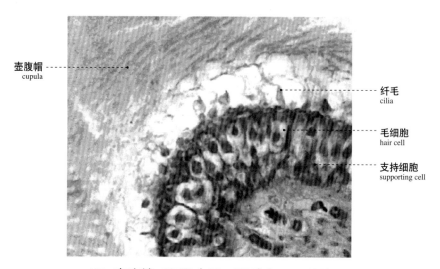

壶腹帽
cupula

纤毛
cilia

毛细胞
hair cell

支持细胞
supporting cell

401. 壶腹嵴（豚鼠内耳，HE 染色，×400）
Crista ampullaris (inner ear of the guinea pig, HE staining, ×400)

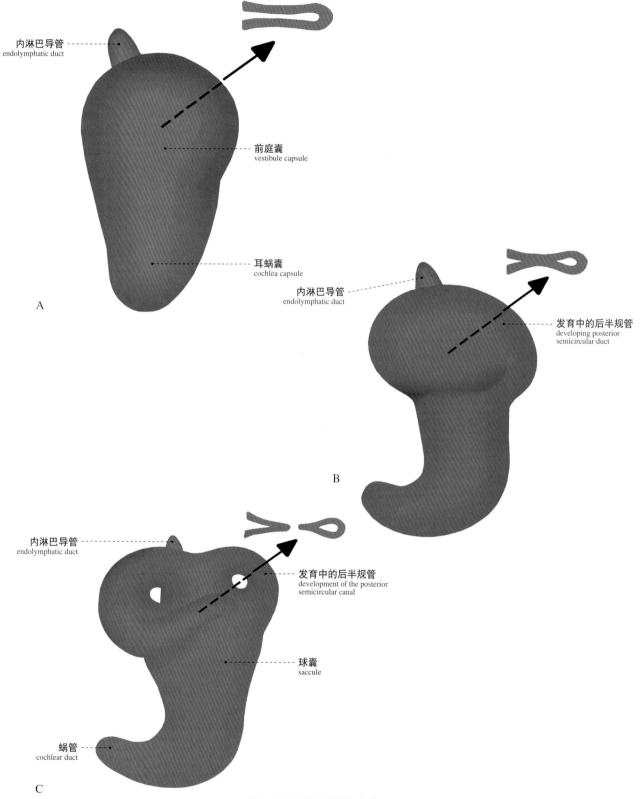

内淋巴导管
endolymphatic duct

前庭囊
vestibule capsule

耳蜗囊
cochlea capsule

A

内淋巴导管
endolymphatic duct

发育中的后半规管
developing posterior
semicircular duct

B

内淋巴导管
endolymphatic duct

发育中的后半规管
development of the posterior
semicircular canal

球囊
saccule

蜗管
cochlear duct

C

402. 内耳膜迷路的发生 1

Development of the membranous labyrinths of the internal ear 1

A ～ C. 第 5 ～ 8 周听泡的发育

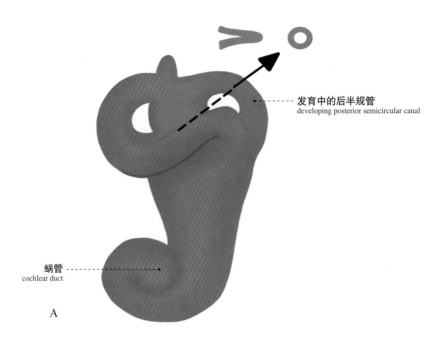

发育中的后半规管
developing posterior semicircular canal

蜗管
cochlear duct

A

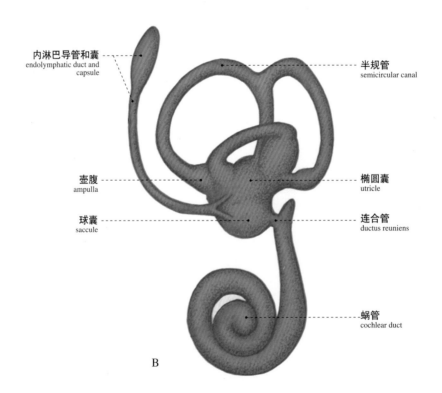

内淋巴导管和囊
endolymphatic duct and capsule

半规管
semicircular canal

壶腹
ampulla

椭圆囊
utricle

球囊
saccule

连合管
ductus reuniens

蜗管
cochlear duct

B

403. 内耳膜迷路的发生 2
Development of the membranous labyrinths of the internal ear 2

A、B. 第 5 ~ 8 周听泡的发育

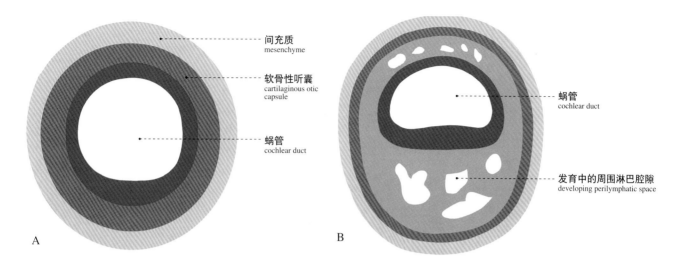

间充质
mesenchyme

软骨性听囊
cartilaginous otic capsule

蜗管
cochlear duct

A

蜗管
cochlear duct

发育中的周围淋巴腔隙
developing perilymphatic space

B

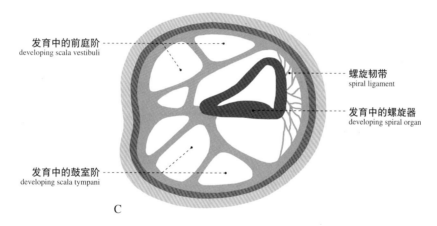

发育中的前庭阶
developing scala vestibuli

螺旋韧带
spiral ligament

发育中的螺旋器
developing spiral organ

发育中的鼓室阶
developing scala tympani

C

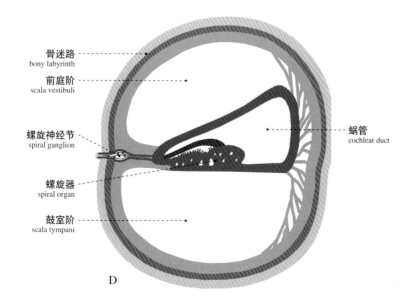

骨迷路
bony labyrinth

前庭阶
scala vestibuli

螺旋神经节
spiral ganglion

蜗管
cochlear duct

螺旋器
spiral organ

鼓室阶
scala tympani

D

404. 内耳骨迷路的发生

Development of the bony labyrinths of the internal ear

A ～ D. 第 8 ～ 12 周通过蜗管切面显示螺旋器的发生

第八章

鼻

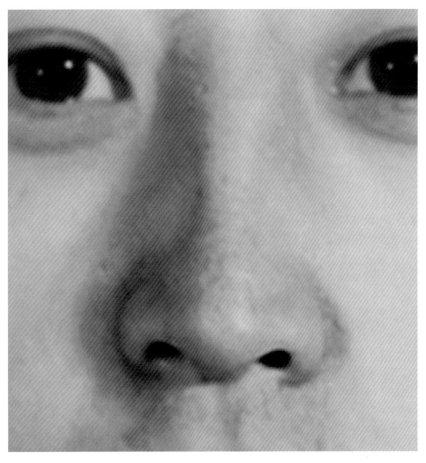

405. 鼻部
Nose

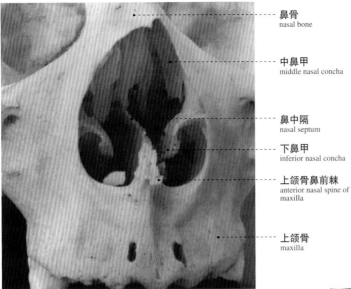

鼻骨
nasal bone

中鼻甲
middle nasal concha

鼻中隔
nasal septum

下鼻甲
inferior nasal concha

上颌骨鼻前棘
anterior nasal spine of maxilla

上颌骨
maxilla

A

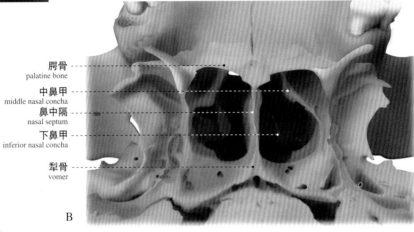

腭骨
palatine bone

中鼻甲
middle nasal concha

鼻中隔
nasal septum

下鼻甲
inferior nasal concha

犁骨
vomer

B

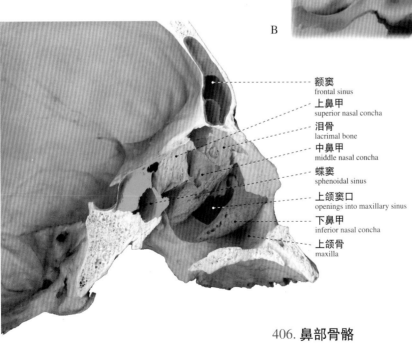

额窦
frontal sinus

上鼻甲
superior nasal concha

泪骨
lacrimal bone

中鼻甲
middle nasal concha

蝶窦
sphenoidal sinus

上颌窦口
openings into maxillary sinus

下鼻甲
inferior nasal concha

上颌骨
maxilla

C

406. 鼻部骨骼

Nasal bones

A. 前面观；B. 后面观；C. 侧面观

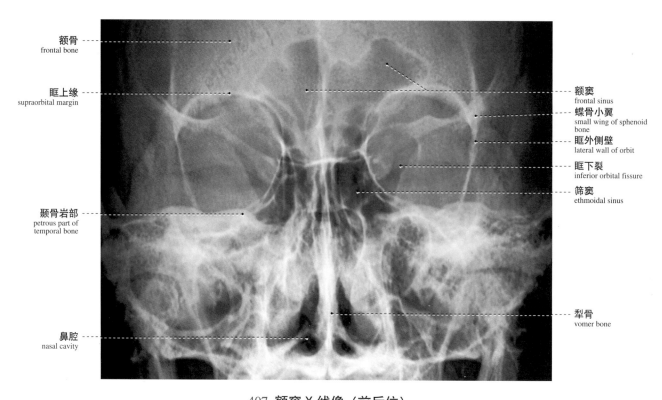

额骨
frontal bone

眶上缘
supraorbital margin

颞骨岩部
petrous part of
temporal bone

鼻腔
nasal cavity

额窦
frontal sinus

蝶骨小翼
small wing of sphenoid
bone

眶外侧壁
lateral wall of orbit

眶下裂
inferior orbital fissure

筛窦
ethmoidal sinus

犁骨
vomer bone

407. 额窦 X 线像（前后位）
Radiograph of the frontal sinus (anteroposterior view)

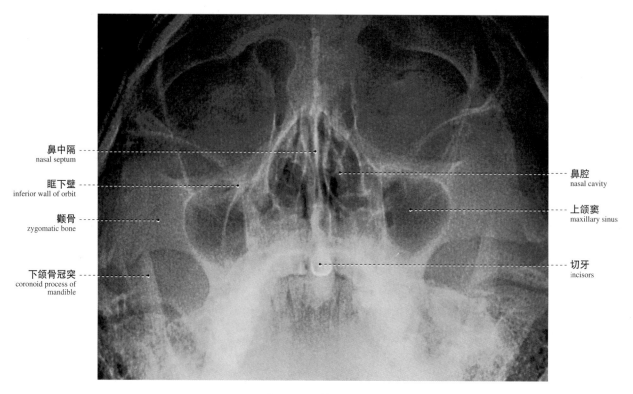

鼻中隔
nasal septum

眶下壁
inferior wall of orbit

颧骨
zygomatic bone

下颌骨冠突
coronoid process of
mandible

鼻腔
nasal cavity

上颌窦
maxillary sinus

切牙
incisors

408. 上颌窦 X 线像（前后位）
Radiograph of the maxillary sinus (anteroposterior view)

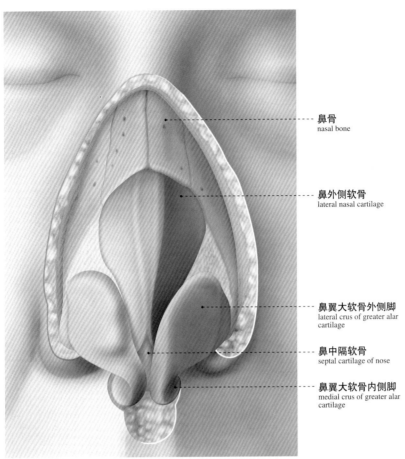

鼻骨
nasal bone

鼻外侧软骨
lateral nasal cartilage

鼻翼大软骨外侧脚
lateral crus of greater alar cartilage

鼻中隔软骨
septal cartilage of nose

鼻翼大软骨内侧脚
medial crus of greater alar cartilage

409. 鼻的骨骼（前面观）
Nose bones (anterior aspect)

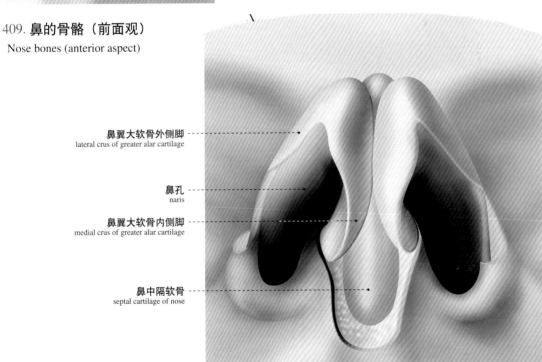

鼻翼大软骨外侧脚
lateral crus of greater alar cartilage

鼻孔
naris

鼻翼大软骨内侧脚
medial crus of greater alar cartilage

鼻中隔软骨
septal cartilage of nose

410. 鼻的骨骼（下面观）
Nose bones (inferior aspect)

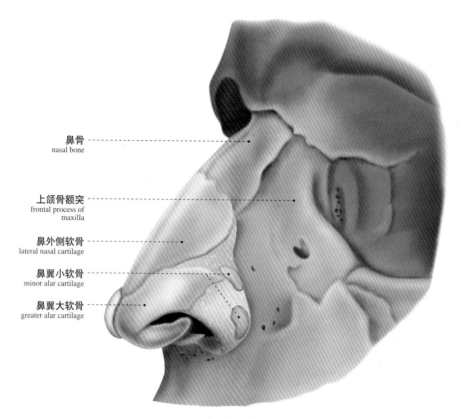

鼻骨
nasal bone

上颌骨额突
frontal process of
maxilla

鼻外侧软骨
lateral nasal cartilage

鼻翼小软骨
minor alar cartilage

鼻翼大软骨
greater alar cartilage

411. 鼻的骨骼（左外侧面观）
Nasal bones (left lateral aspect)

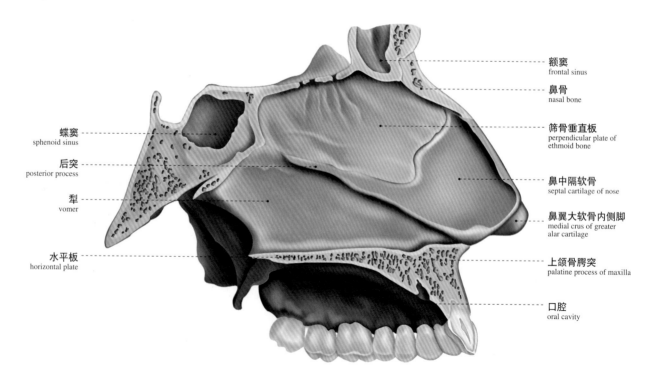

蝶窦
sphenoid sinus

后突
posterior process

犁
vomer

水平板
horizontal plate

额窦
frontal sinus

鼻骨
nasal bone

筛骨垂直板
perpendicular plate of
ethmoid bone

鼻中隔软骨
septal cartilage of nose

鼻翼大软骨内侧脚
medial crus of greater
alar cartilage

上颌骨腭突
palatine process of maxilla

口腔
oral cavity

412. 鼻中隔（右侧面观）
Nasal septum (right lateral aspect)

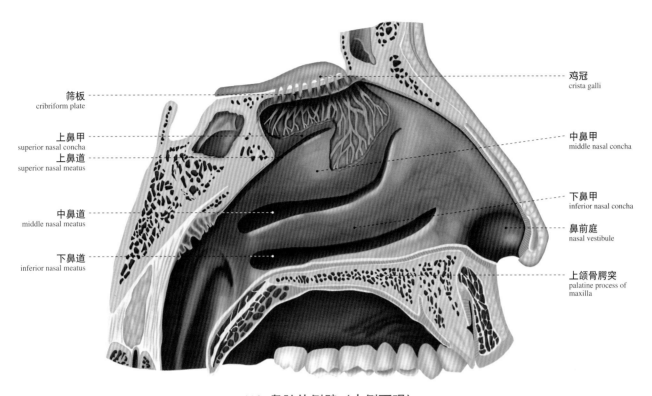

筛板
cribriform plate

上鼻甲
superior nasal concha

上鼻道
superior nasal meatus

中鼻道
middle nasal meatus

下鼻道
inferior nasal meatus

鸡冠
crista galli

中鼻甲
middle nasal concha

下鼻甲
inferior nasal concha

鼻前庭
nasal vestibule

上颌骨腭突
palatine process of maxilla

413. 鼻腔外侧壁（内侧面观）
Lateral wall of the nasal cavity (medial aspect)

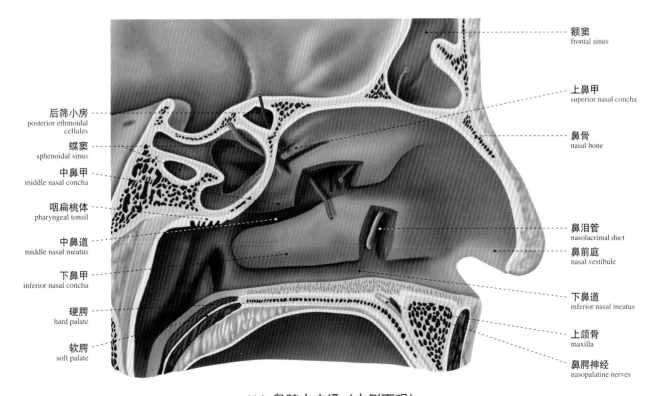

后筛小房
posterior ethmoidal cellules

蝶窦
sphenoidal sinus

中鼻甲
middle nasal concha

咽扁桃体
pharyngeal tonsil

中鼻道
middle nasal meatus

下鼻甲
inferior nasal concha

硬腭
hard palate

软腭
soft palate

额窦
frontal sinus

上鼻甲
superior nasal concha

鼻骨
nasal bone

鼻泪管
nasolacrimal duct

鼻前庭
nasal vestibule

下鼻道
inferior nasal meatus

上颌骨
maxilla

鼻腭神经
nasopalatine nerves

414. 鼻腔内交通（内侧面观）
Traffic of the nasal cavity (medial aspect)

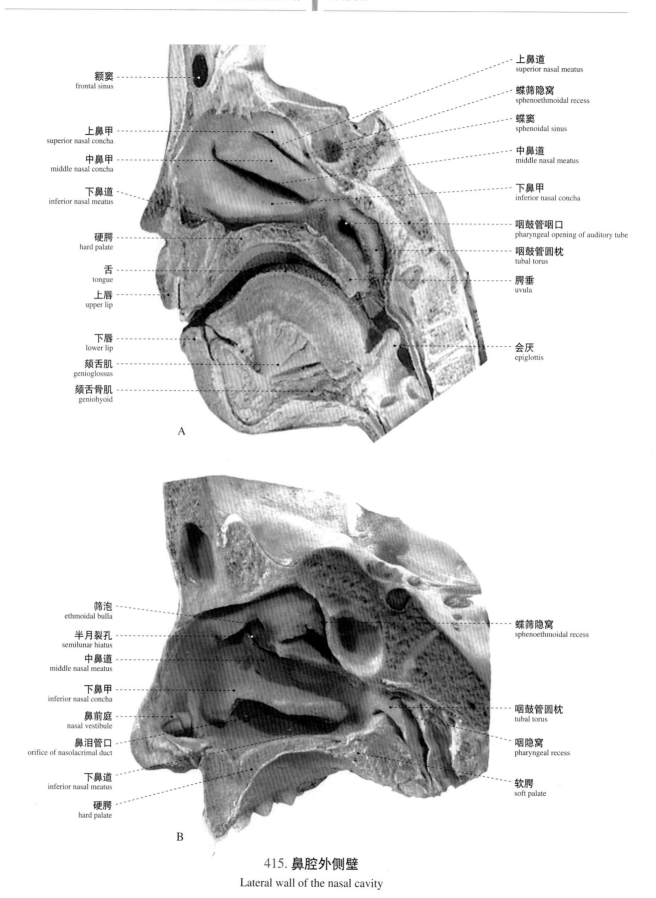

额窦
frontal sinus

上鼻甲
superior nasal concha

中鼻甲
middle nasal concha

下鼻道
inferior nasal meatus

硬腭
hard palate

舌
tongue

上唇
upper lip

下唇
lower lip

颏舌肌
genioglossus

颏舌骨肌
geniohyoid

上鼻道
superior nasal meatus

蝶筛隐窝
sphenoethmoidal recess

蝶窦
sphenoidal sinus

中鼻道
middle nasal meatus

下鼻甲
inferior nasal concha

咽鼓管咽口
pharyngeal opening of auditory tube

咽鼓管圆枕
tubal torus

腭垂
uvula

会厌
epiglottis

A

筛泡
ethmoidal bulla

半月裂孔
semilunar hiatus

中鼻道
middle nasal meatus

下鼻甲
inferior nasal concha

鼻前庭
nasal vestibule

鼻泪管口
orifice of nasolacrimal duct

下鼻道
inferior nasal meatus

硬腭
hard palate

蝶筛隐窝
sphenoethmoidal recess

咽鼓管圆枕
tubal torus

咽隐窝
pharyngeal recess

软腭
soft palate

B

415. 鼻腔外侧壁
Lateral wall of the nasal cavity

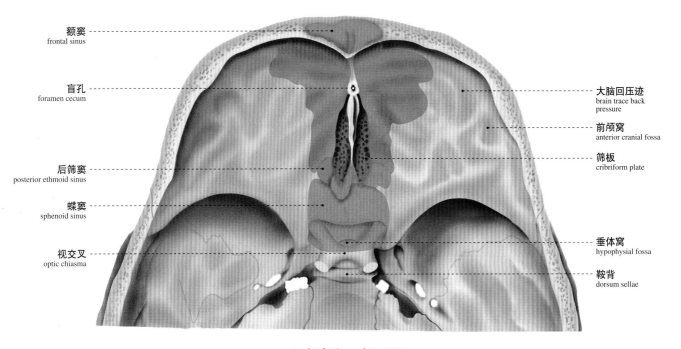

额窦
frontal sinus

盲孔
foramen cecum

后筛窦
posterior ethmoid sinus

蝶窦
sphenoid sinus

视交叉
optic chiasma

大脑回压迹
brain trace back pressure

前颅窝
anterior cranial fossa

筛板
cribriform plate

垂体窝
hypophysial fossa

鞍背
dorsum sellae

416. 鼻旁窦（上面观）
Paranasal sinuses (superior aspect)

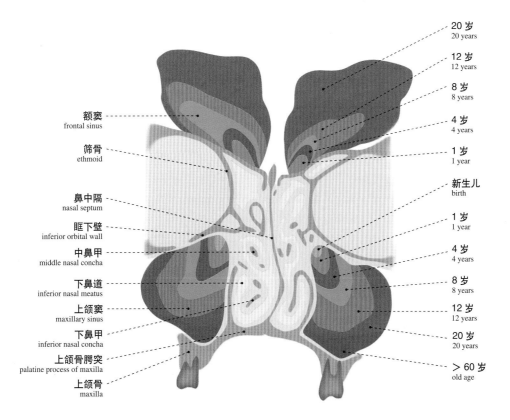

额窦
frontal sinus

筛骨
ethmoid

鼻中隔
nasal septum

眶下壁
inferior orbital wall

中鼻甲
middle nasal concha

下鼻道
inferior nasal meatus

上颌窦
maxillary sinus

下鼻甲
inferior nasal concha

上颌骨腭突
palatine process of maxilla

上颌骨
maxilla

20 岁
20 years

12 岁
12 years

8 岁
8 years

4 岁
4 years

1 岁
1 year

新生儿
birth

1 岁
1 year

4 岁
4 years

8 岁
8 years

12 岁
12 years

20 岁
20 years

> 60 岁
old age

417. 额窦和上颌窦的发育
Growth of frontal and maxillary sinuses

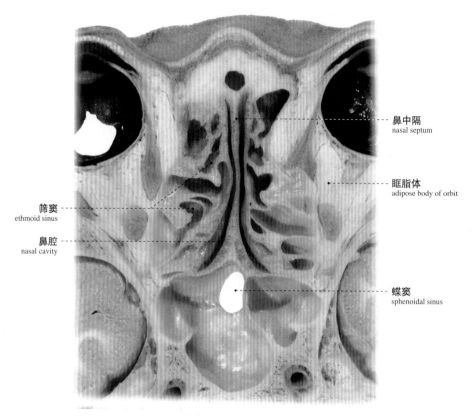

鼻中隔
nasal septum

眶脂体
adipose body of orbit

筛窦
ethmoid sinus

鼻腔
nasal cavity

蝶窦
sphenoidal sinus

418. 鼻部水平断面 1

Horizontal section of the nose 1

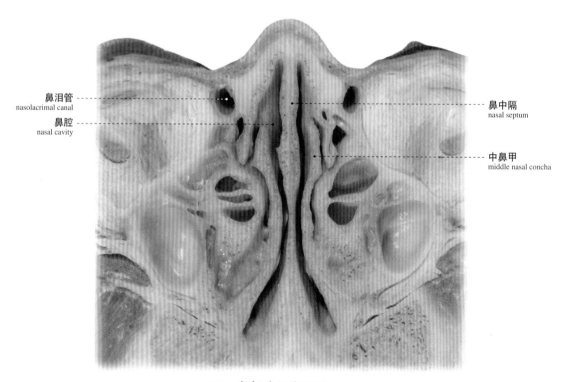

鼻泪管
nasolacrimal canal

鼻腔
nasal cavity

鼻中隔
nasal septum

中鼻甲
middle nasal concha

419. 鼻部水平断面 2

Horizontal section of the nose 2

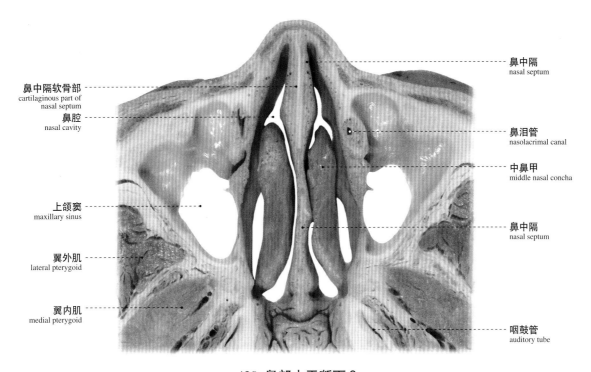

鼻中隔
nasal septum

鼻中隔软骨部
cartilaginous part of
nasal septum

鼻腔
nasal cavity

鼻泪管
nasolacrimal canal

中鼻甲
middle nasal concha

上颌窦
maxillary sinus

鼻中隔
nasal septum

翼外肌
lateral pterygoid

翼内肌
medial pterygoid

咽鼓管
auditory tube

420. 鼻部水平断面 3
Horizontal section of the nose 3

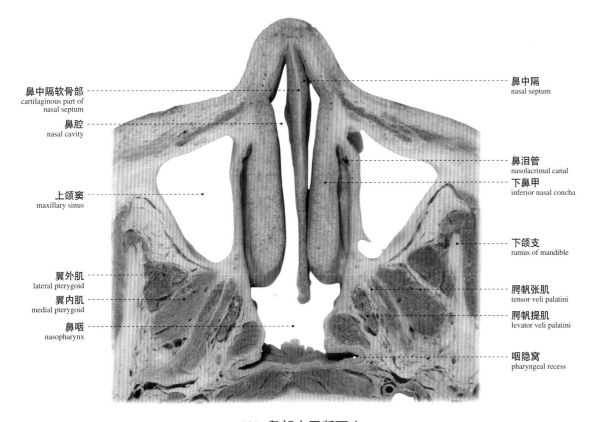

鼻中隔
nasal septum

鼻中隔软骨部
cartilaginous part of
nasal septum

鼻腔
nasal cavity

鼻泪管
nasolacrimal canal

下鼻甲
inferior nasal concha

上颌窦
maxillary sinus

下颌支
ramus of mandible

翼外肌
lateral pterygoid

翼内肌
medial pterygoid

腭帆张肌
tensor veli palatini

鼻咽
nasopharynx

腭帆提肌
levator veli palatini

咽隐窝
pharyngeal recess

421. 鼻部水平断面 4
Horizontal section of the nose 4

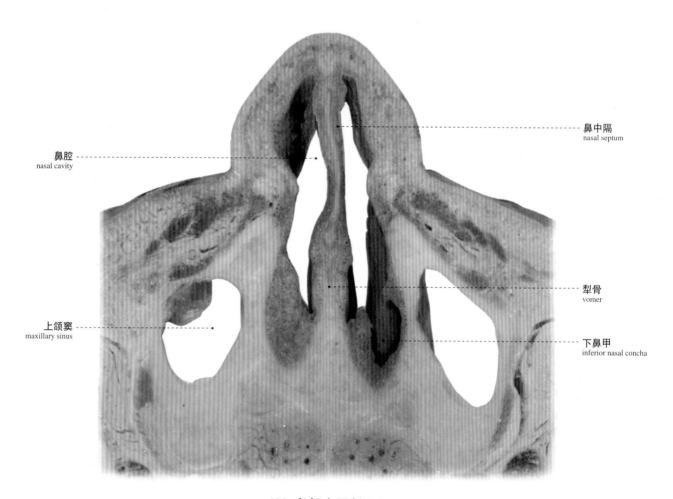

鼻中隔
nasal septum

鼻腔
nasal cavity

犁骨
vomer

上颌窦
maxillary sinus

下鼻甲
inferior nasal concha

422. 鼻部水平断面 5

Horizontal section of the nose 5

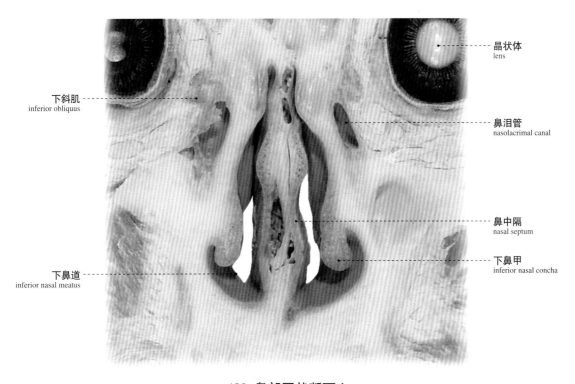

下斜肌
inferior obliquus

晶状体
lens

鼻泪管
nasolacrimal canal

鼻中隔
nasal septum

下鼻甲
inferior nasal concha

下鼻道
inferior nasal meatus

423. 鼻部冠状断面 1
Frontal section of the nose 1

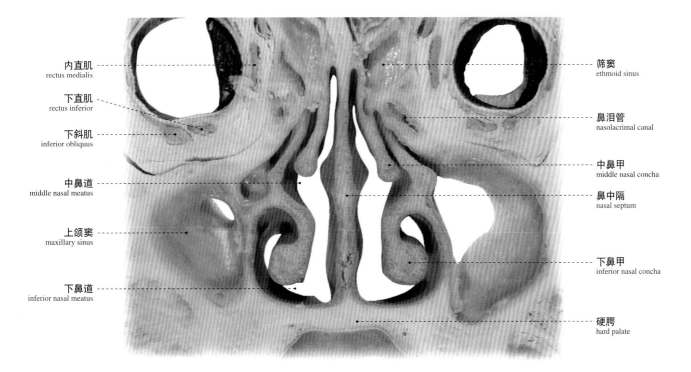

内直肌
rectus medialis

下直肌
rectus inferior

下斜肌
inferior obliquus

中鼻道
middle nasal meatus

上颌窦
maxillary sinus

下鼻道
inferior nasal meatus

筛窦
ethmoid sinus

鼻泪管
nasolacrimal canal

中鼻甲
middle nasal concha

鼻中隔
nasal septum

下鼻甲
inferior nasal concha

硬腭
hard palate

424. 鼻部冠状断面 2
Frontal section of the nose 2

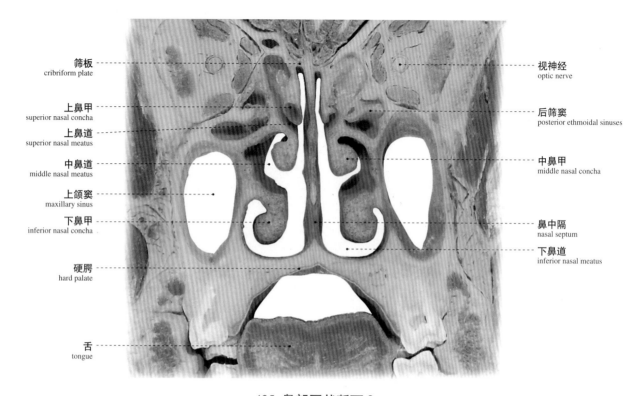

425. 鼻部冠状断面 3

Frontal section of the nose 3

筛板
cribriform plate

上鼻甲
superior nasal concha

上鼻道
superior nasal meatus

中鼻道
middle nasal meatus

上颌窦
maxillary sinus

下鼻甲
inferior nasal concha

硬腭
hard palate

舌
tongue

视神经
optic nerve

后筛窦
posterior ethmoidal sinuses

中鼻甲
middle nasal concha

鼻中隔
nasal septum

下鼻道
inferior nasal meatus

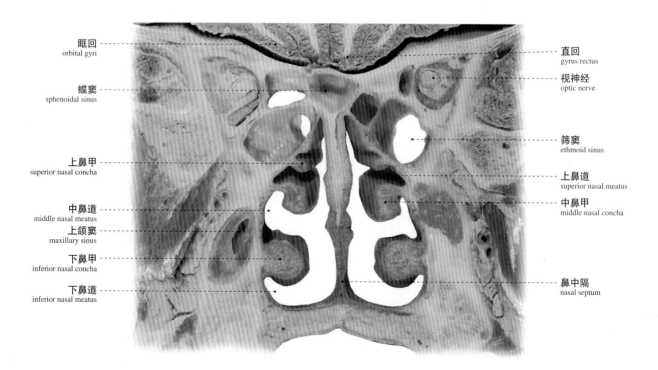

426. 鼻部冠状断面 4

Frontal section of the nose 4

眶回
orbital gyri

蝶窦
sphenoidal sinus

上鼻甲
superior nasal concha

中鼻道
middle nasal meatus

上颌窦
maxillary sinus

下鼻甲
inferior nasal concha

下鼻道
inferior nasal meatus

直回
gyrus rectus

视神经
optic nerve

筛窦
ethmoid sinus

上鼻道
superior nasal meatus

中鼻甲
middle nasal concha

鼻中隔
nasal septum

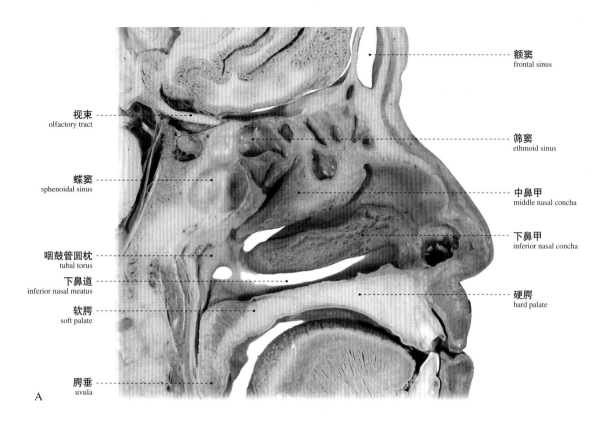

视束
olfactory tract

蝶窦
sphenoidal sinus

咽鼓管圆枕
tubal torus

下鼻道
inferior nasal meatus

软腭
soft palate

腭垂
uvula

额窦
frontal sinus

筛窦
ethmoid sinus

中鼻甲
middle nasal concha

下鼻甲
inferior nasal concha

硬腭
hard palate

A

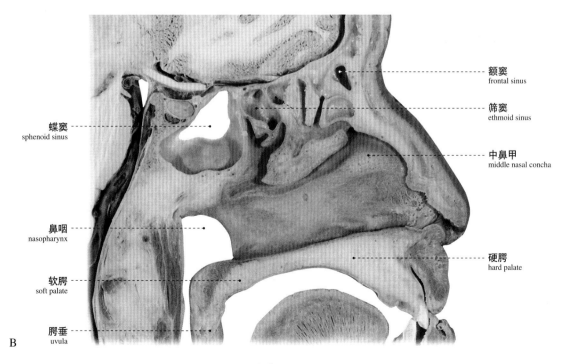

蝶窦
sphenoid sinus

鼻咽
nasopharynx

软腭
soft palate

腭垂
uvula

额窦
frontal sinus

筛窦
ethmoid sinus

中鼻甲
middle nasal concha

硬腭
hard palate

B

427. 鼻部矢状断面
Sagittal section of nose

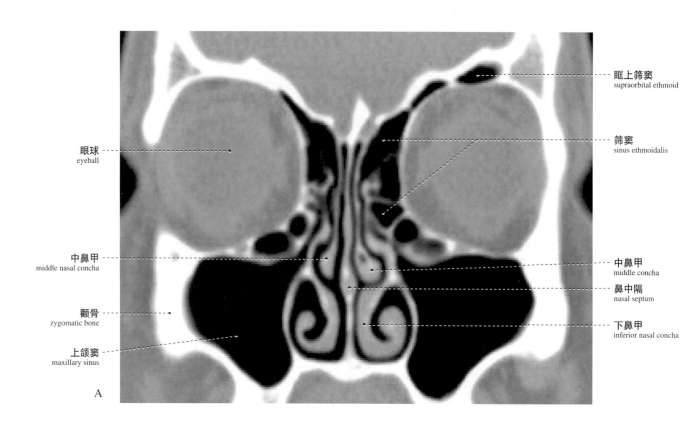

眶上筛窦
supraorbital ethmoid

筛窦
sinus ethmoidalis

眼球
eyeball

中鼻甲
middle nasal concha

中鼻甲
middle concha

鼻中隔
nasal septum

颧骨
zygomatic bone

下鼻甲
inferior nasal concha

上颌窦
maxillary sinus

A

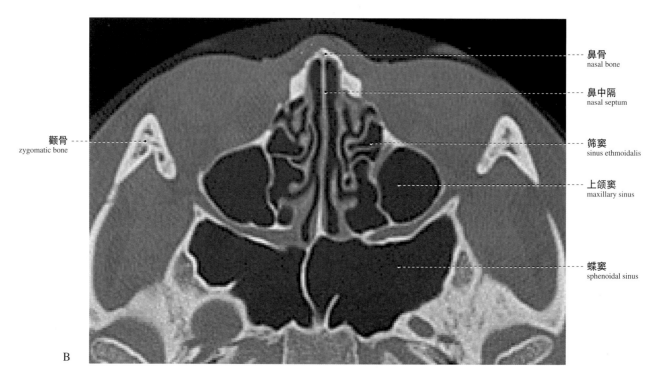

鼻骨
nasal bone

鼻中隔
nasal septum

颧骨
zygomatic bone

筛窦
sinus ethmoidalis

上颌窦
maxillary sinus

蝶窦
sphenoidal sinus

B

428. 鼻旁窦计算机断层摄影
CT of the paranasal sinuses

A. 冠状位；B. 轴位

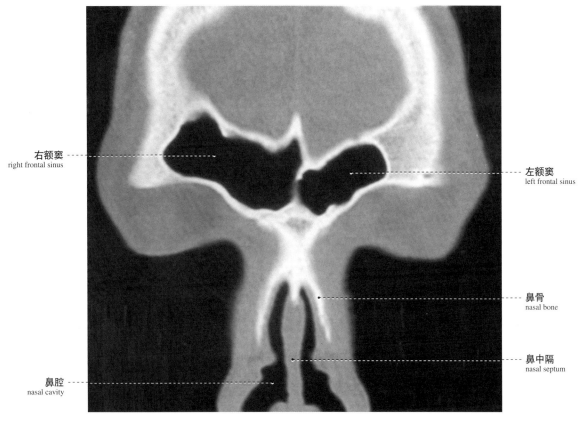

右额窦
right frontal sinus

左额窦
left frontal sinus

鼻骨
nasal bone

鼻中隔
nasal septum

鼻腔
nasal cavity

429. 额窦计算机断层摄影（冠状位）
CT of the frontal sinus (coronal view)

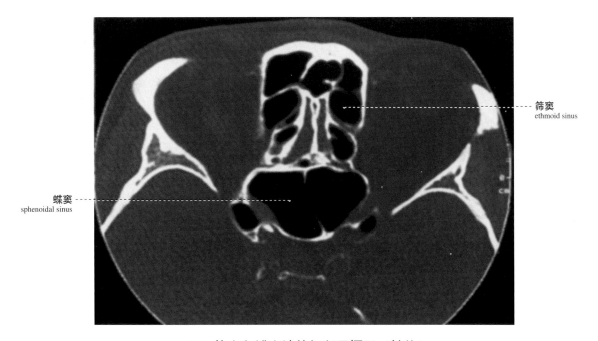

筛窦
ethmoid sinus

蝶窦
sphenoidal sinus

430. 筛窦和蝶窦计算机断层摄影（轴位）
CT of the ethmoid and dish sinus (axial view)

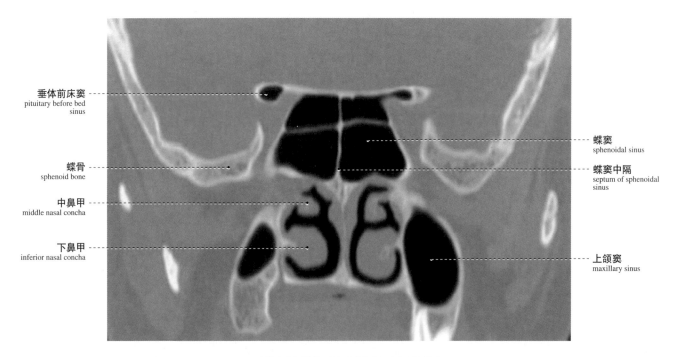

垂体前床窦
pituitary before bed
sinus

蝶骨
sphenoid bone

中鼻甲
middle nasal concha

下鼻甲
inferior nasal concha

蝶窦
sphenoidal sinus

蝶窦中隔
septum of sphenoidal
sinus

上颌窦
maxillary sinus

431. 蝶窦计算机断层摄影（冠状位）
CT of the sphenoidal sinus (coronal view)

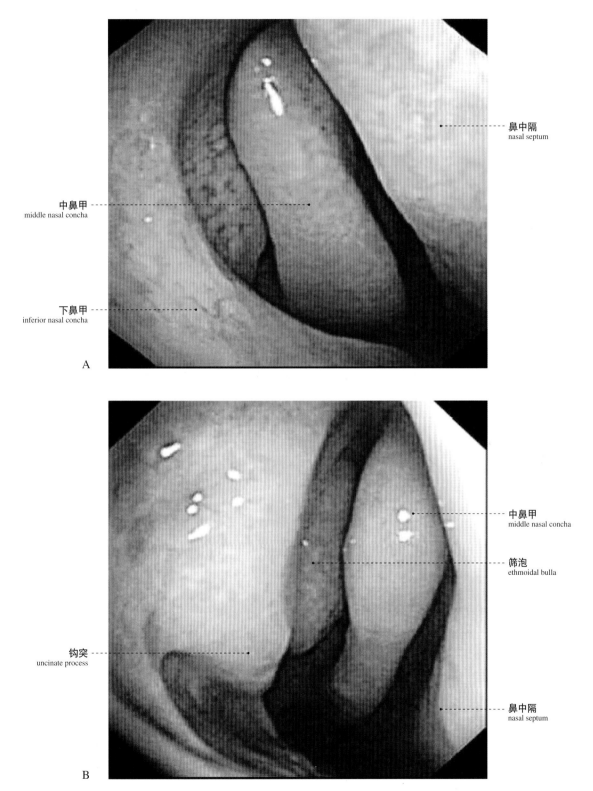

鼻中隔
nasal septum

中鼻甲
middle nasal concha

下鼻甲
inferior nasal concha

A

中鼻甲
middle nasal concha

筛泡
ethmoidal bulla

钩突
uncinate process

鼻中隔
nasal septum

B

432. 鼻腔镜图像（右侧鼻腔）

Conchoscope image (right nasal cavity)

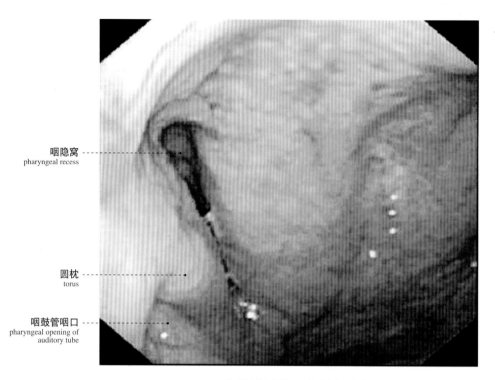

咽隐窝
pharyngeal recess

圆枕
torus

咽鼓管咽口
pharyngeal opening of
auditory tube

433. 鼻腔镜图像（右侧鼻咽部）
Conchoscope image (right nasopharynx)

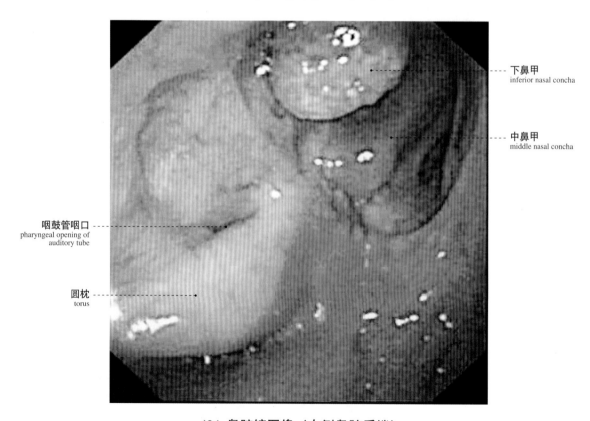

下鼻甲
inferior nasal concha

中鼻甲
middle nasal concha

咽鼓管咽口
pharyngeal opening of
auditory tube

圆枕
torus

434. 鼻腔镜图像（右侧鼻腔后端）
Conchoscope image (right posterior extremity of nasal cavity)

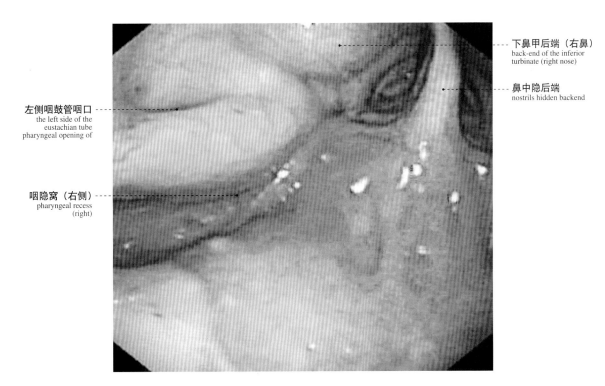

中鼻甲
middle nasal concha

鼻中隔
nasal septum

上颌窦自然口
natural ostium of maxillary sinus

435. 鼻腔镜图像（右侧鼻腔上颌窦口）

Conchoscope image (opening of maxillary sinus of right nasal cavity)

下鼻甲后端（右鼻）
back-end of the inferior
turbinate (right nose)

鼻中隐后端
nostrils hidden backend

左侧咽鼓管咽口
the left side of the
eustachian tube
pharyngeal opening of

咽隐窝（右侧）
pharyngeal recess
(right)

436. 鼻咽镜图像（左侧鼻腔后端）

Nasopharyngoscope image (left posterior extremity of nasal cavity)

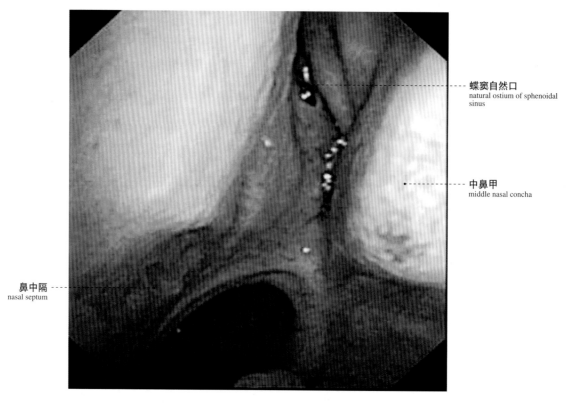

蝶窦自然口
natural ostium of sphenoidal sinus

中鼻甲
middle nasal concha

鼻中隔
nasal septum

437. 鼻腔镜图像（左侧鼻腔蝶窦）
Conchoscope image (sphenoidal sinus of left nasal cavity)

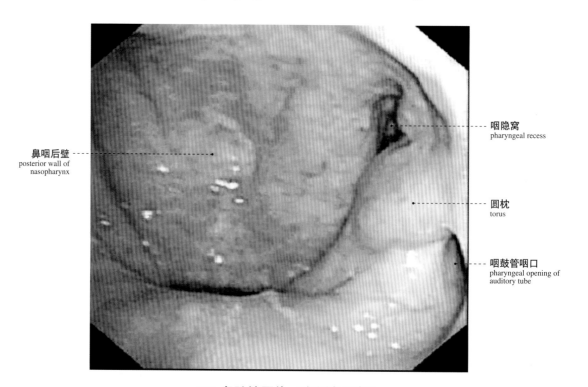

咽隐窝
pharyngeal recess

鼻咽后壁
posterior wall of nasopharynx

圆枕
torus

咽鼓管咽口
pharyngeal opening of auditory tube

438. 鼻腔镜图像（左侧鼻咽部）
Conchoscope image (left nasopharynx)

第九章

喉

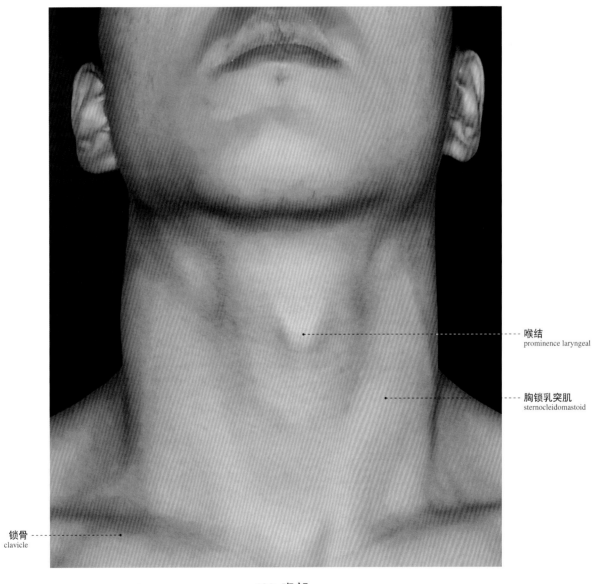

喉结
prominence laryngeal

胸锁乳突肌
sternocleidomastoid

锁骨
clavicle

439. 喉部
Laryngeal

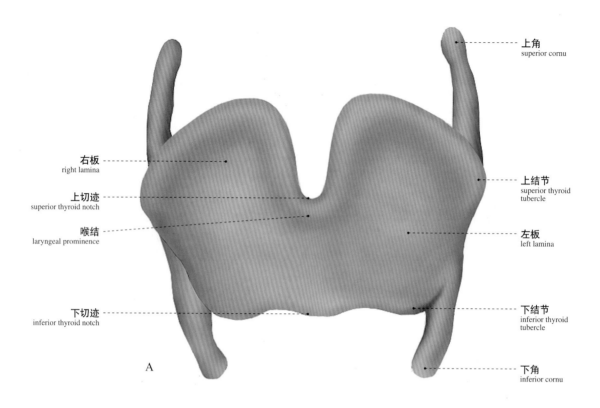

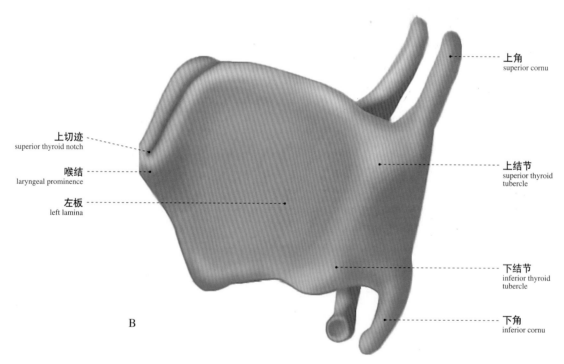

右板
right lamina

上切迹
superior thyroid notch

喉结
laryngeal prominence

下切迹
inferior thyroid notch

上角
superior cornu

上结节
superior thyroid tubercle

左板
left lamina

下结节
inferior thyroid tubercle

下角
inferior cornu

A

上切迹
superior thyroid notch

喉结
laryngeal prominence

左板
left lamina

上角
superior cornu

上结节
superior thyroid tubercle

下结节
inferior thyroid tubercle

下角
inferior cornu

B

440. 甲状软骨
Thyroid cartilage
A. 前面观；B. 外侧面观

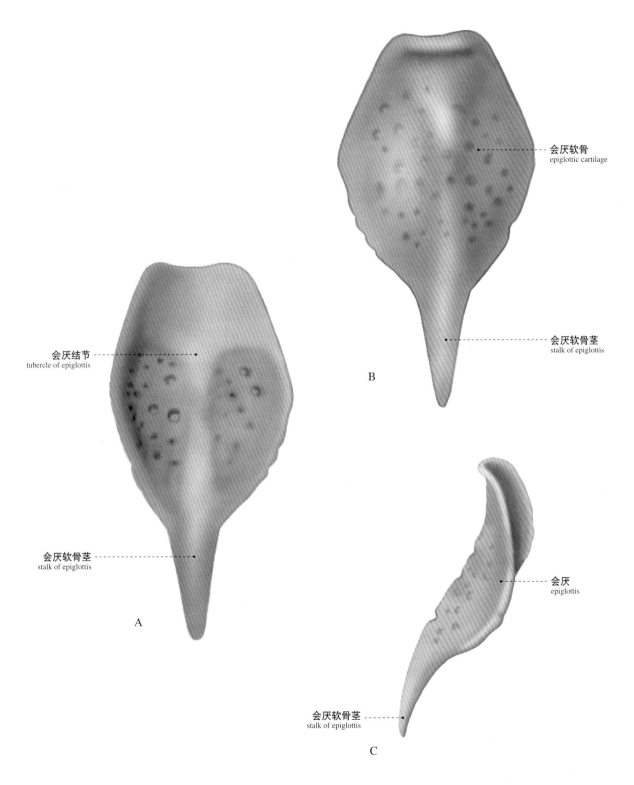

会厌软骨
epiglottic cartilage

会厌软骨茎
stalk of epiglottis

B

会厌结节
tubercle of epiglottis

会厌软骨茎
stalk of epiglottis

A

会厌
epiglottis

会厌软骨茎
stalk of epiglottis

C

441. 会厌软骨
Epiglottic cartilage

A. 后面观；B. 前面观；C. 侧面观

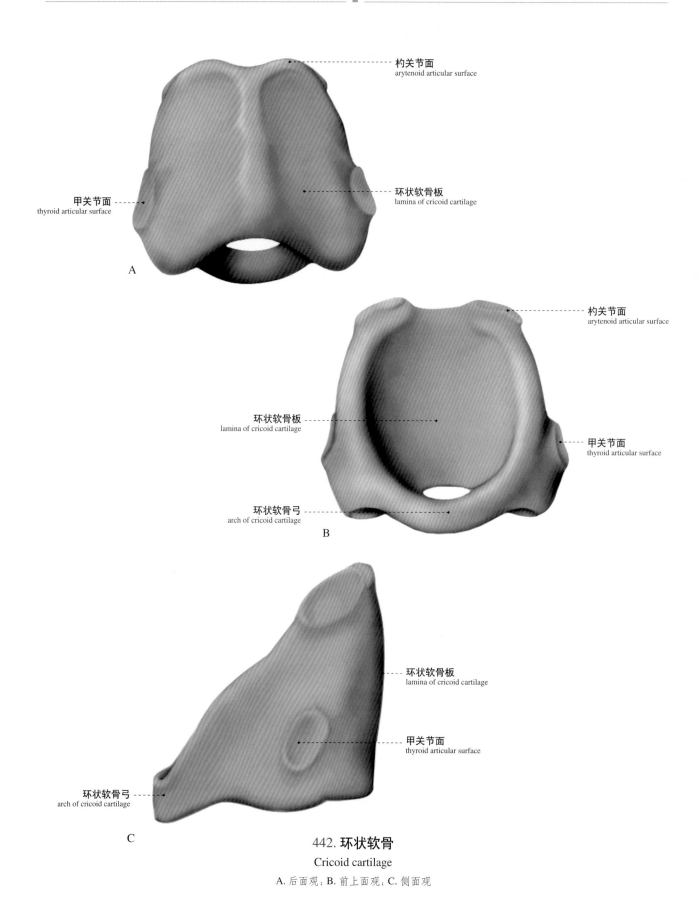

杓关节面
arytenoid articular surface

甲关节面
thyroid articular surface

环状软骨板
lamina of cricoid cartilage

A

杓关节面
arytenoid articular surface

环状软骨板
lamina of cricoid cartilage

甲关节面
thyroid articular surface

环状软骨弓
arch of cricoid cartilage

B

环状软骨板
lamina of cricoid cartilage

甲关节面
thyroid articular surface

环状软骨弓
arch of cricoid cartilage

C

442. 环状软骨
Cricoid cartilage
A. 后面观；B. 前上面观；C. 侧面观

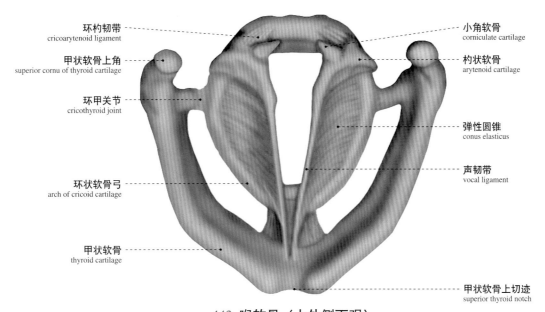

环杓韧带
cricoarytenoid ligament

甲状软骨上角
superior cornu of thyroid cartilage

环甲关节
cricothyroid joint

环状软骨弓
arch of cricoid cartilage

甲状软骨
thyroid cartilage

小角软骨
corniculate cartilage

杓状软骨
arytenoid cartilage

弹性圆锥
conus elasticus

声韧带
vocal ligament

甲状软骨上切迹
superior thyroid notch

443. 喉软骨（上外侧面观）
Laryngeal cartilage (superior lateral aspect)

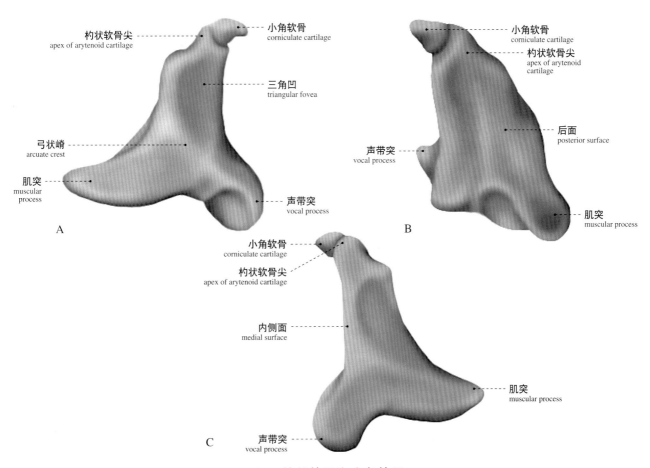

杓状软骨尖
apex of arytenoid cartilage

小角软骨
corniculate cartilage

三角凹
triangular fovea

弓状嵴
arcuate crest

肌突
muscular process

声带突
vocal process

A

小角软骨
corniculate cartilage

杓状软骨尖
apex of arytenoid cartilage

后面
posterior surface

声带突
vocal process

肌突
muscular process

B

小角软骨
corniculate cartilage

杓状软骨尖
apex of arytenoid cartilage

内侧面
medial surface

肌突
muscular process

声带突
vocal process

C

444. 杓状软骨和小角软骨
Arytenoid cartilage and corniculate cartilage

A. 外侧面观；B. 后面观；C. 内面观

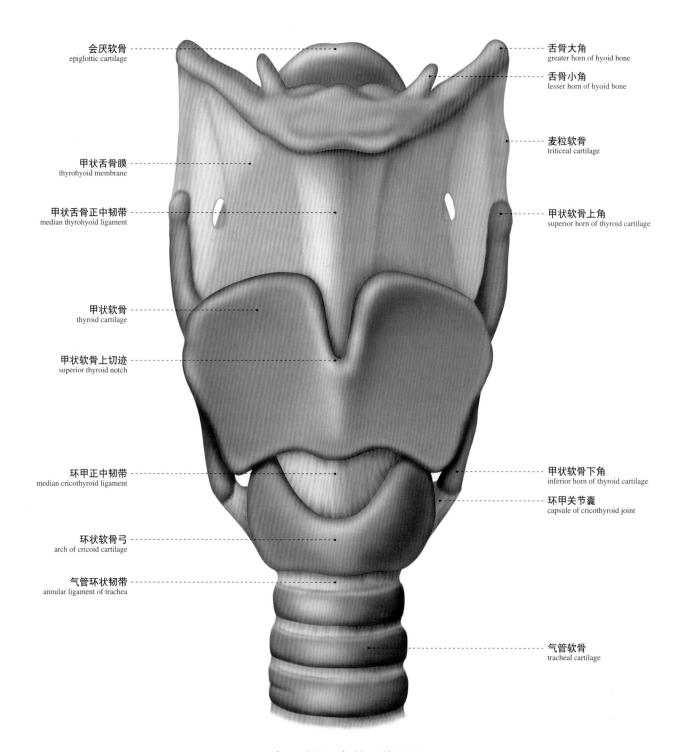

会厌软骨
epiglottic cartilage

甲状舌骨膜
thyrohyoid membrane

甲状舌骨正中韧带
median thyrohyoid ligament

甲状软骨
thyroid cartilage

甲状软骨上切迹
superior thyroid notch

环甲正中韧带
median cricothyroid ligament

环状软骨弓
arch of cricoid cartilage

气管环状韧带
annular ligament of trachea

舌骨大角
greater horn of hyoid bone

舌骨小角
lesser horn of hyoid bone

麦粒软骨
triticeal cartilage

甲状软骨上角
superior horn of thyroid cartilage

甲状软骨下角
inferior horn of thyroid cartilage

环甲关节囊
capsule of cricothyroid joint

气管软骨
tracheal cartilage

445. 喉，舌骨，气管（前面观）
Larynx, hyoid bone, trachea (anterior aspect)

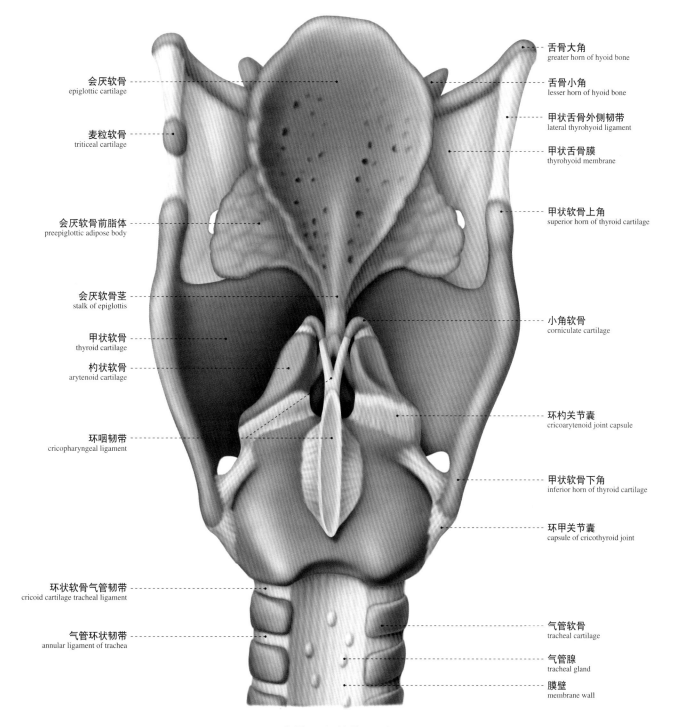

会厌软骨
epiglottic cartilage

麦粒软骨
triticeal cartilage

会厌软骨前脂体
preepiglottic adipose body

会厌软骨茎
stalk of epiglottis

甲状软骨
thyroid cartilage

杓状软骨
arytenoid cartilage

环咽韧带
cricopharyngeal ligament

环状软骨气管韧带
cricoid cartilage tracheal ligament

气管环状韧带
annular ligament of trachea

舌骨大角
greater horn of hyoid bone

舌骨小角
lesser horn of hyoid bone

甲状舌骨外侧韧带
lateral thyrohyoid ligament

甲状舌骨膜
thyrohyoid membrane

甲状软骨上角
superior horn of thyroid cartilage

小角软骨
corniculate cartilage

环杓关节囊
cricoarytenoid joint capsule

甲状软骨下角
inferior horn of thyroid cartilage

环甲关节囊
capsule of cricothyroid joint

气管软骨
tracheal cartilage

气管腺
tracheal gland

膜壁
membrane wall

446. 喉软骨和关节（后面观）
Laryngeal cartilage and joints (posterior aspect)

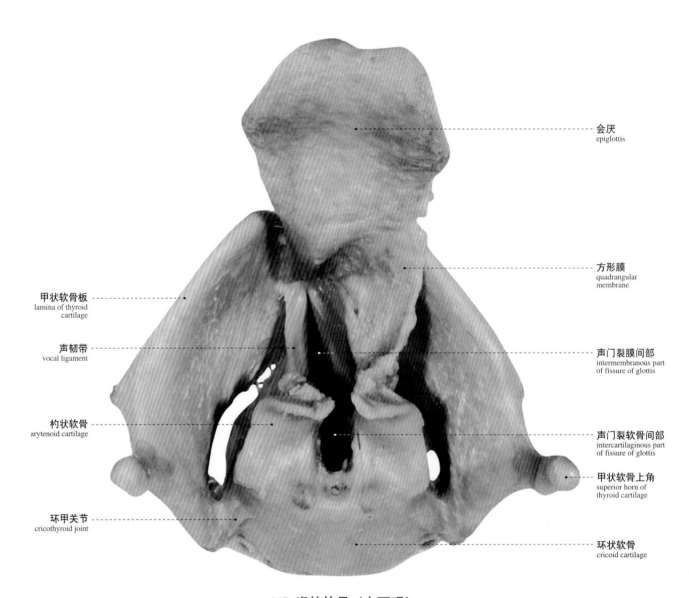

会厌
epiglottis

方形膜
quadrangular
membrane

甲状软骨板
lamina of thyroid
cartilage

声韧带
vocal ligament

声门裂膜间部
intermembranous part
of fissure of glottis

杓状软骨
arytenoid cartilage

声门裂软骨间部
intercartilaginous part
of fissure of glottis

甲状软骨上角
superior horn of
thyroid cartilage

环甲关节
cricothyroid joint

环状软骨
cricoid cartilage

447. 喉的软骨（上面观）
Cartilages of the larynx (superior aspect)

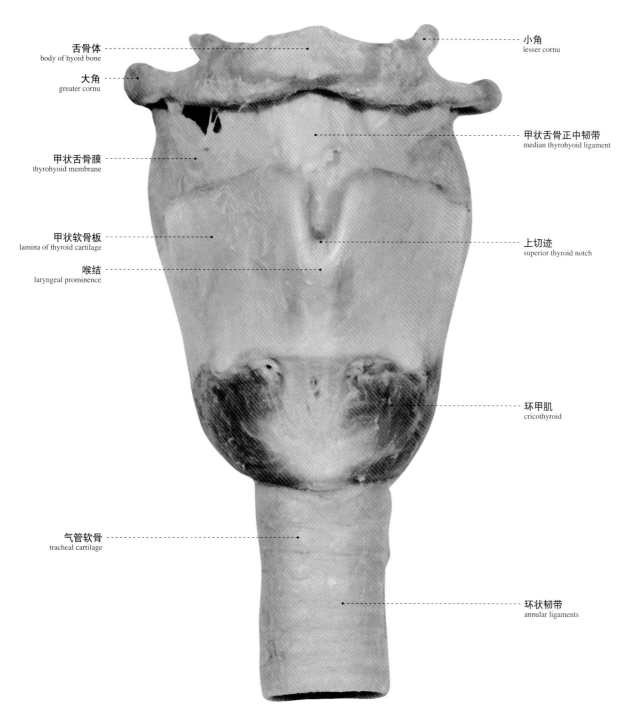

舌骨体
body of hyoid bone

大角
greater cornu

甲状舌骨膜
thyrohyoid membrane

甲状软骨板
lamina of thyroid cartilage

喉结
laryngeal prominence

气管软骨
tracheal cartilage

小角
lesser cornu

甲状舌骨正中韧带
median thyrohyoid ligament

上切迹
superior thyroid notch

环甲肌
cricothyroid

环状韧带
annular ligaments

448. 喉肌（前面观）
Laryngeal muscles (anterior aspect)

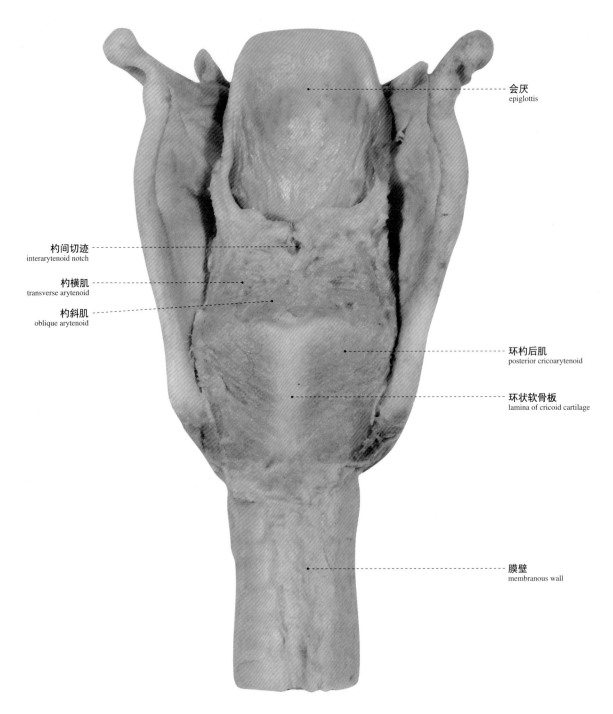

会厌
epiglottis

杓间切迹
interarytenoid notch

杓横肌
transverse arytenoid

杓斜肌
oblique arytenoid

环杓后肌
posterior cricoarytenoid

环状软骨板
lamina of cricoid cartilage

膜壁
membranous wall

449. 喉肌（后面观）
Laryngeal muscles (posterior aspect)

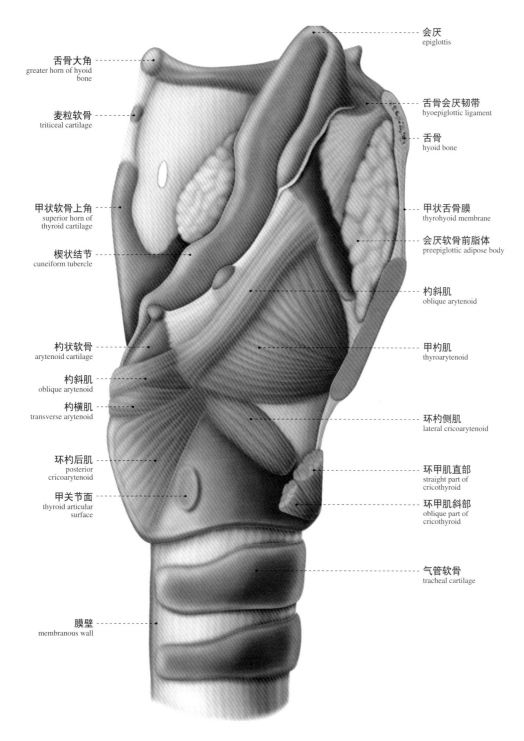

会厌
epiglottis

舌骨大角
greater horn of hyoid
bone

麦粒软骨
triticeal cartilage

舌骨会厌韧带
hyoepiglottic ligament

舌骨
hyoid bone

甲状软骨上角
superior horn of
thyroid cartilage

甲状舌骨膜
thyrohyoid membrane

会厌软骨前脂体
preepiglottic adipose body

楔状结节
cuneiform tubercle

杓斜肌
oblique arytenoid

杓状软骨
arytenoid cartilage

甲杓肌
thyroarytenoid

杓斜肌
oblique arytenoid

杓横肌
transverse arytenoid

环杓侧肌
lateral cricoarytenoid

环杓后肌
posterior
cricoarytenoid

环甲肌直部
straight part of
cricothyroid

甲关节面
thyroid articular
surface

环甲肌斜部
oblique part of
cricothyroid

气管软骨
tracheal cartilage

膜壁
membranous wall

450. 喉肌（后斜面观）
Laryngeal muscles (after oblique aspect)

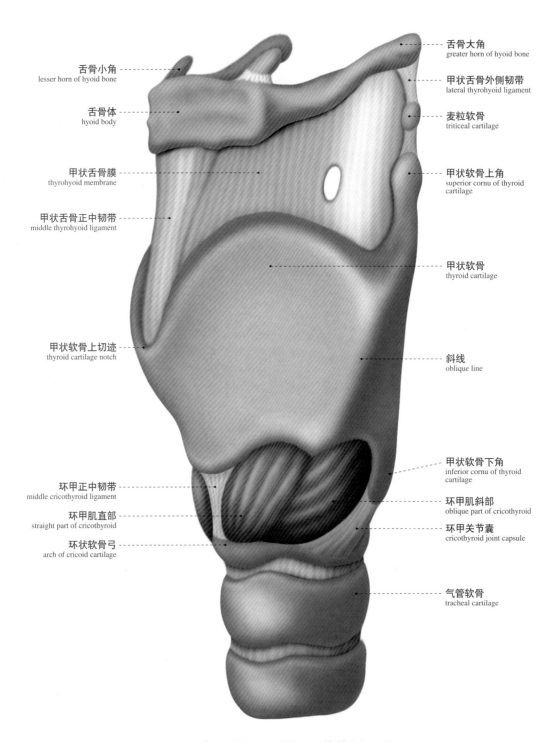

舌骨小角
lesser horn of hyoid bone

舌骨体
hyoid body

甲状舌骨膜
thyrohyoid membrane

甲状舌骨正中韧带
middle thyrohyoid ligament

甲状软骨上切迹
thyroid cartilage notch

环甲正中韧带
middle cricothyroid ligament

环甲肌直部
straight part of cricothyroid

环状软骨弓
arch of cricoid cartilage

舌骨大角
greater horn of hyoid bone

甲状舌骨外侧韧带
lateral thyrohyoid ligament

麦粒软骨
triticeal cartilage

甲状软骨上角
superior cornu of thyroid cartilage

甲状软骨
thyroid cartilage

斜线
oblique line

甲状软骨下角
inferior cornu of thyroid cartilage

环甲肌斜部
oblique part of cricothyroid

环甲关节囊
cricothyroid joint capsule

气管软骨
tracheal cartilage

451. 喉，舌骨，环甲肌（前外侧面观）

Larynx, hyoid bone, cricothyroid muscle (anterolateral aspect)

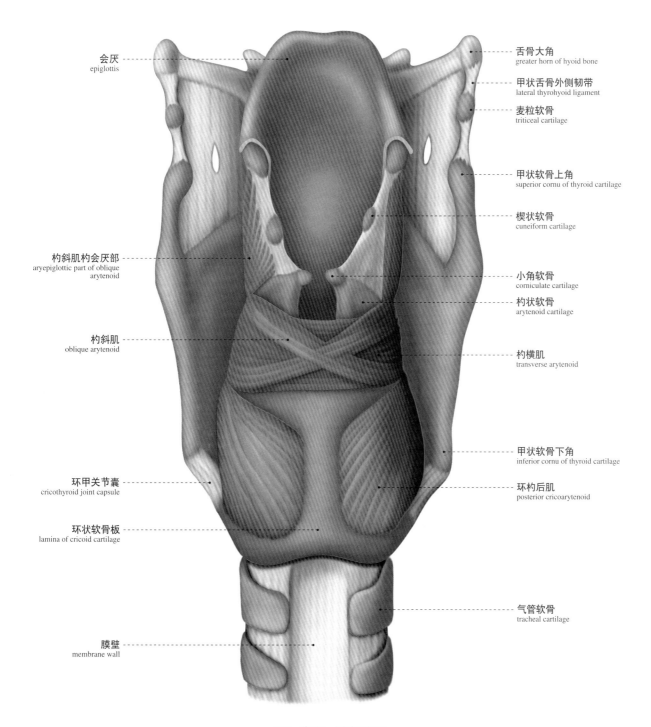

会厌
epiglottis

舌骨大角
greater horn of hyoid bone

甲状舌骨外侧韧带
lateral thyrohyoid ligament

麦粒软骨
triticeal cartilage

甲状软骨上角
superior cornu of thyroid cartilage

楔状软骨
cuneiform cartilage

杓斜肌杓会厌部
aryepiglottic part of oblique
arytenoid

小角软骨
corniculate cartilage

杓状软骨
arytenoid cartilage

杓斜肌
oblique arytenoid

杓横肌
transverse arytenoid

甲状软骨下角
inferior cornu of thyroid cartilage

环甲关节囊
cricothyroid joint capsule

环杓后肌
posterior cricoarytenoid

环状软骨板
lamina of cricoid cartilage

气管软骨
tracheal cartilage

膜壁
membrane wall

452. 喉肌（后面观）

Laryngeal muscles (posterior aspect)

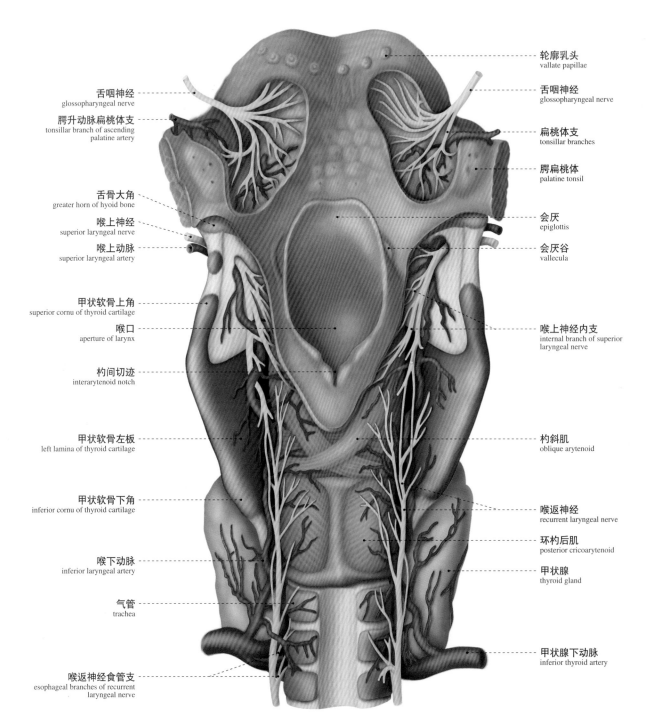

轮廓乳头
vallate papillae

舌咽神经
glossopharyngeal nerve

扁桃体支
tonsillar branches

腭扁桃体
palatine tonsil

会厌
epiglottis

会厌谷
vallecula

喉上神经内支
internal branch of superior laryngeal nerve

杓斜肌
oblique arytenoid

喉返神经
recurrent laryngeal nerve

环杓后肌
posterior cricoarytenoid

甲状腺
thyroid gland

甲状腺下动脉
inferior thyroid artery

舌咽神经
glossopharyngeal nerve

腭升动脉扁桃体支
tonsillar branch of ascending palatine artery

舌骨大角
greater horn of hyoid bone

喉上神经
superior laryngeal nerve

喉上动脉
superior laryngeal artery

甲状软骨上角
superior cornu of thyroid cartilage

喉口
aperture of larynx

杓间切迹
interarytenoid notch

甲状软骨左板
left lamina of thyroid cartilage

甲状软骨下角
inferior cornu of thyroid cartilage

喉下动脉
inferior laryngeal artery

气管
trachea

喉返神经食管支
esophageal branches of recurrent laryngeal nerve

453. 喉和舌的动脉和神经（后面观）
Arteries and nerves of the larynx and tongue (posterior aspect)

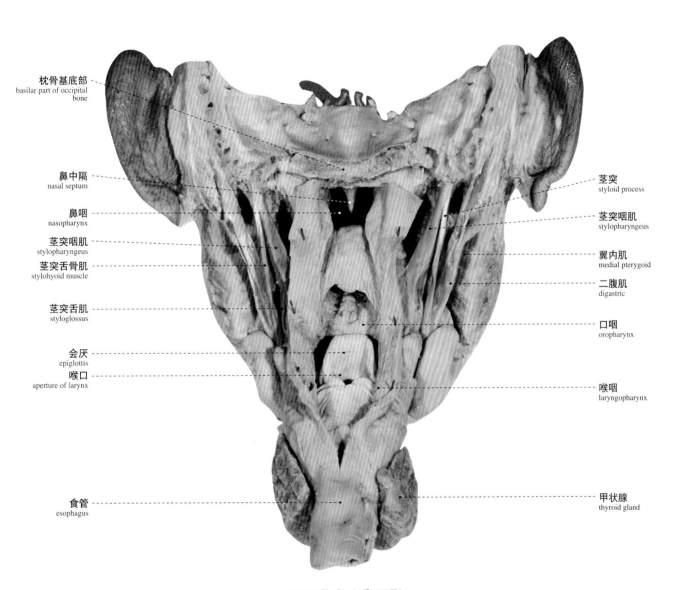

枕骨基底部
basilar part of occipital bone

鼻中隔
nasal septum

鼻咽
nasopharynx

茎突咽肌
stylopharyngeus

茎突舌骨肌
stylohyoid muscle

茎突舌肌
styloglossus

会厌
epiglottis

喉口
aperture of larynx

食管
esophagus

茎突
styloid process

茎突咽肌
stylopharyngeus

翼内肌
medial pterygoid

二腹肌
digastric

口咽
oropharynx

喉咽
laryngopharynx

甲状腺
thyroid gland

454. 咽腔（后面观）
Cavity of the pharynx (posterior aspect)

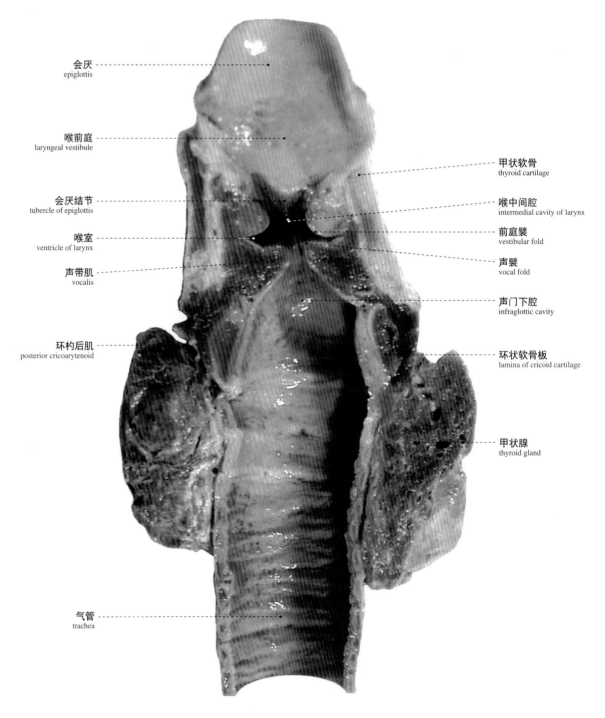

会厌
epiglottis

喉前庭
laryngeal vestibule

会厌结节
tubercle of epiglottis

喉室
ventricle of larynx

声带肌
vocalis

环杓后肌
posterior cricoarytenoid

气管
trachea

甲状软骨
thyroid cartilage

喉中间腔
intermedial cavity of larynx

前庭襞
vestibular fold

声襞
vocal fold

声门下腔
infraglottic cavity

环状软骨板
lamina of cricoid cartilage

甲状腺
thyroid gland

455. 喉冠状切面（后面观）
Coronal section of the larynx (posterior aspect)

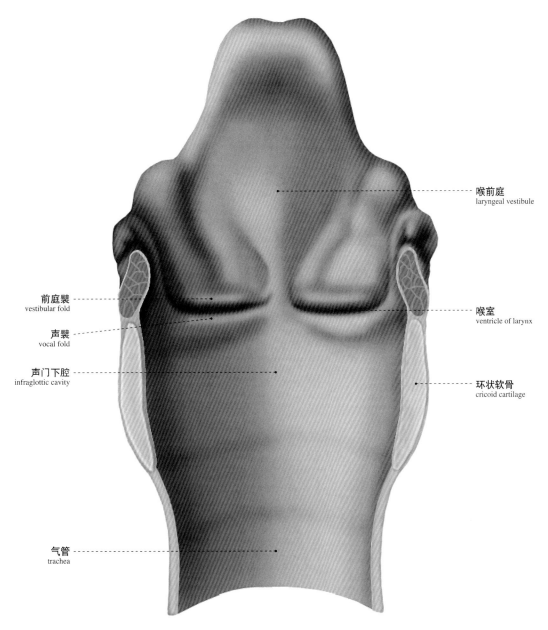

喉前庭
laryngeal vestibule

前庭襞
vestibular fold

声襞
vocal fold

声门下腔
infraglottic cavity

喉室
ventricle of larynx

环状软骨
cricoid cartilage

气管
trachea

456. 喉腔（后面观）
Laryngeal cavity (posterior aspect)

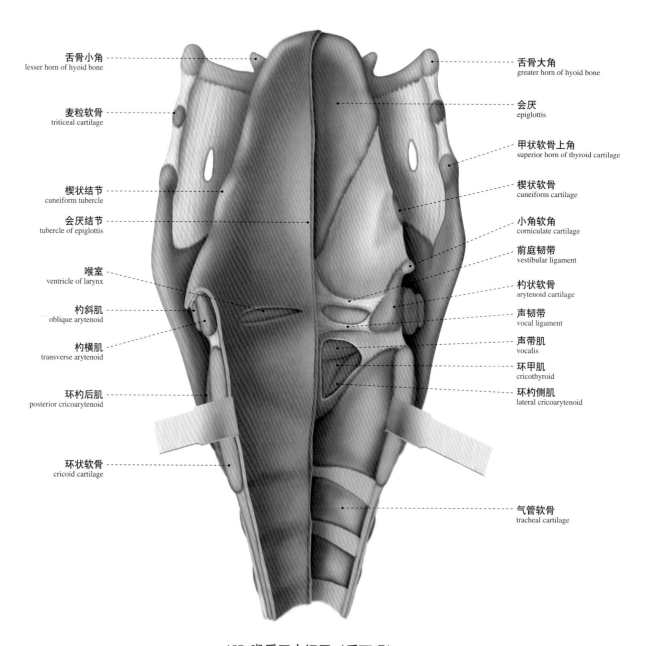

舌骨小角
lesser horn of hyoid bone

麦粒软骨
triticeal cartilage

楔状结节
cuneiform tubercle

会厌结节
tubercle of epiglottis

喉室
ventricle of larynx

杓斜肌
oblique arytenoid

杓横肌
transverse arytenoid

环杓后肌
posterior cricoarytenoid

环状软骨
cricoid cartilage

舌骨大角
greater horn of hyoid bone

会厌
epiglottis

甲状软骨上角
superior horn of thyroid cartilage

楔状软骨
cuneiform cartilage

小角软角
corniculate cartilage

前庭韧带
vestibular ligament

杓状软骨
arytenoid cartilage

声韧带
vocal ligament

声带肌
vocalis

环甲肌
cricothyroid

环杓侧肌
lateral cricoarytenoid

气管软骨
tracheal cartilage

457. 喉后正中切开（后面观）
Laryngeal posterior midline incision (posterior aspect)

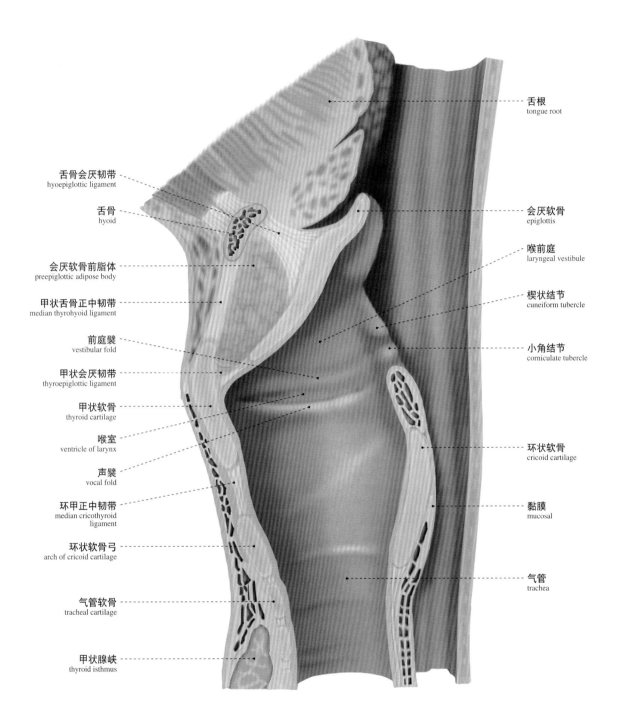

舌骨会厌韧带
hyoepiglottic ligament

舌骨
hyoid

会厌软骨前脂体
preepiglottic adipose body

甲状舌骨正中韧带
median thyrohyoid ligament

前庭襞
vestibular fold

甲状会厌韧带
thyroepiglottic ligament

甲状软骨
thyroid cartilage

喉室
ventricle of larynx

声襞
vocal fold

环甲正中韧带
median cricothyroid
ligament

环状软骨弓
arch of cricoid cartilage

气管软骨
tracheal cartilage

甲状腺峡
thyroid isthmus

舌根
tongue root

会厌软骨
epiglottis

喉前庭
laryngeal vestibule

楔状结节
cuneiform tubercle

小角结节
corniculate tubercle

环状软骨
cricoid cartilage

黏膜
mucosal

气管
trachea

458. 喉矢状切面（内侧面观1）
Sagittal section of the larynx (medial aspect 1)

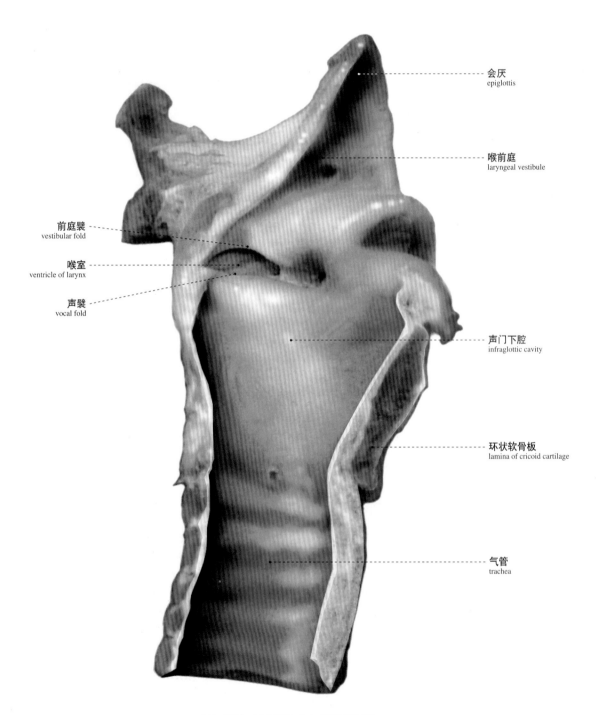

会厌
epiglottis

喉前庭
laryngeal vestibule

前庭襞
vestibular fold

喉室
ventricle of larynx

声襞
vocal fold

声门下腔
infraglottic cavity

环状软骨板
lamina of cricoid cartilage

气管
trachea

459. 喉矢状切面（内侧面观 2）

Sagittal section of the larynx (medial aspect 2)

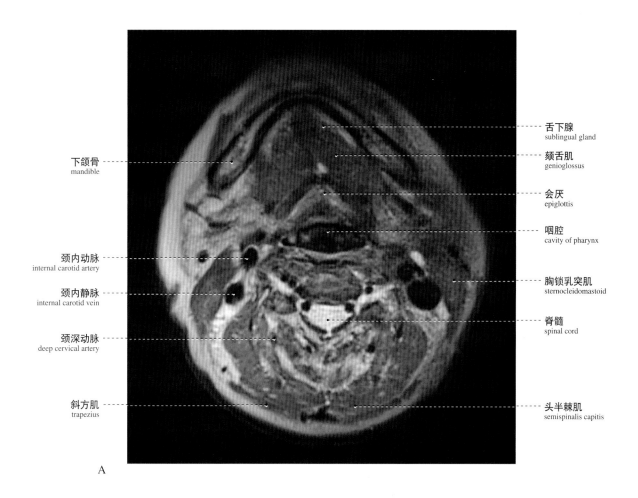

下颌骨
mandible

颈内动脉
internal carotid artery

颈内静脉
internal carotid vein

颈深动脉
deep cervical artery

斜方肌
trapezius

舌下腺
sublingual gland

颏舌肌
genioglossus

会厌
epiglottis

咽腔
cavity of pharynx

胸锁乳突肌
sternocleidomastoid

脊髓
spinal cord

头半棘肌
semispinalis capitis

A

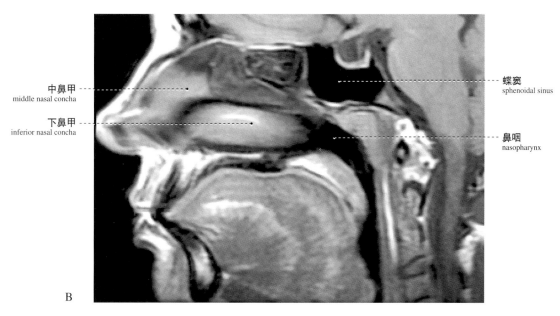

中鼻甲
middle nasal concha

下鼻甲
inferior nasal concha

蝶窦
sphenoidal sinus

鼻咽
nasopharynx

B

460. 喉部磁共振成像
MRI of the Larynx

A. 轴位；B. 矢状位

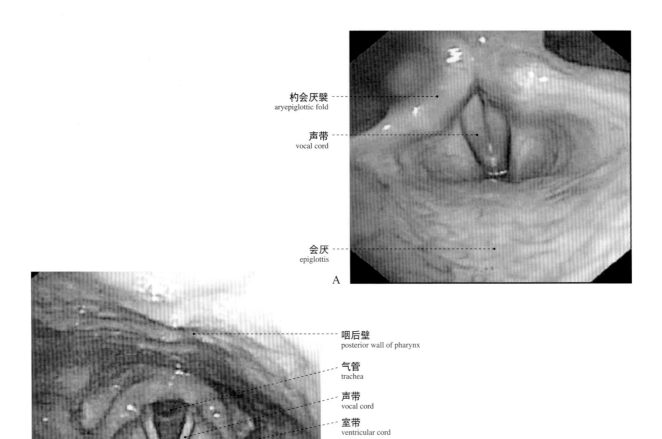

杓会厌襞
aryepiglottic fold

声带
vocal cord

会厌
epiglottis

A

咽后壁
posterior wall of pharynx

气管
trachea

声带
vocal cord

室带
ventricular cord

杓会厌襞
aryepiglottic fold

会厌
epiglottis

B

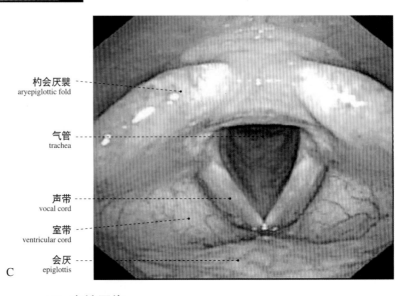

杓会厌襞
aryepiglottic fold

气管
trachea

声带
vocal cord

室带
ventricular cord

会厌
epiglottis

C

461. 喉镜图像
Laryngoscope image

第十章

甲状腺

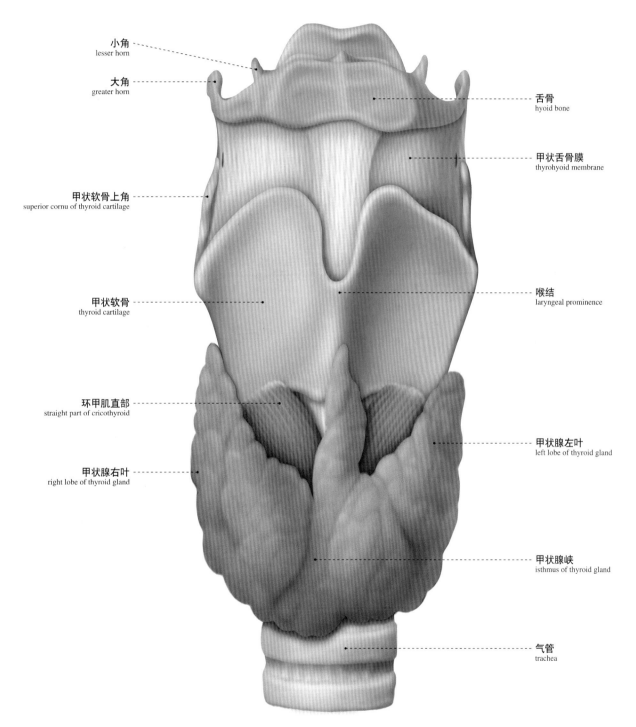

小角
lesser horn

大角
greater horn

甲状软骨上角
superior cornu of thyroid cartilage

甲状软骨
thyroid cartilage

环甲肌直部
straight part of cricothyroid

甲状腺右叶
right lobe of thyroid gland

舌骨
hyoid bone

甲状舌骨膜
thyrohyoid membrane

喉结
laryngeal prominence

甲状腺左叶
left lobe of thyroid gland

甲状腺峡
isthmus of thyroid gland

气管
trachea

462. 甲状腺（前面观）
Thyroid gland (anterior aspect)

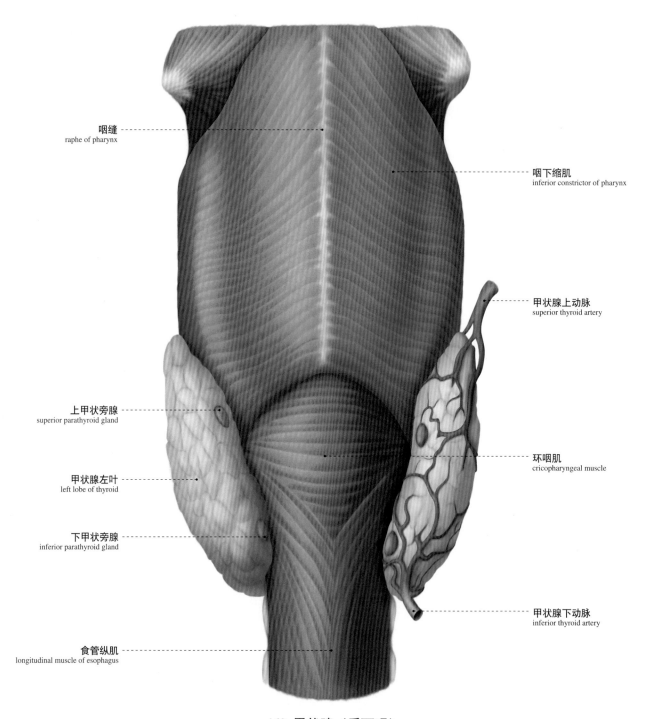

咽缝
raphe of pharynx

咽下缩肌
inferior constrictor of pharynx

甲状腺上动脉
superior thyroid artery

上甲状旁腺
superior parathyroid gland

环咽肌
cricopharyngeal muscle

甲状腺左叶
left lobe of thyroid

下甲状旁腺
inferior parathyroid gland

甲状腺下动脉
inferior thyroid artery

食管纵肌
longitudinal muscle of esophagus

463. 甲状腺（后面观）
Thyroid gland (posterior aspect)

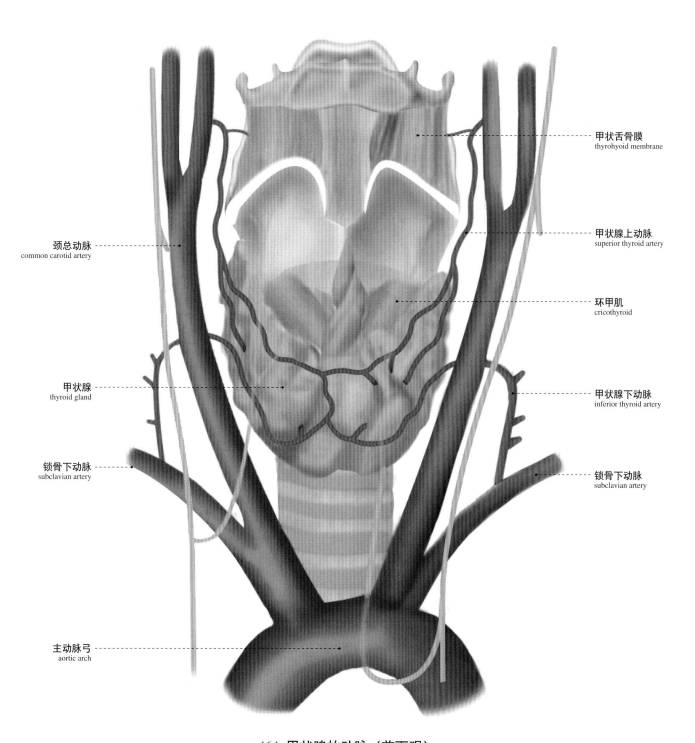

甲状舌骨膜
thyrohyoid membrane

甲状腺上动脉
superior thyroid artery

环甲肌
cricothyroid

甲状腺下动脉
inferior thyroid artery

锁骨下动脉
subclavian artery

颈总动脉
common carotid artery

甲状腺
thyroid gland

锁骨下动脉
subclavian artery

主动脉弓
aortic arch

464. 甲状腺的动脉（前面观）
Arteries of the thyroid gland (anterior aspect)

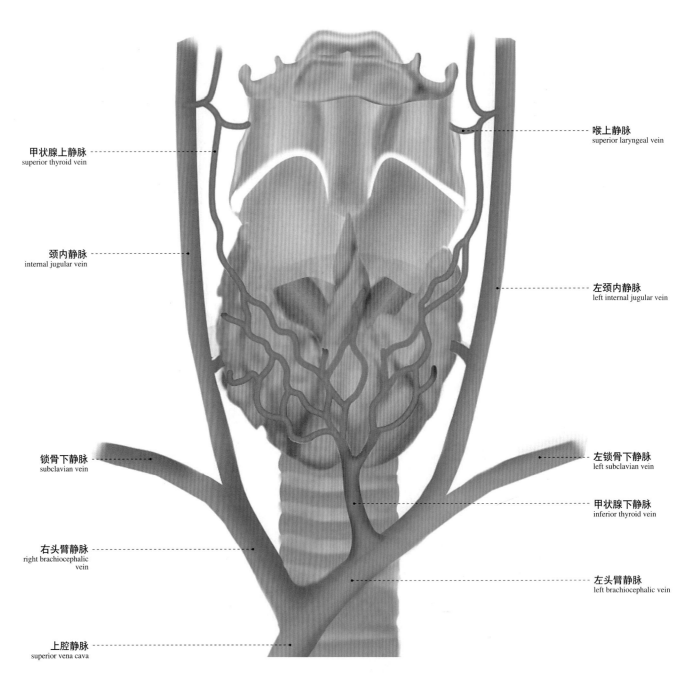

喉上静脉
superior laryngeal vein

甲状腺上静脉
superior thyroid vein

颈内静脉
internal jugular vein

左颈内静脉
left internal jugular vein

锁骨下静脉
subclavian vein

左锁骨下静脉
left subclavian vein

甲状腺下静脉
inferior thyroid vein

右头臂静脉
right brachiocephalic vein

左头臂静脉
left brachiocephalic vein

上腔静脉
superior vena cava

465. 甲状腺的静脉（前面观）
Veins of the thyroid gland (anterior aspect)

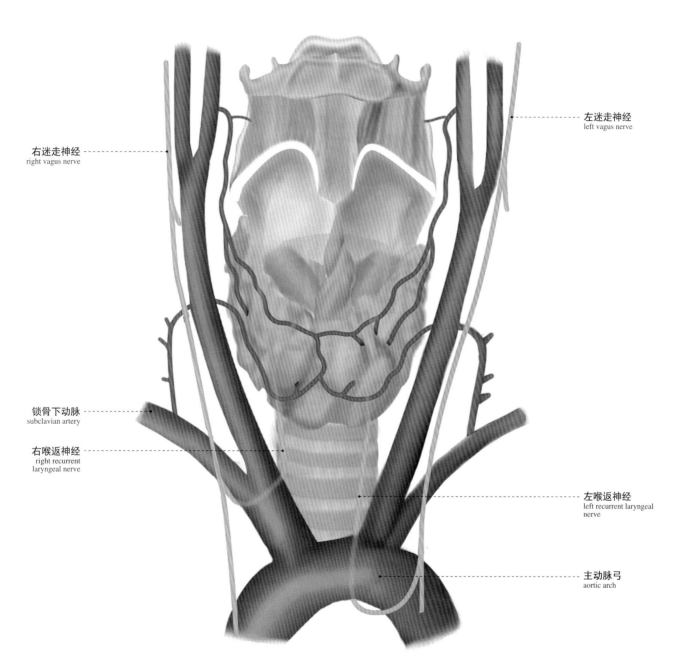

右迷走神经
right vagus nerve

左迷走神经
left vagus nerve

锁骨下动脉
subclavian artery

右喉返神经
right recurrent
laryngeal nerve

左喉返神经
left recurrent laryngeal
nerve

主动脉弓
aortic arch

466. 甲状腺的神经（前面观）
Nerves of the thyroid gland (anterior aspect)

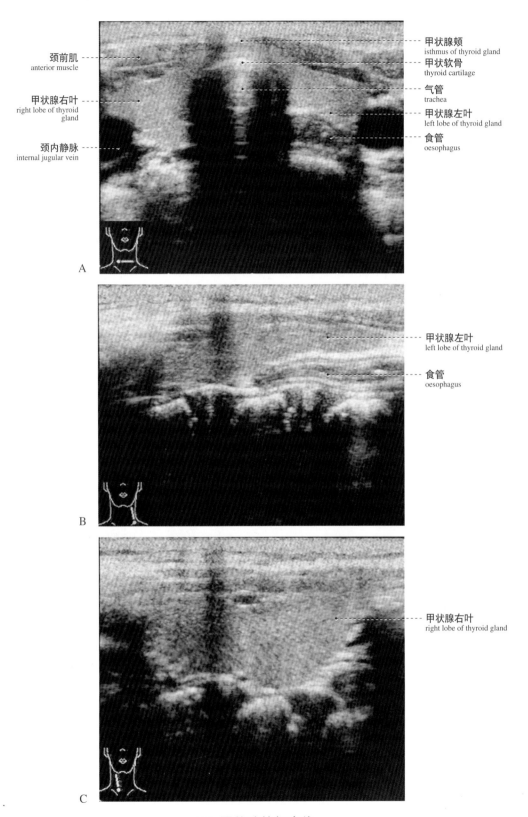

颈前肌
anterior muscle

甲状腺右叶
right lobe of thyroid gland

颈内静脉
internal jugular vein

甲状腺颊
isthmus of thyroid gland

甲状软骨
thyroid cartilage

气管
trachea

甲状腺左叶
left lobe of thyroid gland

食管
oesophagus

A

甲状腺左叶
left lobe of thyroid gland

食管
oesophagus

B

甲状腺右叶
right lobe of thyroid gland

C

467. 甲状腺的超声像

Thyroid ultrasound image

A. 颈部横切面观；B. 左颈部斜切面观；C. 右颈部斜切面观

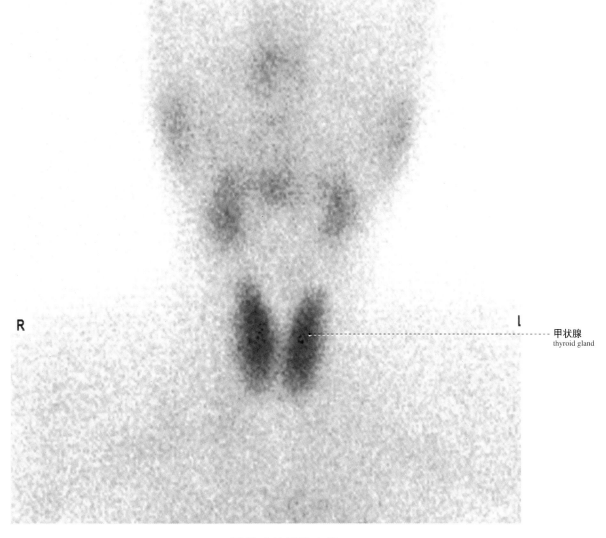

R   L

甲状腺
thyroid gland

468. 甲状腺的同位素像
Isotope image of the thyroid gland

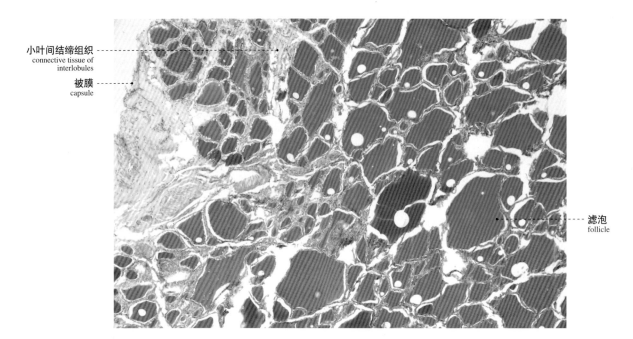

小叶间结缔组织
connective tissue of interlobules

被膜
capsule

滤泡
follicle

469. 甲状腺（人甲状腺，HE 染色，×40）
Thyroid gland (human thyroid gland, HE staining, ×40)

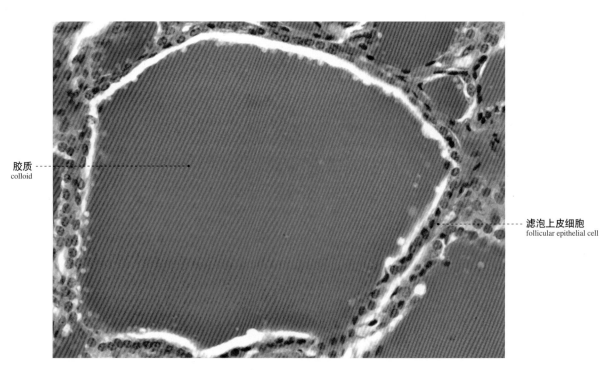

胶质
colloid

滤泡上皮细胞
follicular epithelial cell

470. 滤泡（人甲状腺，HE 染色，×100）
Follicle (human thyroid gland, HE staining, ×100)

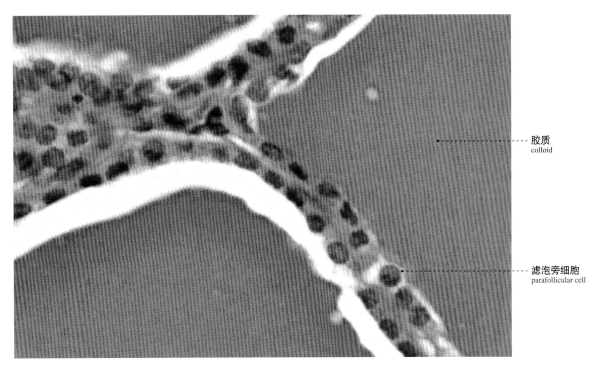

胶质
colloid

滤泡旁细胞
parafollicular cell

471. 滤泡旁细胞（人甲状腺，HE 染色，×400）

Parafollicular cell (human thyroid gland, HE staining, ×400)

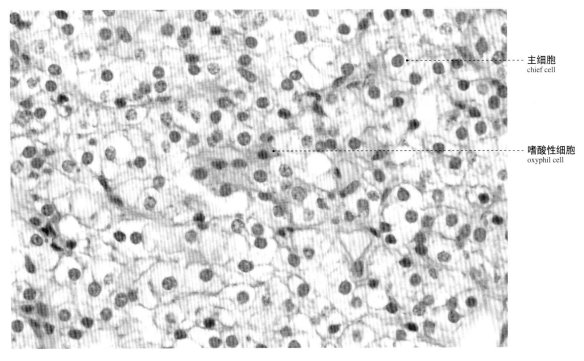

主细胞
chief cell

嗜酸性细胞
oxyphil cell

472. 甲状旁腺（人甲状旁腺，HE 染色，×400）

Parathyroid gland (human parathyroid gland, HE staining, ×400)

第十一章

口 部

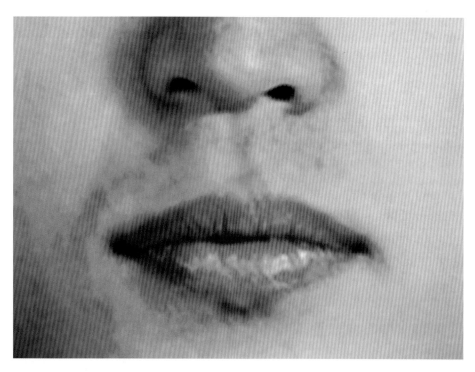

473. 口部体表
Mouth surface

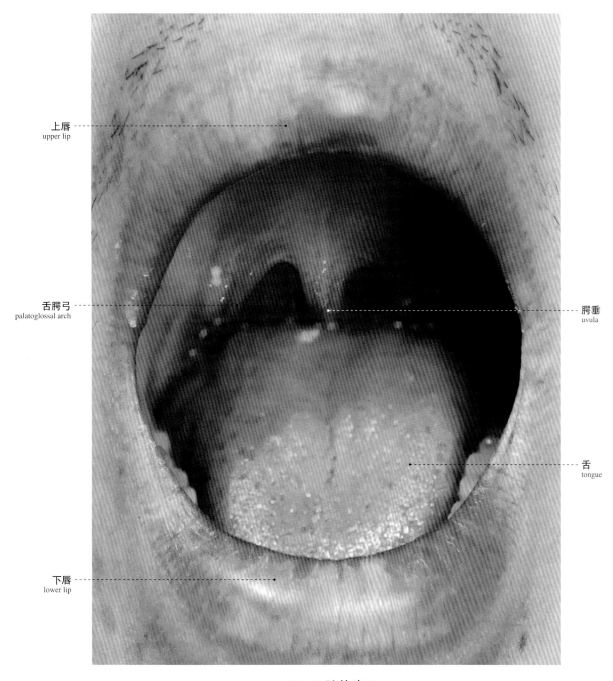

上唇
upper lip

舌腭弓
palatoglossal arch

腭垂
uvula

舌
tongue

下唇
lower lip

474. 口腔体表 1
Surface of the oral cavity 1

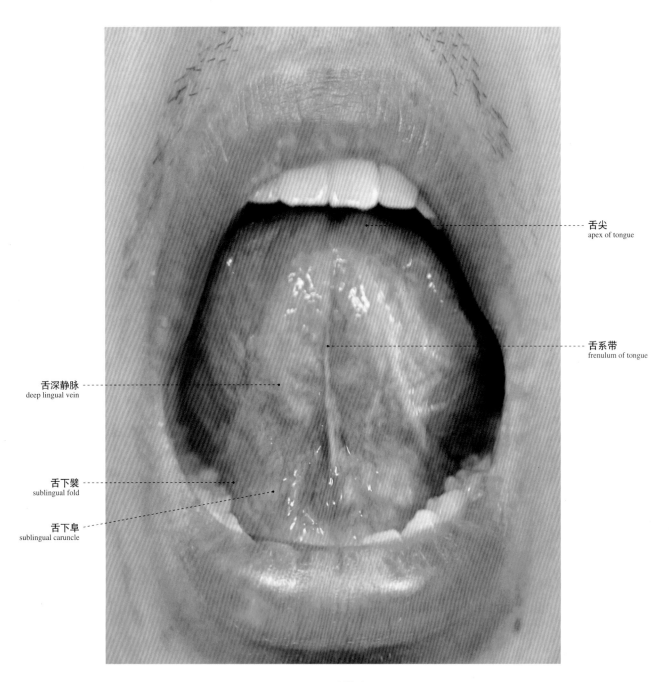

舌尖
apex of tongue

舌系带
frenulum of tongue

舌深静脉
deep lingual vein

舌下襞
sublingual fold

舌下阜
sublingual caruncle

475. 口腔体表 2
Surface of the oral cavity 2

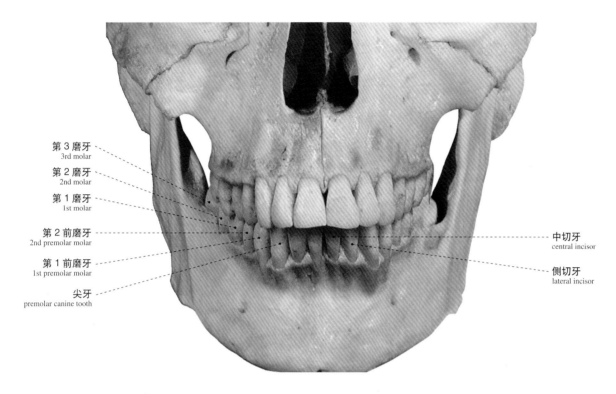

第 3 磨牙
3rd molar

第 2 磨牙
2nd molar

第 1 磨牙
1st molar

第 2 前磨牙
2nd premolar molar

第 1 前磨牙
1st premolar molar

尖牙
premolar canine tooth

中切牙
central incisor

侧切牙
lateral incisor

476. 牙齿（前面观）
Tooth (anterior aspect)

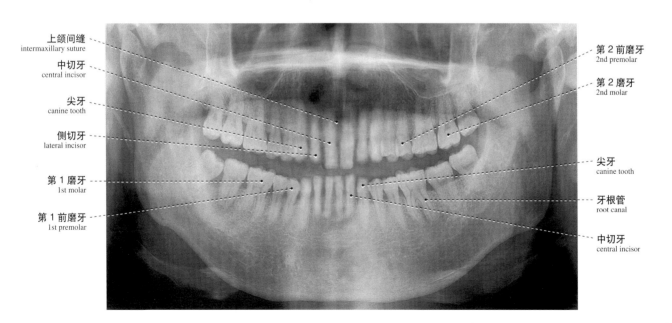

上颌间缝
intermaxillary suture

中切牙
central incisor

尖牙
canine tooth

侧切牙
lateral incisor

第 1 磨牙
1st molar

第 1 前磨牙
1st premolar

第 2 前磨牙
2nd premolar

第 2 磨牙
2nd molar

尖牙
canine tooth

牙根管
root canal

中切牙
central incisor

477. 牙齿 X 线像（前后位）
Radiograph of the tooth (anteroposterior view)

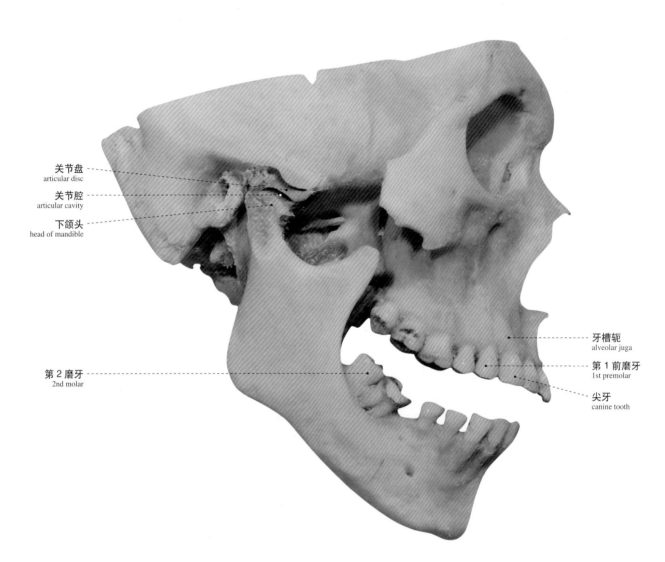

关节盘
articular disc

关节腔
articular cavity

下颌头
head of mandible

第 2 磨牙
2nd molar

牙槽轭
alveolar juga

第 1 前磨牙
1st premolar

尖牙
canine tooth

478. 口腔骨骼及牙齿（侧面观）
Oral bones and tooth (lateral aspect)

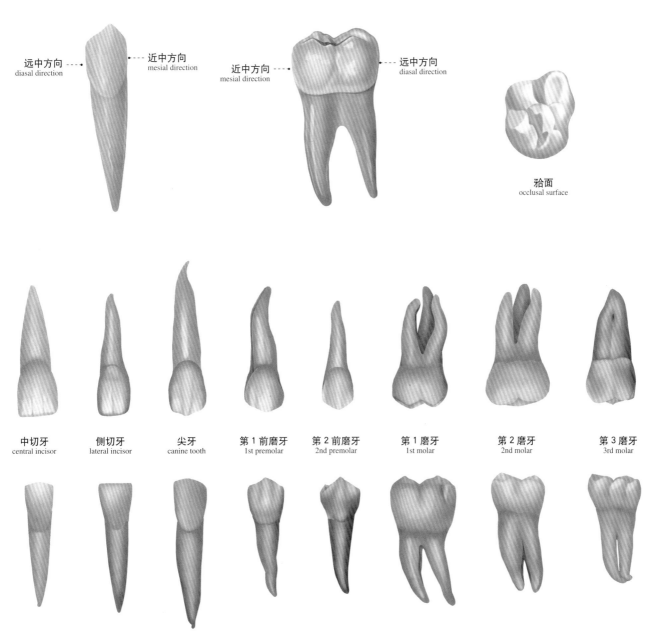

远中方向
diasal direction

近中方向
mesial direction

近中方向
mesial direction

远中方向
diasal direction

𬌗面
occlusal surface

中切牙
central incisor

侧切牙
lateral incisor

尖牙
canine tooth

第1前磨牙
1st premolar

第2前磨牙
2nd premolar

第1磨牙
1st molar

第2磨牙
2nd molar

第3磨牙
3rd molar

479. 上下颌恒牙（左侧）
Maxillary and mandibular permanent tooth (left)

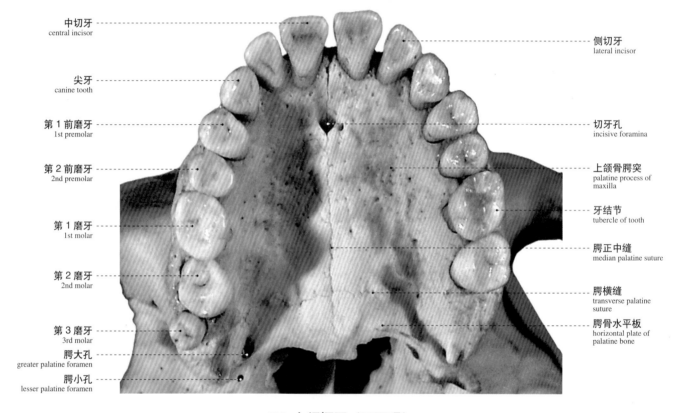

中切牙
central incisor

尖牙
canine tooth

第 1 前磨牙
1st premolar

第 2 前磨牙
2nd premolar

第 1 磨牙
1st molar

第 2 磨牙
2nd molar

第 3 磨牙
3rd molar

腭大孔
greater palatine foramen

腭小孔
lesser palatine foramen

侧切牙
lateral incisor

切牙孔
incisive foramina

上颌骨腭突
palatine process of maxilla

牙结节
tubercle of tooth

腭正中缝
median palatine suture

腭横缝
transverse palatine suture

腭骨水平板
horizontal plate of palatine bone

480. 上颌恒牙（下面观）
Maxillary permanent tooth (inferior aspect)

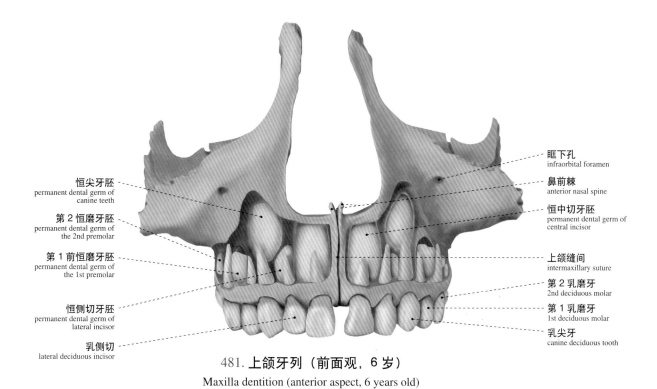

恒尖牙胚
permanent dental germ of
canine teeth

第 2 恒磨牙胚
permanent dental germ of
the 2nd premolar

第 1 前恒磨牙胚
permanent dental germ of
the 1st premolar

恒侧切牙胚
permanent dental germ of
lateral incisor

乳侧切
lateral deciduous incisor

眶下孔
infraorbital foramen

鼻前棘
anterior nasal spine

恒中切牙胚
permanent dental germ of
central incisor

上颌缝间
intermaxillary suture

第 2 乳磨牙
2nd deciduous molar

第 1 乳磨牙
1st deciduous molar

乳尖牙
canine deciduous tooth

481. 上颌牙列（前面观，6 岁）
Maxilla dentition (anterior aspect, 6 years old)

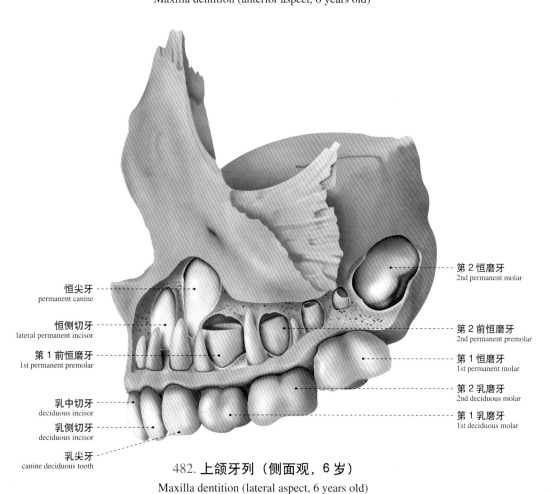

恒尖牙
permanent canine

恒侧切牙
lateral permanent incisor

第 1 前恒磨牙
1st permanent premolar

乳中切牙
deciduous incisor

乳侧切牙
deciduous incisor

乳尖牙
canine deciduous tooth

第 2 恒磨牙
2nd permanent molar

第 2 前恒磨牙
2nd permanent premolar

第 1 恒磨牙
1st permanent molar

第 2 乳磨牙
2nd deciduous molar

第 1 乳磨牙
1st deciduous molar

482. 上颌牙列（侧面观，6 岁）
Maxilla dentition (lateral aspect, 6 years old)

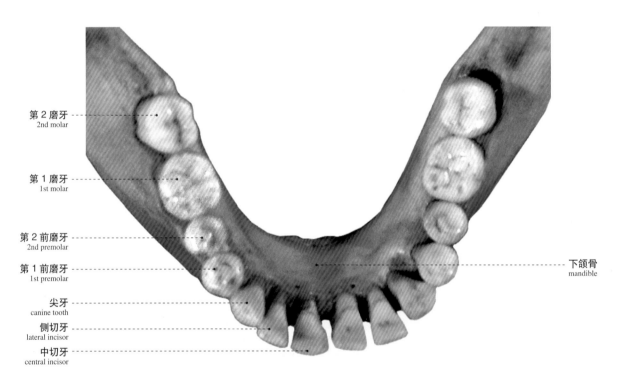

第2磨牙
2nd molar

第1磨牙
1st molar

第2前磨牙
2nd premolar

第1前磨牙
1st premolar

尖牙
canine tooth

侧切牙
lateral incisor

中切牙
central incisor

下颌骨
mandible

483. 下颌恒牙（上面观）
Mandibular permanent tooth (superior aspect)

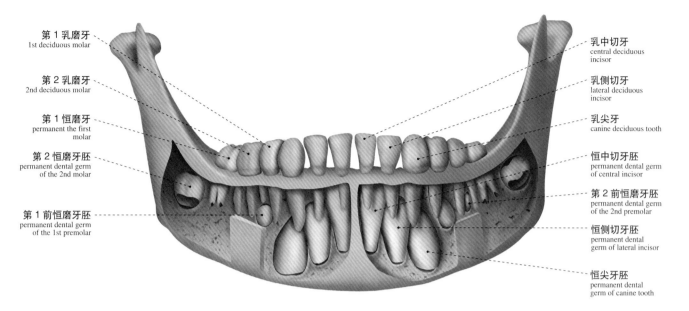

第 1 乳磨牙
1st deciduous molar

第 2 乳磨牙
2nd deciduous molar

第 1 恒磨牙
permanent the first
molar

第 2 恒磨牙胚
permanent dental germ
of the 2nd molar

第 1 前恒磨牙胚
permanent dental germ
of the 1st premolar

乳中切牙
central deciduous
incisor

乳侧切牙
lateral deciduous
incisor

乳尖牙
canine deciduous tooth

恒中切牙胚
permanent dental germ
of central incisor

第 2 前恒磨牙胚
permanent dental germ
of the 2nd premolar

恒侧切牙胚
permanent dental
germ of lateral incisor

恒尖牙胚
permanent dental
germ of canine tooth

484. 下颌牙列（前面观，6 岁）
Mandible dentition (anterior aspect, 6 years old)

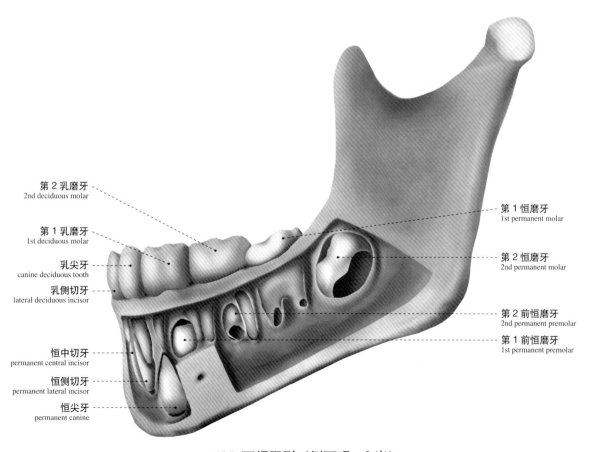

第 2 乳磨牙
2nd deciduous molar

第 1 乳磨牙
1st deciduous molar

乳尖牙
canine deciduous tooth

乳侧切牙
lateral deciduous incisor

恒中切牙
permanent central incisor

恒侧切牙
permanent lateral incisor

恒尖牙
permanent canine

第 1 恒磨牙
1st permanent molar

第 2 恒磨牙
2nd permanent molar

第 2 前恒磨牙
2nd permanent premolar

第 1 前恒磨牙
1st permanent premolar

485. 下颌牙列（侧面观，6 岁）
Mandible dentition (lateral aspect, 6 years old)

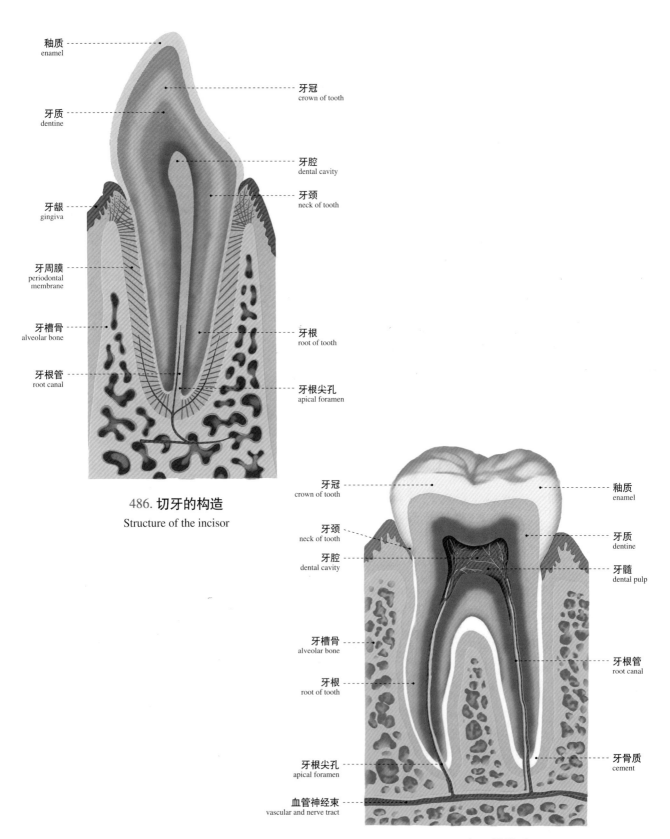

釉质
enamel

牙质
dentine

牙龈
gingiva

牙周膜
periodontal
membrane

牙槽骨
alveolar bone

牙根管
root canal

牙冠
crown of tooth

牙腔
dental cavity

牙颈
neck of tooth

牙根
root of tooth

牙根尖孔
apical foramen

486. 切牙的构造
Structure of the incisor

牙冠
crown of tooth

牙颈
neck of tooth

牙腔
dental cavity

牙槽骨
alveolar bone

牙根
root of tooth

牙根尖孔
apical foramen

血管神经束
vascular and nerve tract

釉质
enamel

牙质
dentine

牙髓
dental pulp

牙根管
root canal

牙骨质
cement

487. 磨牙的构造
Structure of the molar

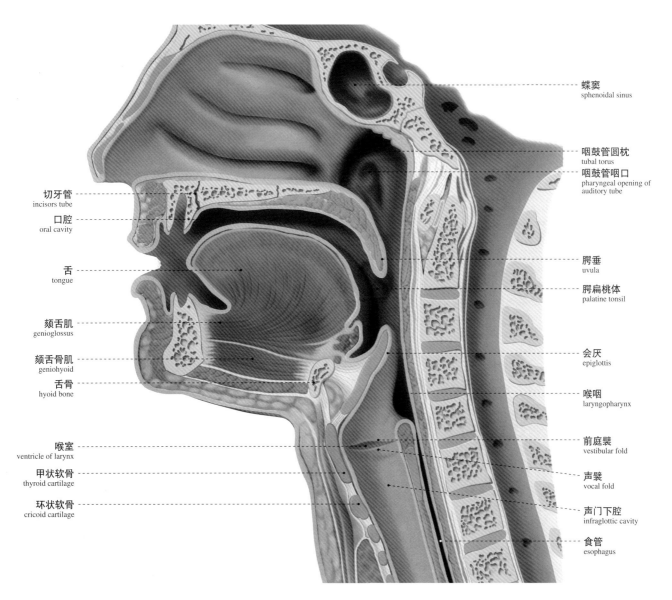

切牙管
incisors tube

口腔
oral cavity

舌
tongue

颏舌肌
genioglossus

颏舌骨肌
geniohyoid

舌骨
hyoid bone

喉室
ventricle of larynx

甲状软骨
thyroid cartilage

环状软骨
cricoid cartilage

蝶窦
sphenoidal sinus

咽鼓管圆枕
tubal torus

咽鼓管咽口
pharyngeal opening of
auditory tube

腭垂
uvula

腭扁桃体
palatine tonsil

会厌
epiglottis

喉咽
laryngopharynx

前庭襞
vestibular fold

声襞
vocal fold

声门下腔
infraglottic cavity

食管
esophagus

488. 口腔肌肉（正中矢状断面观）
Oral muscles (midsagittal section aspect)

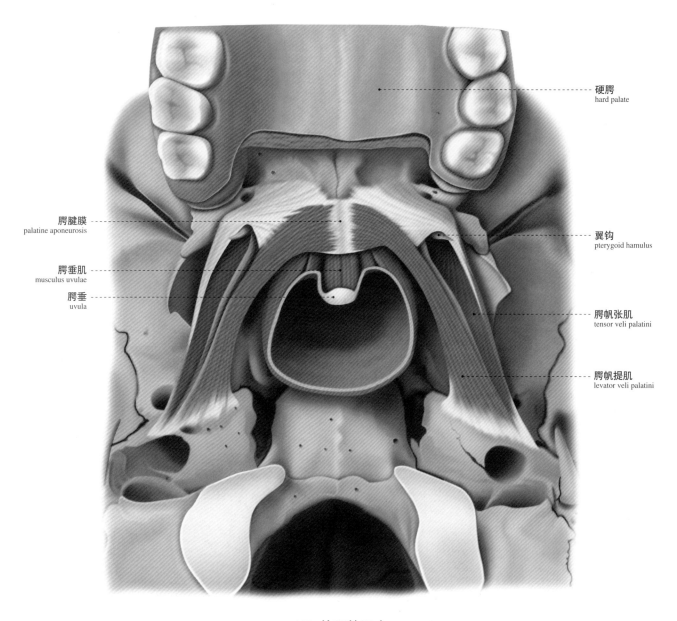

硬腭
hard palate

腭腱膜
palatine aponeurosis

腭垂肌
musculus uvulae

腭垂
uvula

翼钩
pterygoid hamulus

腭帆张肌
tensor veli palatini

腭帆提肌
levator veli palatini

489. 软腭的肌肉
Muscles of the soft palate

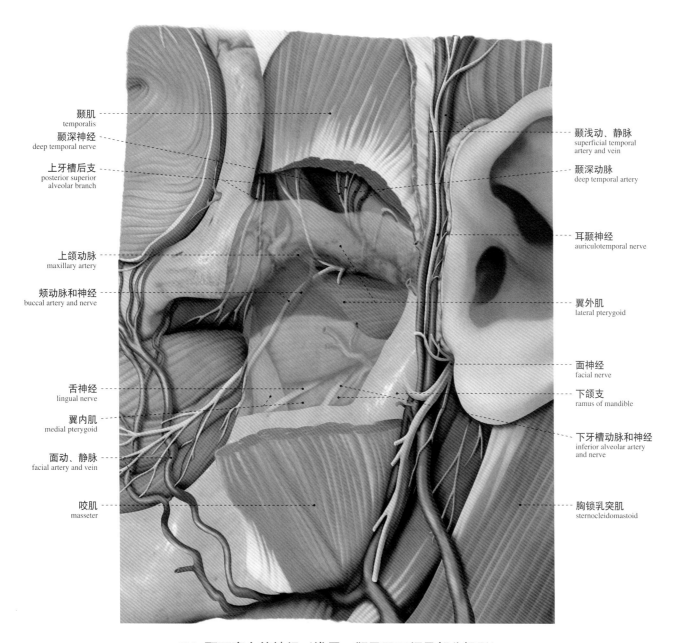

颞肌
temporalis

颞深神经
deep temporal nerve

上牙槽后支
posterior superior
alveolar branch

上颌动脉
maxillary artery

颊动脉和神经
buccal artery and nerve

舌神经
lingual nerve

翼内肌
medial pterygoid

面动、静脉
facial artery and vein

咬肌
masseter

颞浅动、静脉
superficial temporal
artery and vein

颞深动脉
deep temporal artery

耳颞神经
auriculotemporal nerve

翼外肌
lateral pterygoid

面神经
facial nerve

下颌支
ramus of mandible

下牙槽动脉和神经
inferior alveolar artery
and nerve

胸锁乳突肌
sternocleidomastoid

490. 颞下窝血管神经（浅层，颧弓及下颌骨部分投影）

Blood vessels and nerves of infratemporal fossa (superficial layer, the part projection of the zygomatic arch and mandibular)

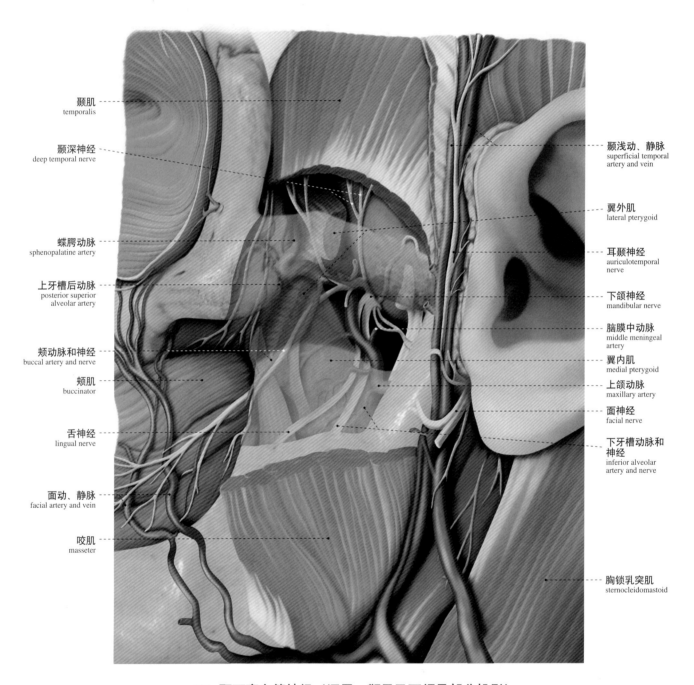

颞肌
temporalis

颞深神经
deep temporal nerve

蝶腭动脉
sphenopalatine artery

上牙槽后动脉
posterior superior
alveolar artery

颊动脉和神经
buccal artery and nerve

颊肌
buccinator

舌神经
lingual nerve

面动、静脉
facial artery and vein

咬肌
masseter

颞浅动、静脉
superficial temporal
artery and vein

翼外肌
lateral pterygoid

耳颞神经
auriculotemporal
nerve

下颌神经
mandibular nerve

脑膜中动脉
middle meningeal
artery

翼内肌
medial pterygoid

上颌动脉
maxillary artery

面神经
facial nerve

下牙槽动脉和
神经
inferior alveolar
artery and nerve

胸锁乳突肌
sternocleidomastoid

491. 颞下窝血管神经（深层，颧弓及下颌骨部分投影）

Blood vessels and nerves of infratemporal fossa (deep layer, the part projection of the zygomatic arch and mandibular)

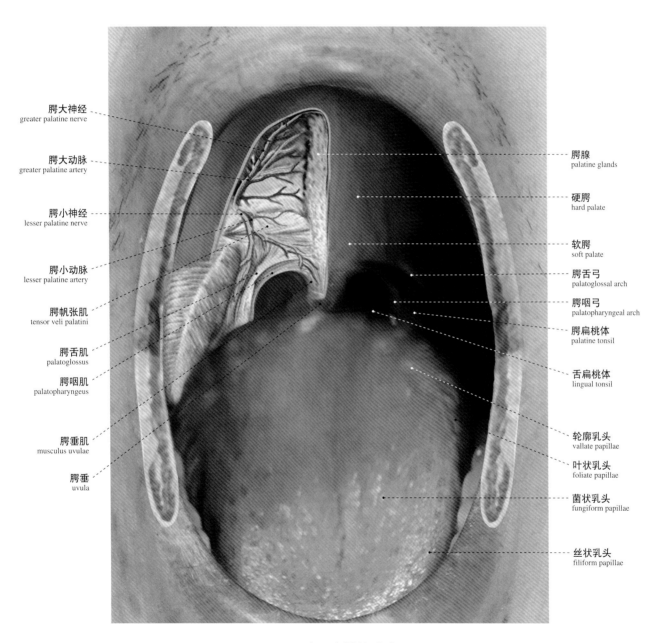

腭大神经
greater palatine nerve

腭大动脉
greater palatine artery

腭小神经
lesser palatine nerve

腭小动脉
lesser palatine artery

腭帆张肌
tensor veli palatini

腭舌肌
palatoglossus

腭咽肌
palatopharyngeus

腭垂肌
musculus uvulae

腭垂
uvula

腭腺
palatine glands

硬腭
hard palate

软腭
soft palate

腭舌弓
palatoglossal arch

腭咽弓
palatopharyngeal arch

腭扁桃体
palatine tonsil

舌扁桃体
lingual tonsil

轮廓乳头
vallate papillae

叶状乳头
foliate papillae

菌状乳头
fungiform papillae

丝状乳头
filiform papillae

492. 口腔及扁桃体动脉
Oral cavity and the arteries of the palatine tonsil

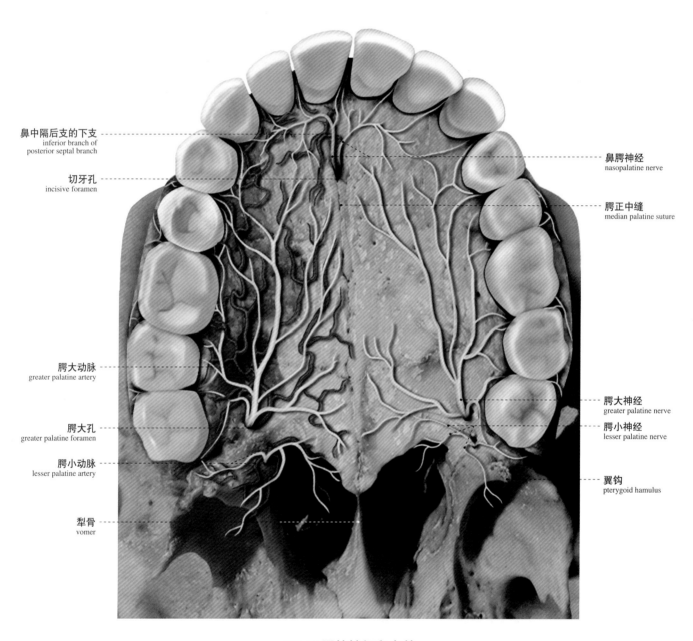

鼻中隔后支的下支
inferior branch of
posterior septal branch

切牙孔
incisive foramen

腭大动脉
greater palatine artery

腭大孔
greater palatine foramen

腭小动脉
lesser palatine artery

犁骨
vomer

鼻腭神经
nasopalatine nerve

腭正中缝
median palatine suture

腭大神经
greater palatine nerve

腭小神经
lesser palatine nerve

翼钩
pterygoid hamulus

493. 硬腭的神经和血管

Nerves and blood vessels of the hard palate

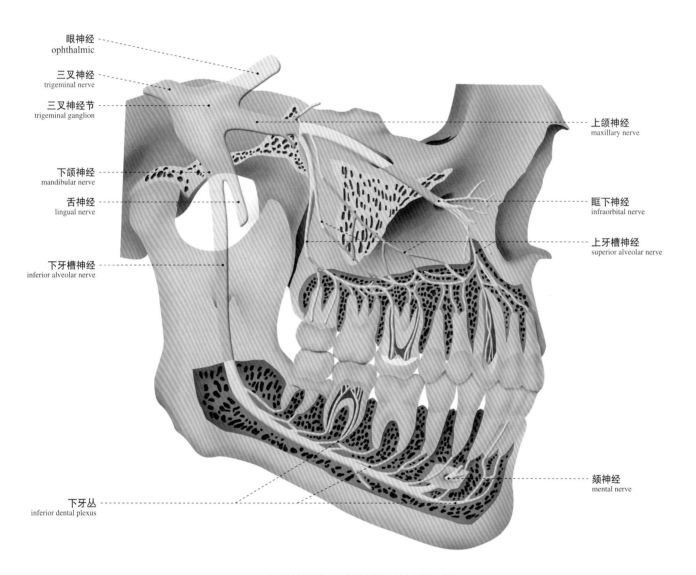

眼神经
ophthalmic

三叉神经
trigeminal nerve

三叉神经节
trigeminal ganglion

下颌神经
mandibular nerve

舌神经
lingual nerve

下牙槽神经
inferior alveolar nerve

下牙丛
inferior dental plexus

上颌神经
maxillary nerve

眶下神经
infraorbital nerve

上牙槽神经
superior alveolar nerve

颏神经
mental nerve

494. 上颌神经和下颌神经（外侧面观）
Maxillary nerves and mandibular nerves (lateral aspect)

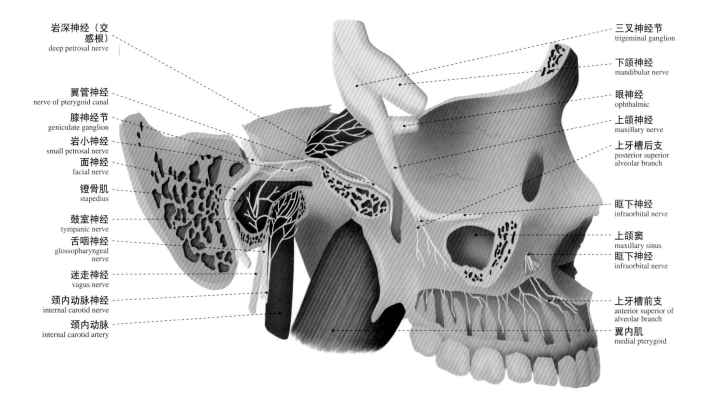

岩深神经（交
感根）
deep petrosal nerve

翼管神经
nerve of pterygoid canal

膝神经节
geniculate ganglion

岩小神经
small petrosal nerve

面神经
facial nerve

镫骨肌
stapedius

鼓室神经
tympanic nerve

舌咽神经
glossopharyngeal
nerve

迷走神经
vagus nerve

颈内动脉神经
internal carotid nerve

颈内动脉
internal carotid artery

三叉神经节
trigeminal ganglion

下颌神经
mandibular nerve

眼神经
ophthalmic

上颌神经
maxillary nerve

上牙槽后支
posterior superior
alveolar branch

眶下神经
infraorbital nerve

上颌窦
maxillary sinus

眶下神经
infraorbital nerve

上牙槽前支
anterior superior of
alveolar branch

翼内肌
medial pterygoid

495. 翼腭神经节的根（外侧面观）
Root of the pterygopalatine ganglion (lateral aspect)

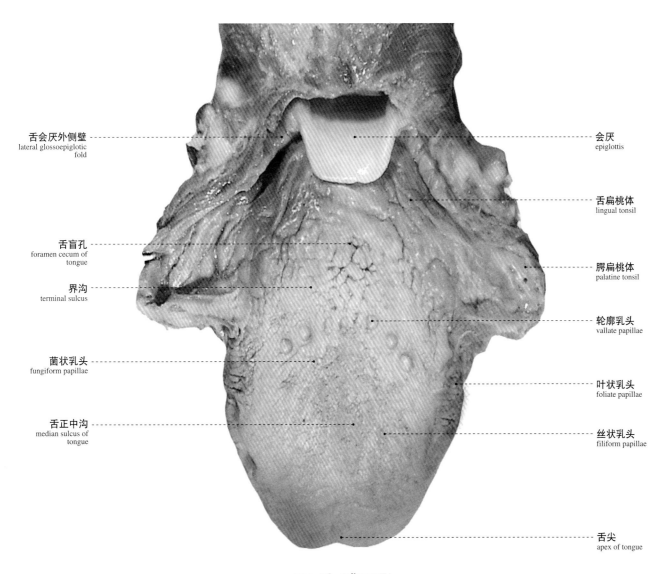

舌会厌外侧壁
lateral glossoepiglotic fold

会厌
epiglottis

舌盲孔
foramen cecum of tongue

舌扁桃体
lingual tonsil

界沟
terminal sulcus

腭扁桃体
palatine tonsil

轮廓乳头
vallate papillae

菌状乳头
fungiform papillae

叶状乳头
foliate papillae

舌正中沟
median sulcus of tongue

丝状乳头
filiform papillae

舌尖
apex of tongue

496. 舌（背面观）
Tongue (dorsal aspect)

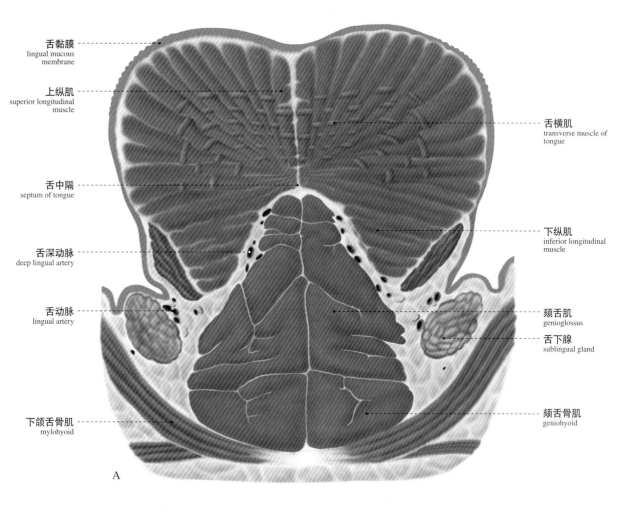

舌黏膜
lingual mucous membrane

上纵肌
superior longitudinal muscle

舌中隔
septum of tongue

舌深动脉
deep lingual artery

舌动脉
lingual artery

下颌舌骨肌
mylohyoid

舌横肌
transverse muscle of tongue

下纵肌
inferior longitudinal muscle

颏舌肌
genioglossus

舌下腺
sublingual gland

颏舌骨肌
geniohyoid

A

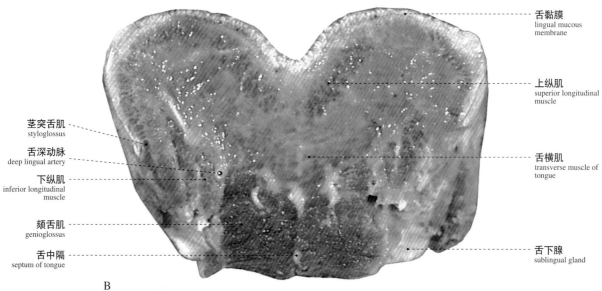

舌黏膜
lingual mucous membrane

上纵肌
superior longitudinal muscle

舌横肌
transverse muscle of tongue

茎突舌肌
styloglossus

舌深动脉
deep lingual artery

下纵肌
inferior longitudinal muscle

颏舌肌
genioglossus

舌中隔
septum of tongue

舌下腺
sublingual gland

B

497. 舌（冠状切面）
Tongue (coronal section)

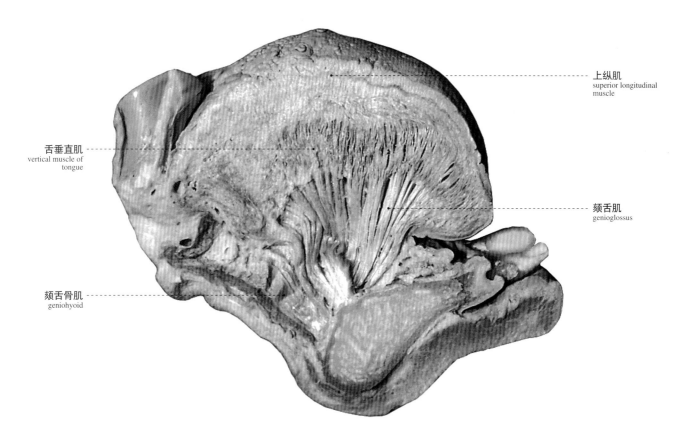

舌垂直肌
vertical muscle of
tongue

颏舌骨肌
geniohyoid

上纵肌
superior longitudinal
muscle

颏舌肌
genioglossus

498. 舌（矢状切面）
Tongue (sagittal section)

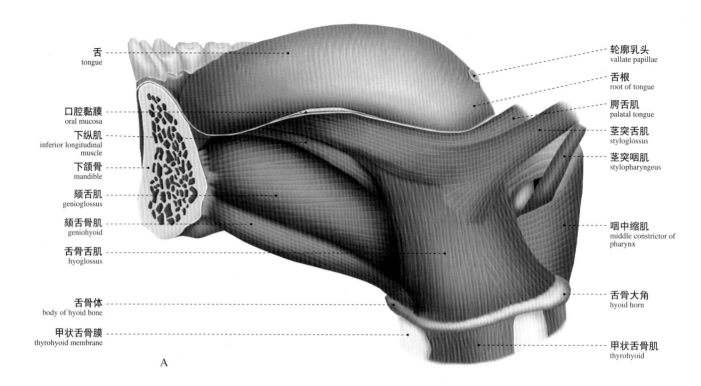

舌
tongue

口腔黏膜
oral mucosa

下纵肌
inferior longitudinal
muscle

下颌骨
mandible

颏舌肌
genioglossus

颏舌骨肌
geniohyoid

舌骨舌肌
hyoglossus

舌骨体
body of hyoid bone

甲状舌骨膜
thyrohyoid membrane

轮廓乳头
vallate papillae

舌根
root of tongue

腭舌肌
palatal tongue

茎突舌肌
styloglossus

茎突咽肌
stylopharyngeus

咽中缩肌
middle constrictor of
pharynx

舌骨大角
hyoid horn

甲状舌骨肌
thyrohyoid

A

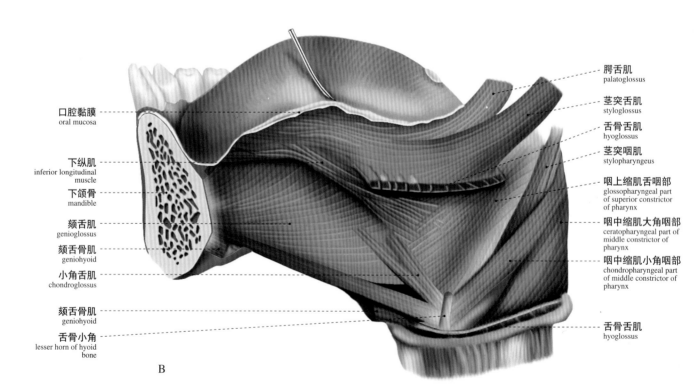

口腔黏膜
oral mucosa

下纵肌
inferior longitudinal
muscle

下颌骨
mandible

颏舌肌
genioglossus

颏舌骨肌
geniohyoid

小角舌肌
chondroglossus

颏舌骨肌
geniohyoid

舌骨小角
lesser horn of hyoid
bone

腭舌肌
palatoglossus

茎突舌肌
styloglossus

舌骨舌肌
hyoglossus

茎突咽肌
stylopharyngeus

咽上缩肌舌咽部
glossopharyngeal part
of superior constrictor
of pharynx

咽中缩肌大角咽部
ceratopharyngeal part of
middle constrictor of
pharynx

咽中缩肌小角咽部
chondropharyngeal part
of middle constrictor of
pharynx

舌骨舌肌
hyoglossus

B

499. 舌肌（外侧面观）
Muscles of the tongue (lateral aspect)

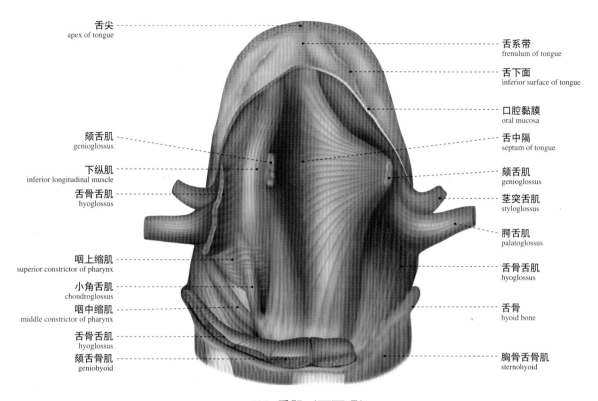

舌尖
apex of tongue

舌系带
frenulum of tongue

舌下面
inferior surface of tongue

口腔黏膜
oral mucosa

颏舌肌
genioglossus

舌中隔
septum of tongue

下纵肌
inferior longitudinal muscle

颏舌肌
genioglossus

舌骨舌肌
hyoglossus

茎突舌肌
styloglossus

腭舌肌
palatoglossus

咽上缩肌
superior constrictor of pharynx

舌骨舌肌
hyoglossus

小角舌肌
chondroglossus

咽中缩肌
middle constrictor of pharynx

舌骨
hyoid bone

舌骨舌肌
hyoglossus

颏舌骨肌
geniohyoid

胸骨舌骨肌
sternohyoid

500. 舌肌（下面观）
Muscles of the tongue (inferior aspect)

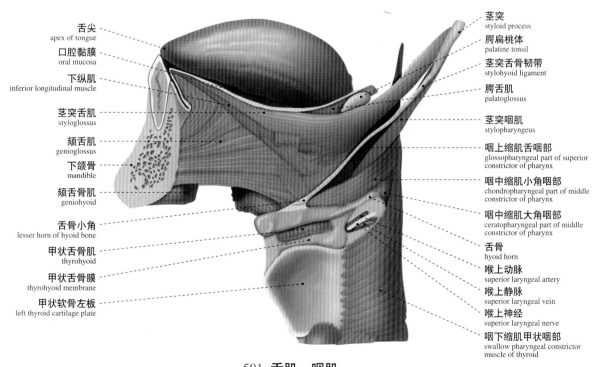

舌尖
apex of tongue

茎突
styloid process

口腔黏膜
oral mucosa

腭扁桃体
palatine tonsil

下纵肌
inferior longitudinal muscle

茎突舌骨韧带
stylohyoid ligament

腭舌肌
palatoglossus

茎突舌肌
styloglossus

茎突咽肌
stylopharyngeus

颏舌肌
genioglossus

咽上缩肌舌咽部
glossopharyngeal part of superior constrictor of pharynx

下颌骨
mandible

咽中缩肌小角咽部
chondropharyngeal part of middle constrictor of pharynx

颏舌骨肌
geniohyoid

咽中缩肌大角咽部
ceratopharyngeal part of middle constrictor of pharynx

舌骨小角
lesser horn of hyoid bone

舌骨
hyoid horn

甲状舌骨肌
thyrohyoid

喉上动脉
superior laryngeal artery

甲状舌骨膜
thyrohyoid membrane

喉上静脉
superior laryngeal vein

甲状软骨左板
left thyroid cartilage plate

喉上神经
superior laryngeal nerve

咽下缩肌甲状咽部
swallow pharyngeal constrictor muscle of thyroid

501. 舌肌、咽肌
Muscles of the tongue and pharynx

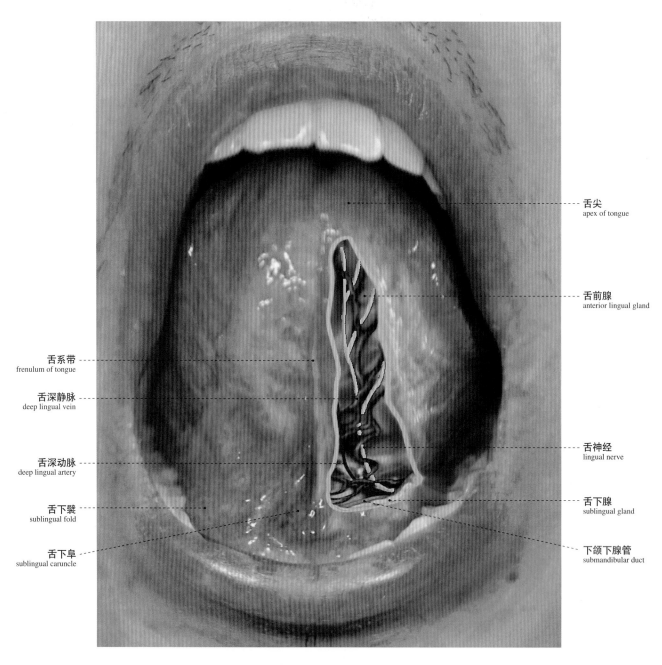

舌尖
apex of tongue

舌前腺
anterior lingual gland

舌系带
frenulum of tongue

舌深静脉
deep lingual vein

舌深动脉
deep lingual artery

舌下襞
sublingual fold

舌下阜
sublingual caruncle

舌神经
lingual nerve

舌下腺
sublingual gland

下颌下腺管
submandibular duct

502. 舌的血管神经
Blood vessels and nerves of the tongue

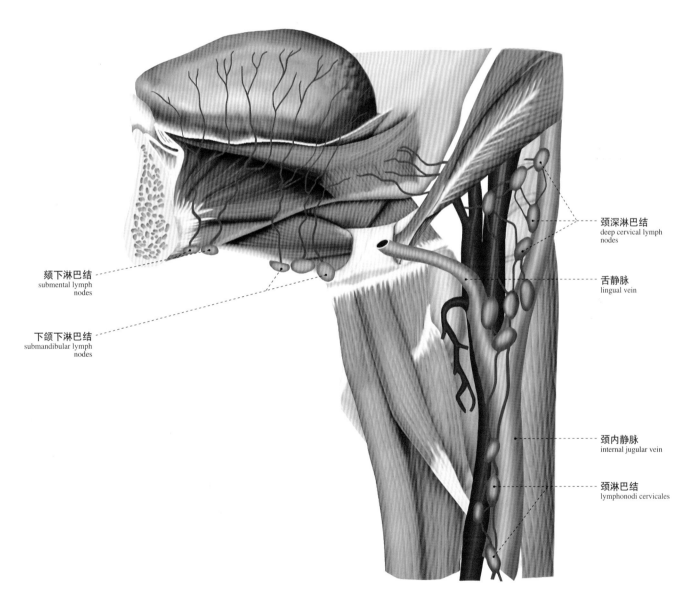

颈深淋巴结
deep cervical lymph
nodes

舌静脉
lingual vein

颏下淋巴结
submental lymph
nodes

下颌下淋巴结
submandibular lymph
nodes

颈内静脉
internal jugular vein

颈淋巴结
lymphonodi cervicales

503. 舌与口腔底淋巴（侧面观）
Lymph of the tongue and oral floor (lateral aspect)

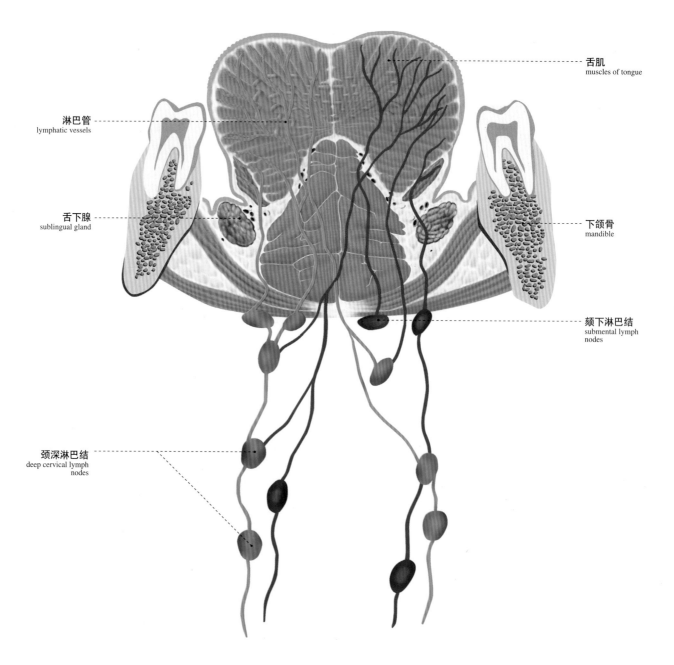

淋巴管
lymphatic vessels

舌下腺
sublingual gland

颈深淋巴结
deep cervical lymph nodes

舌肌
muscles of tongue

下颌骨
mandible

颏下淋巴结
submental lymph nodes

504. 舌与口腔底淋巴（前面观）
Lymph of the tongue and oral floor (anterior aspect)

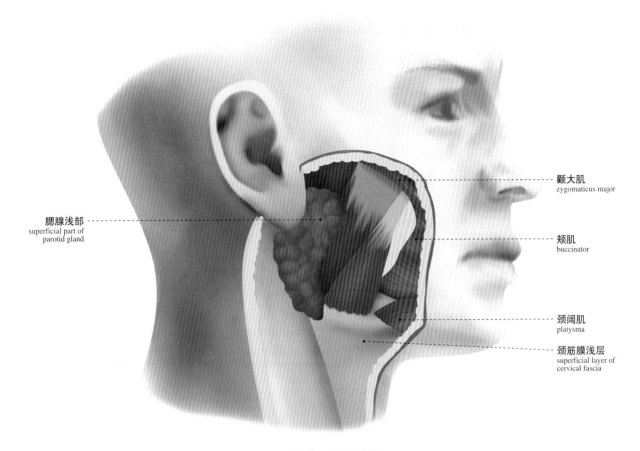

颧大肌
zygomaticus major

颊肌
buccinator

腮腺浅部
superficial part of
parotid gland

颈阔肌
platysma

颈筋膜浅层
superficial layer of
cervical fascia

505. 腮腺（侧面观）
Parotid gland (lateral aspect)

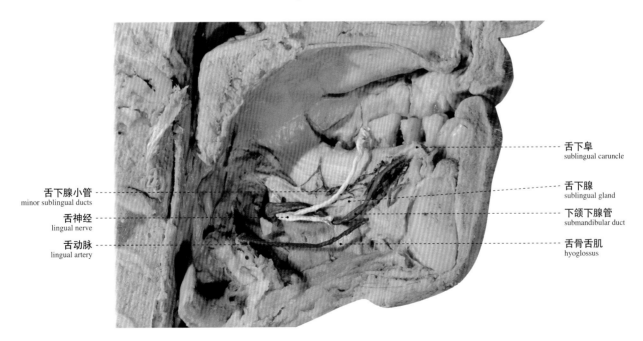

舌下阜
sublingual caruncle

舌下腺小管
minor sublingual ducts

舌神经
lingual nerve

舌动脉
lingual artery

舌下腺
sublingual gland

下颌下腺管
submandibular duct

舌骨舌肌
hyoglossus

506. 口腔腺（内侧面观）
Oral glands (medial aspect)

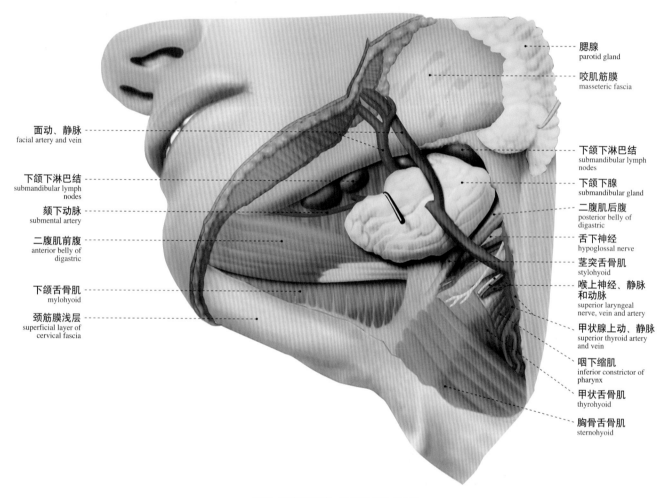

面动、静脉
facial artery and vein

下颌下淋巴结
submandibular lymph nodes

颏下动脉
submental artery

二腹肌前腹
anterior belly of digastric

下颌舌骨肌
mylohyoid

颈筋膜浅层
superficial layer of cervical fascia

腮腺
parotid gland

咬肌筋膜
masseteric fascia

下颌下淋巴结
submandibular lymph nodes

下颌下腺
submandibular gland

二腹肌后腹
posterior belly of digastric

舌下神经
hypoglossal nerve

茎突舌骨肌
stylohyoid

喉上神经、静脉和动脉
superior laryngeal nerve, vein and artery

甲状腺上动、静脉
superior thyroid artery and vein

咽下缩肌
inferior constrictor of pharynx

甲状舌骨肌
thyrohyoid

胸骨舌骨肌
sternohyoid

507. 下颌下腺（下外侧面观）
Submandibular gland (inferolateral aspect)

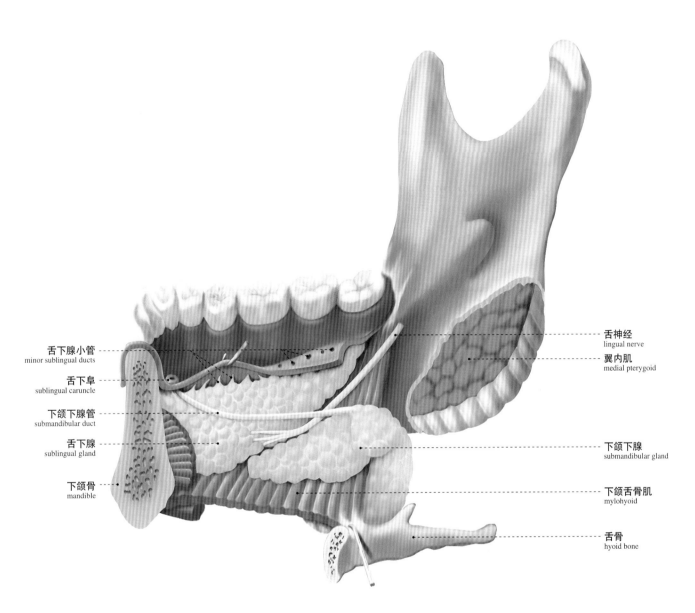

舌下腺小管
minor sublingual ducts

舌下阜
sublingual caruncle

下颌下腺管
submandibular duct

舌下腺
sublingual gland

下颌骨
mandible

舌神经
lingual nerve

翼内肌
medial pterygoid

下颌下腺
submandibular gland

下颌舌骨肌
mylohyoid

舌骨
hyoid bone

508. 下颌下腺和舌下腺（内侧面观）
Submandibular gland and sublingual gland (medial aspect)

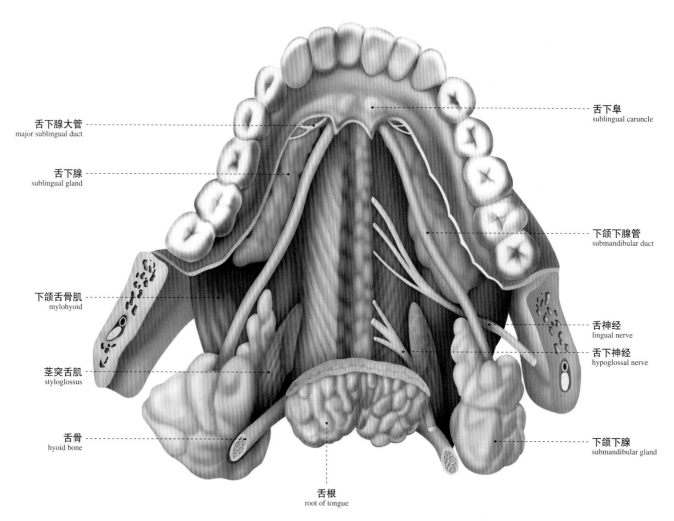

舌下腺大管
major sublingual duct

舌下腺
sublingual gland

下颌舌骨肌
mylohyoid

茎突舌肌
styloglossus

舌骨
hyoid bone

舌下阜
sublingual caruncle

下颌下腺管
submandibular duct

舌神经
lingual nerve

舌下神经
hypoglossal nerve

下颌下腺
submandibular gland

舌根
root of tongue

509. 下颌下腺和舌下腺（上面观）
Submandibular gland and sublingual gland (superior aspect)

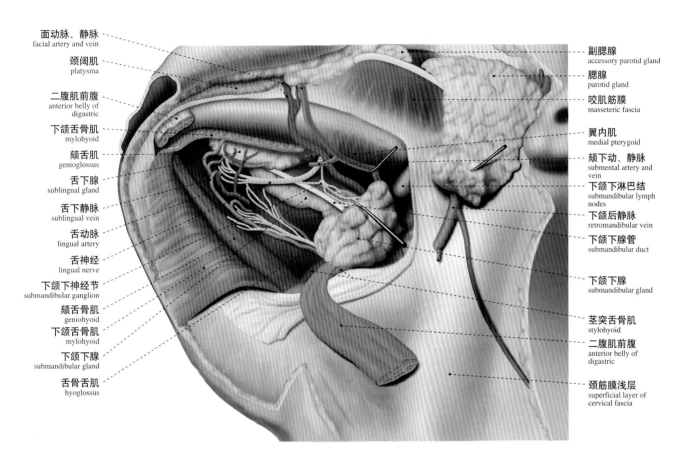

面动脉、静脉
facial artery and vein

颈阔肌
platysma

二腹肌前腹
anterior belly of digastric

下颌舌骨肌
mylohyoid

颏舌肌
genioglossus

舌下腺
sublingual gland

舌下静脉
sublingual vein

舌动脉
lingual artery

舌神经
lingual nerve

下颌下神经节
submandibular ganglion

颏舌骨肌
geniohyoid

下颌舌骨肌
mylohyoid

下颌下腺
submandibular gland

舌骨舌肌
hyoglossus

副腮腺
accessory parotid gland

腮腺
parotid gland

咬肌筋膜
masseteric fascia

翼内肌
medial pterygoid

颏下动、静脉
submental artery and vein

下颌下淋巴结
submandibular lymph nodes

下颌后静脉
retromandibular vein

下颌下腺管
submandibular duct

下颌下腺
submandibular gland

茎突舌骨肌
stylohyoid

二腹肌前腹
anterior belly of digastric

颈筋膜浅层
superficial layer of cervical fascia

510. 口腔腺（下外侧面观）
Oral glands (inferolateral aspect)

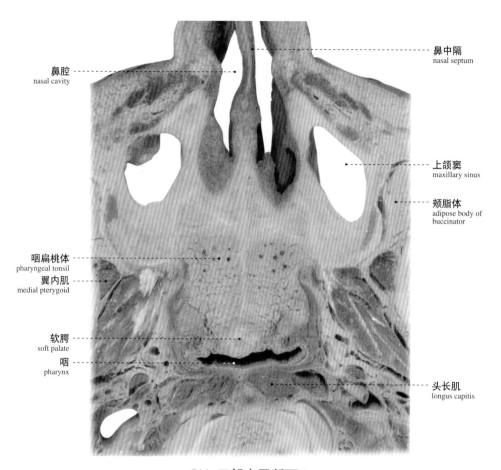

鼻腔
nasal cavity

鼻中隔
nasal septum

上颌窦
maxillary sinus

颊脂体
adipose body of buccinator

咽扁桃体
pharyngeal tonsil

翼内肌
medial pterygoid

软腭
soft palate

咽
pharynx

头长肌
longus capitis

511. 口部水平断面 1
Horizontal section of the mouth 1

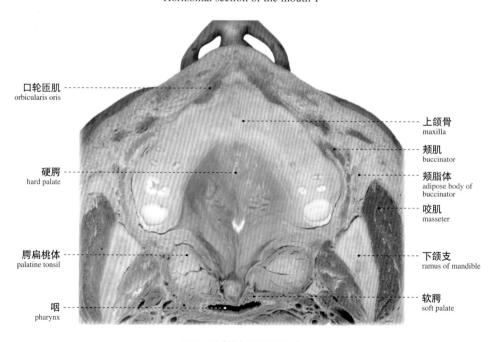

口轮匝肌
orbicularis oris

上颌骨
maxilla

颊肌
buccinator

颊脂体
adipose body of buccinator

硬腭
hard palate

咬肌
masseter

腭扁桃体
palatine tonsil

下颌支
ramus of mandible

咽
pharynx

软腭
soft palate

512. 口部水平断面 2
Horizontal section of the mouth 2

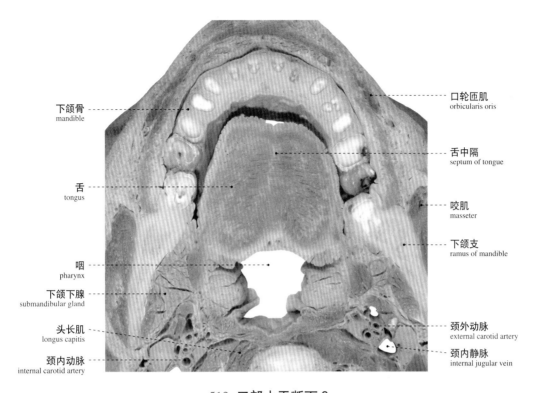

口轮匝肌
orbicularis oris

舌中隔
septum of tongue

咬肌
masseter

下颌支
ramus of mandible

颈外动脉
external carotid artery

颈内静脉
internal jugular vein

下颌骨
mandible

舌
tongus

咽
pharynx

下颌下腺
submandibular gland

头长肌
longus capitis

颈内动脉
internal carotid artery

513. 口部水平断面 3
Horizontal section of the mouth 3

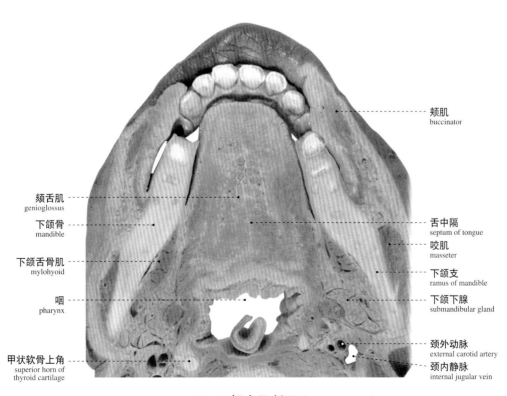

颊肌
buccinator

舌中隔
septum of tongue

咬肌
masseter

下颌支
ramus of mandible

下颌下腺
submandibular gland

颈外动脉
external carotid artery

颈内静脉
internal jugular vein

颏舌肌
genioglossus

下颌骨
mandible

下颌舌骨肌
mylohyoid

咽
pharynx

甲状软骨上角
superior horn of
thyroid cartilage

514. 口部水平断面 4
Horizontal section of the mouth 4

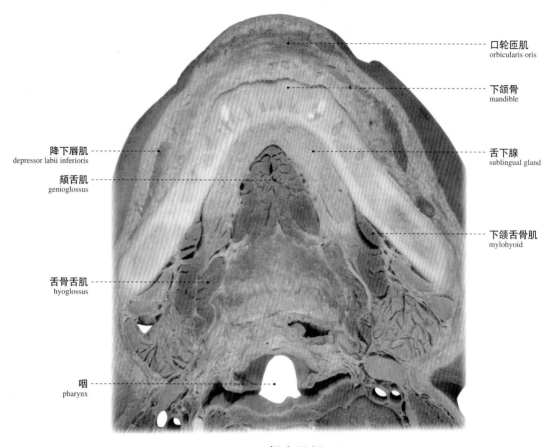

口轮匝肌
orbicularis oris

下颌骨
mandible

降下唇肌
depressor labii inferioris

舌下腺
sublingual gland

颏舌肌
genioglossus

下颌舌骨肌
mylohyoid

舌骨舌肌
hyoglossus

咽
pharynx

515. 口部水平断面 5

Horizontal section of the mouth 5

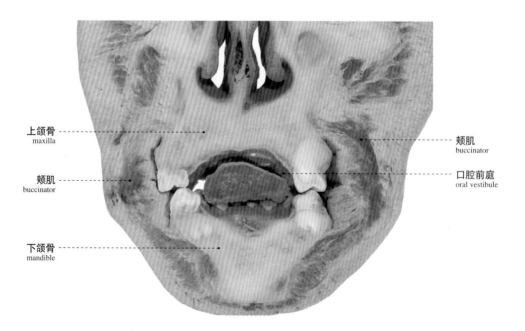

上颌骨
maxilla

颊肌
buccinator

颊肌
buccinator

口腔前庭
oral vestibule

下颌骨
mandible

516. 口部冠状断面 1

Coronal section of the mouth 1

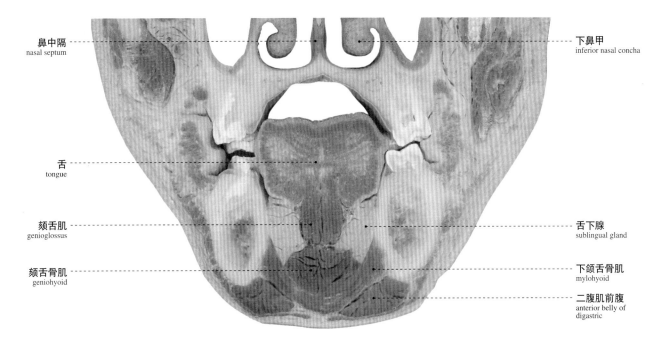

鼻中隔
nasal septum

舌
tongue

颏舌肌
genioglossus

颏舌骨肌
geniohyoid

下鼻甲
inferior nasal concha

舌下腺
sublingual gland

下颌舌骨肌
mylohyoid

二腹肌前腹
anterior belly of digastric

517. 口部冠状断面 2
Coronal section of the mouth 2

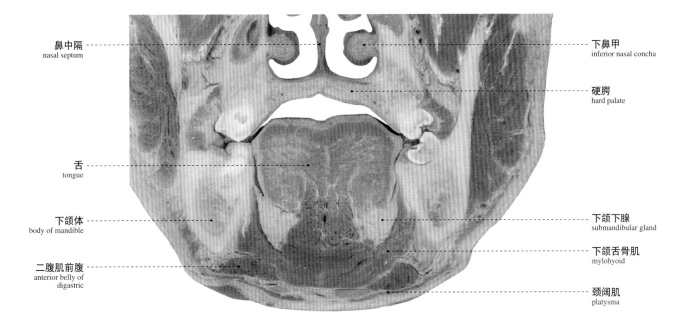

鼻中隔
nasal septum

舌
tongue

下颌体
body of mandible

二腹肌前腹
anterior belly of digastric

下鼻甲
inferior nasal concha

硬腭
hard palate

下颌下腺
submandibular gland

下颌舌骨肌
mylohyoid

颈阔肌
platysma

518. 口部冠状断面 3
Coronal section of the mouth 3

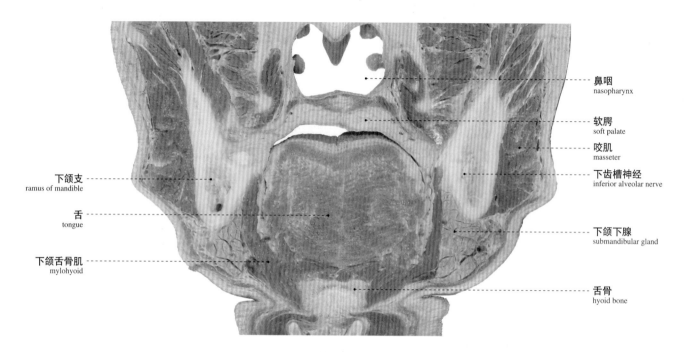

鼻咽
nasopharynx

软腭
soft palate

咬肌
masseter

下颌支
ramus of mandible

下齿槽神经
inferior alveolar nerve

舌
tongue

下颌下腺
submandibular gland

下颌舌骨肌
mylohyoid

舌骨
hyoid bone

519. 口部冠状断面 4
Coronal section of the mouth 4

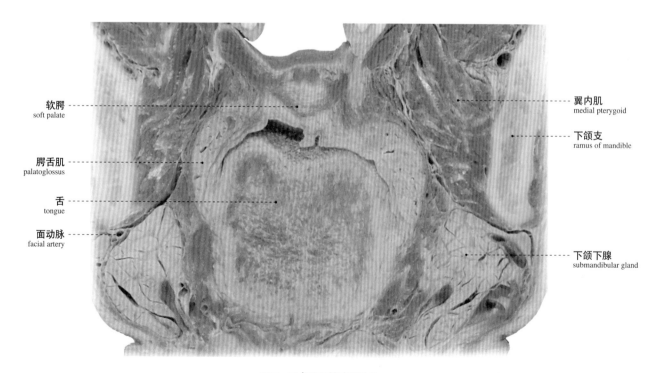

软腭
soft palate

翼内肌
medial pterygoid

下颌支
ramus of mandible

腭舌肌
palatoglossus

舌
tongue

面动脉
facial artery

下颌下腺
submandibular gland

520. 口部冠状断面 5
Coronal section of the mouth 5

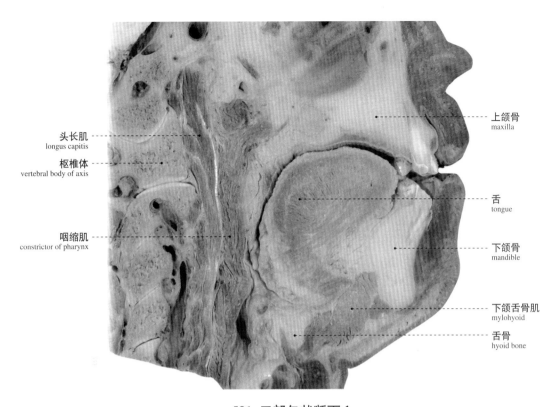

头长肌
longus capitis

枢椎体
vertebral body of axis

咽缩肌
constrictor of pharynx

上颌骨
maxilla

舌
tongue

下颌骨
mandible

下颌舌骨肌
mylohyoid

舌骨
hyoid bone

521. 口部矢状断面 1

Sagittal section of the mouth 1

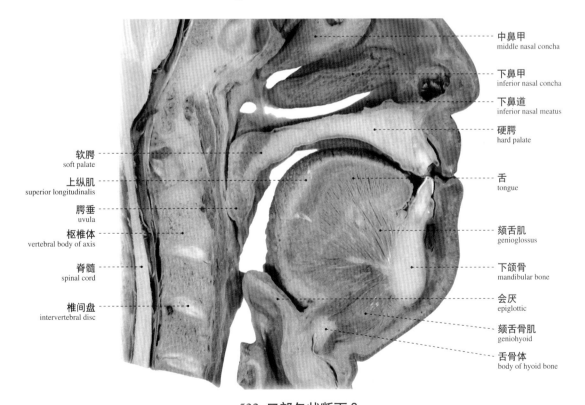

软腭
soft palate

上纵肌
superior longitudinalis

腭垂
uvula

枢椎体
vertebral body of axis

脊髓
spinal cord

椎间盘
intervertebral disc

中鼻甲
middle nasal concha

下鼻甲
inferior nasal concha

下鼻道
inferior nasal meatus

硬腭
hard palate

舌
tongue

颏舌肌
genioglossus

下颌骨
mandibular bone

会厌
epiglottic

颏舌骨肌
geniohyoid

舌骨体
body of hyoid bone

522. 口部矢状断面 2

Sagittal section of the mouth 2

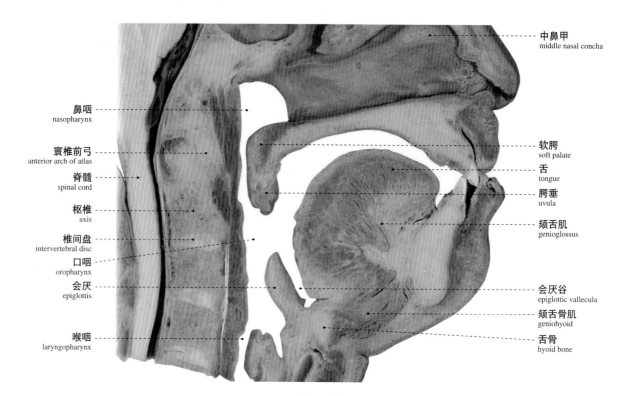

中鼻甲
middle nasal concha

鼻咽
nasopharynx

寰椎前弓
anterior arch of atlas

脊髓
spinal cord

枢椎
axis

椎间盘
intervertebral disc

口咽
oropharynx

会厌
epiglottis

喉咽
laryngopharynx

软腭
soft palate

舌
tongue

腭垂
uvula

颏舌肌
genioglossus

会厌谷
epiglottic vallecula

颏舌骨肌
geniohyoid

舌骨
hyoid bone

523. 口部矢状断面 3
Sagittal section of the mouth 3

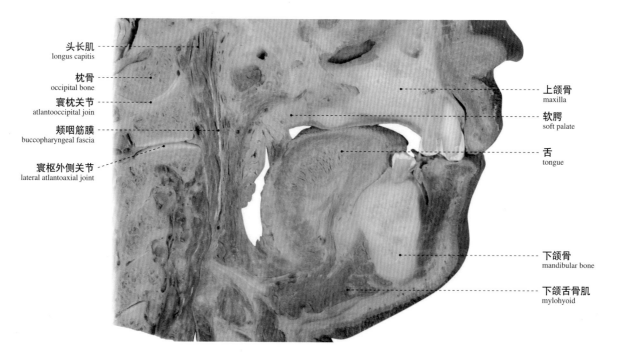

头长肌
longus capitis

枕骨
occipital bone

寰枕关节
atlantooccipital join

颊咽筋膜
buccopharyngeal fascia

寰枢外侧关节
lateral atlantoaxial joint

上颌骨
maxilla

软腭
soft palate

舌
tongue

下颌骨
mandibular bone

下颌舌骨肌
mylohyoid

524. 口部矢状断面 4
Sagittal section of the mouth 4

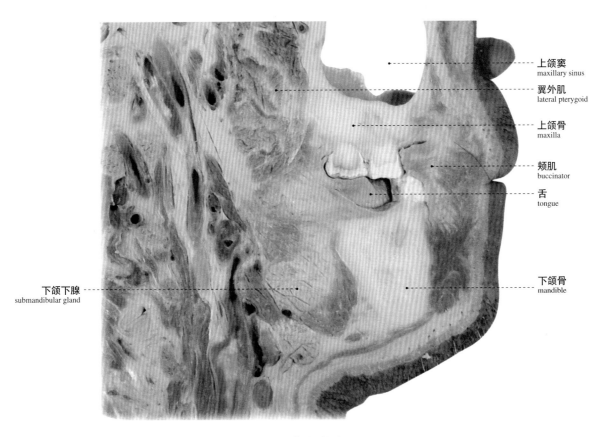

上颌窦
maxillary sinus

翼外肌
lateral pterygoid

上颌骨
maxilla

颊肌
buccinator

舌
tongue

下颌骨
mandible

下颌下腺
submandibular gland

525. 口部矢状断面 5
Sagittal section of the mouth 5

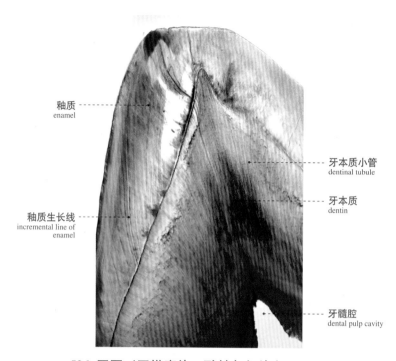

釉质
enamel

牙本质小管
dentinal tubule

牙本质
dentin

釉质生长线
incremental line of
enamel

牙髓腔
dental pulp cavity

526. 牙冠（牙纵磨片，酸性复红染色，×40）
Crown of tooth (longitudinal ground section of tooth, acid fuchsin staining, ×40)

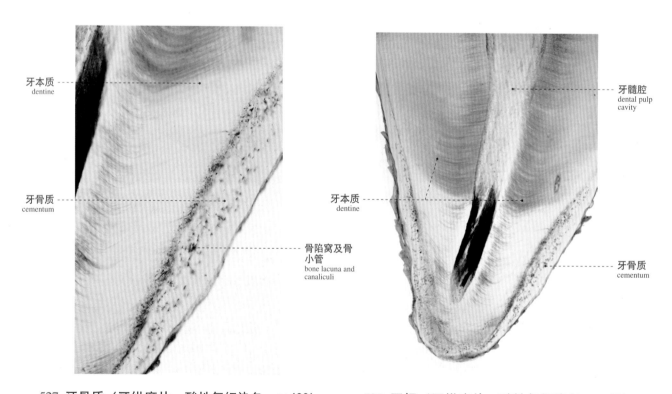

牙本质
dentine

牙骨质
cementum

骨陷窝及骨
小管
bone lacuna and
canaliculi

牙髓腔
dental pulp
cavity

牙本质
dentine

牙骨质
cementum

527. 牙骨质（牙纵磨片，酸性复红染色，×400）
Cementum (longitudinal ground section of tooth, acid fuchsin
staining, ×400)

528. 牙根（牙纵磨片，酸性复红染色，×40）
Root of tooth (longitudinal ground section of tooth, acid fuchsin
staining, ×40)

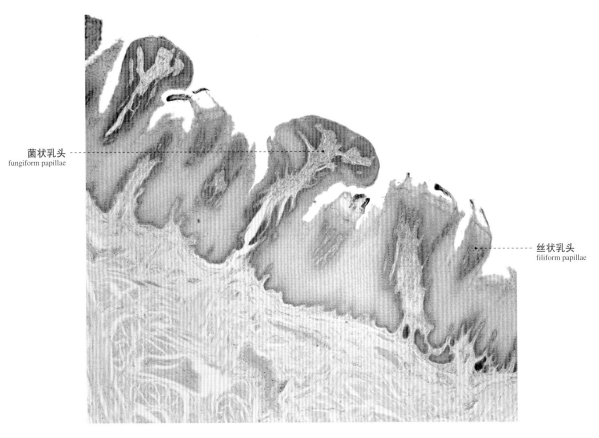

菌状乳头
fungiform papillae

丝状乳头
filiform papillae

529. 菌状乳头和丝状乳头（人舌，HE 染色，×40）
Fungiform papillae and filiform papillae (human tongue, HE staining, ×40)

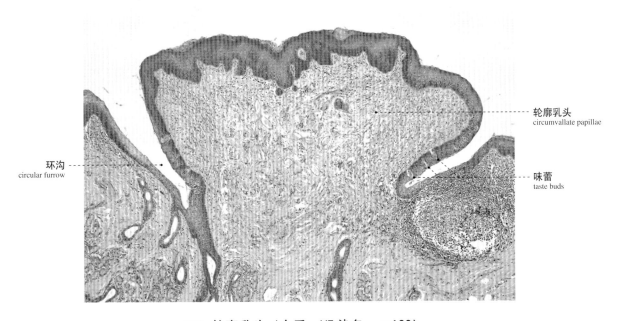

环沟
circular furrow

轮廓乳头
circumvallate papillae

味蕾
taste buds

530. 轮廓乳头（人舌，HE 染色，×100）
Circumvallate papillae (human tongue, HE staining, ×100)

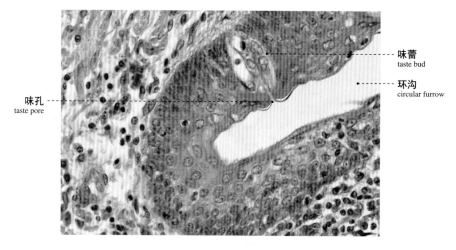

味蕾
taste bud

环沟
circular furrow

味孔
taste pore

531. 味蕾（人舌，HE 染色，×400）
Taste bud (human tongue, HE staining, ×400)

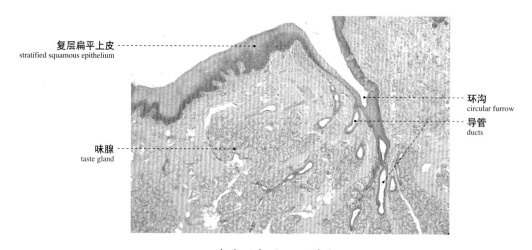

复层扁平上皮
stratified squamous epithelium

环沟
circular furrow

导管
ducts

味腺
taste gland

532. 味腺（人舌，HE 染色，×100）
Taste gland (human tongue, HE staining, ×100)

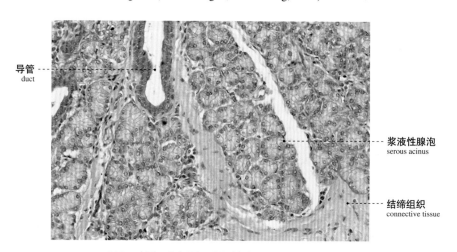

导管
duct

浆液性腺泡
serous acinus

结缔组织
connective tissue

533. 味腺（人舌，HE 染色，×400）
Taste gland (human tongue, HE staining, ×400)

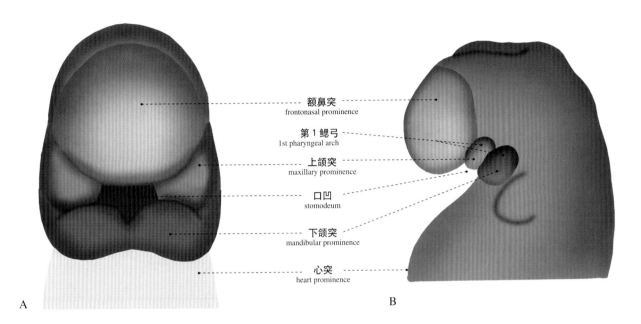

额鼻突
frontonasal prominence

第 1 鳃弓
1st pharyngeal arch

上颌突
maxillary prominence

口凹
stomodeum

下颌突
mandibular prominence

心突
heart prominence

A

B

534. 人颜面的发生（24±1 天）
Development of the human face (24±1 days)

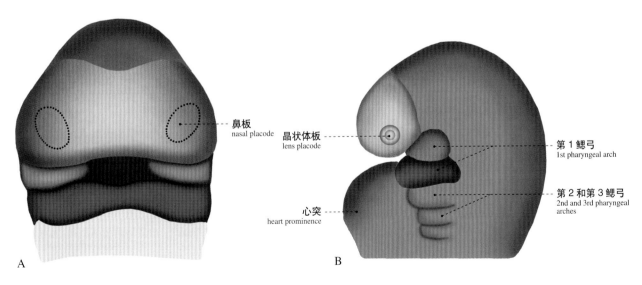

鼻板
nasal placode

晶状体板
lens placode

第 1 鳃弓
1st pharyngeal arch

第 2 和第 3 鳃弓
2nd and 3rd pharyngeal arches

心突
heart prominence

A

B

535. 人颜面的发生（28±1 天）
Development of the human face (28±1 days)

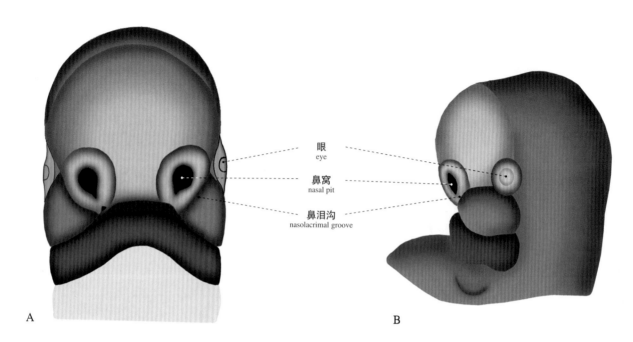

眼
eye

鼻窝
nasal pit

鼻泪沟
nasolacrimal groove

A   B

536. 人颜面的发生（31±1 天）
Development of the human face (31±1 days)

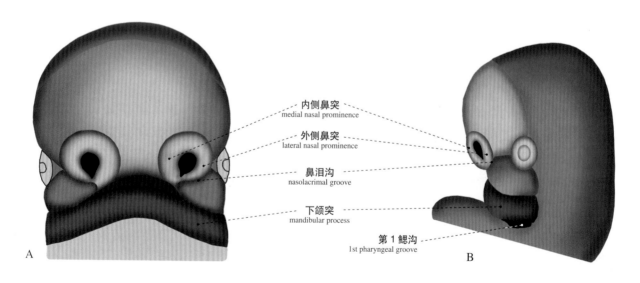

内侧鼻突
medial nasal prominence

外侧鼻突
lateral nasal prominence

鼻泪沟
nasolacrimal groove

下颌突
mandibular process

第 1 鳃沟
1st pharyngeal groove

A   B

537. 人颜面的发生（33±1 天）
Development of the human face (33±1 days)

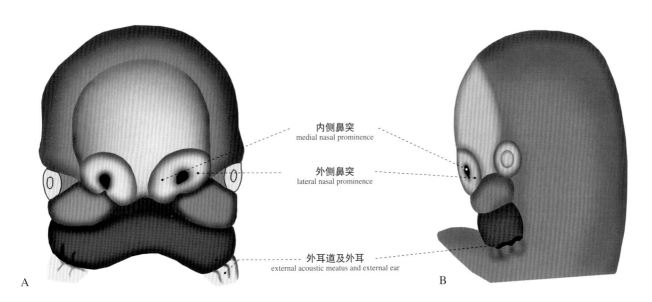

内侧鼻突
medial nasal prominence

外侧鼻突
lateral nasal prominence

外耳道及外耳
external acoustic meatus and external ear

A
B

538. 人颜面的发生（35±1 天）
Development of the human face (35±1 days)

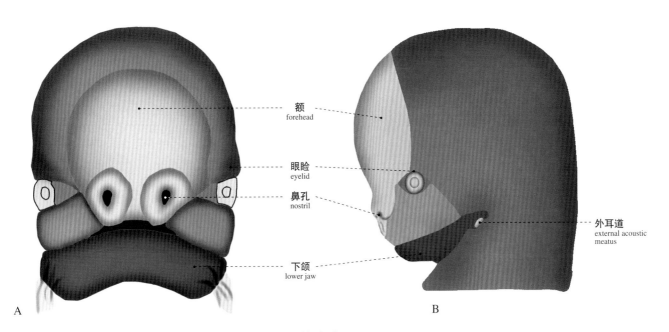

额
forehead

眼睑
eyelid

鼻孔
nostril

下颌
lower jaw

外耳道
external acoustic
meatus

A
B

539. 人颜面的发生（40±1 天）
Development of the human face (40±1 days)

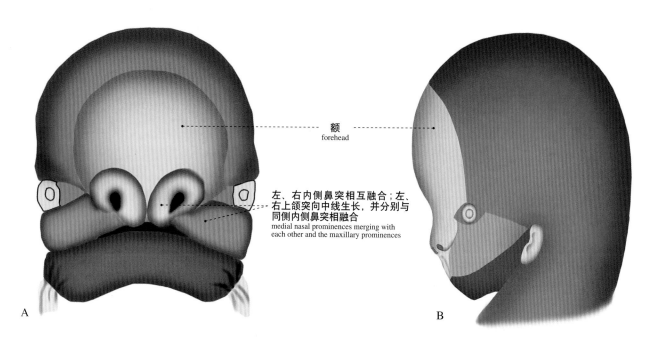

额
forehead

左、右内侧鼻突相互融合；左、右上颌突向中线生长，并分别与同侧内侧鼻突相互融合
medial nasal prominences merging with each other and the maxillary prominences

A

B

540. 人颜面的发生（48±1 天）
Development of the human face (48±1 days)

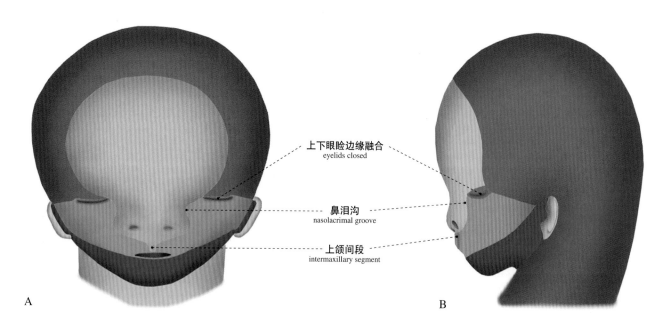

上下眼睑边缘融合
eyelids closed

鼻泪沟
nasolacrimal groove

上颌间段
intermaxillary segment

A

B

541. 人颜面的发生（10 周 ±1 天）
Development of the human face (10 weeks±1 days)

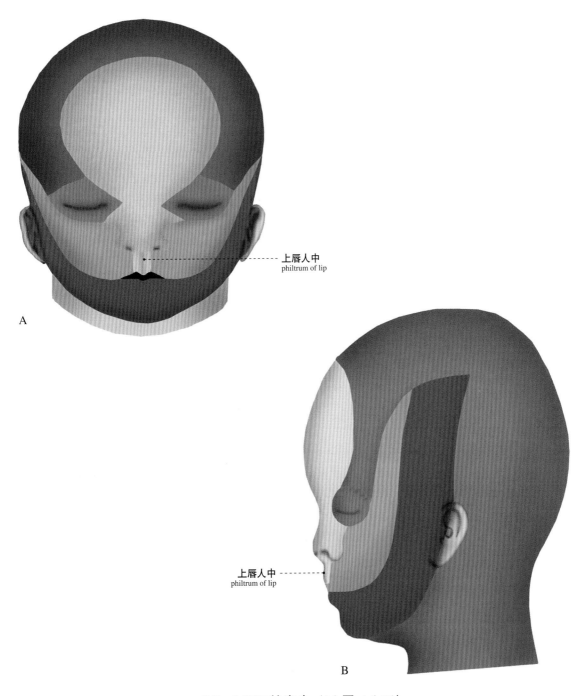

上唇人中
philtrum of lip

A

上唇人中
philtrum of lip

B

542. 人颜面的发生（14 周 ±1 天）
Development of the human face (14 weeks±1 days)

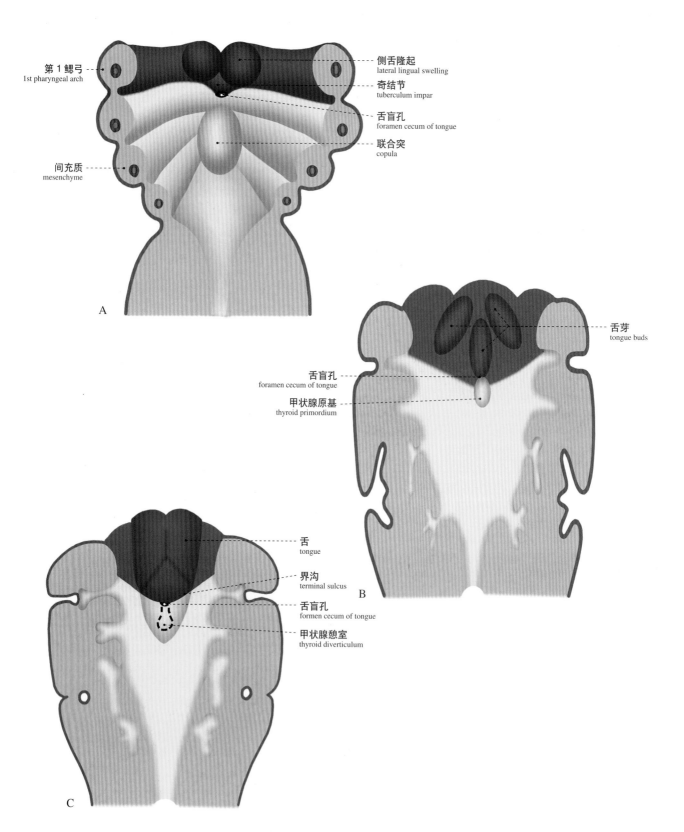

第 1 鳃弓
1st pharyngeal arch

间充质
mesenchyme

侧舌隆起
lateral lingual swelling

奇结节
tuberculum impar

舌盲孔
foramen cecum of tongue

联合突
copula

A

舌芽
tongue buds

舌盲孔
foramen cecum of tongue

甲状腺原基
thyroid primordium

B

舌
tongue

界沟
terminal sulcus

舌盲孔
formen cecum of tongue

甲状腺憩室
thyroid diverticulum

C

543. 舌的发生
Development of the tongue

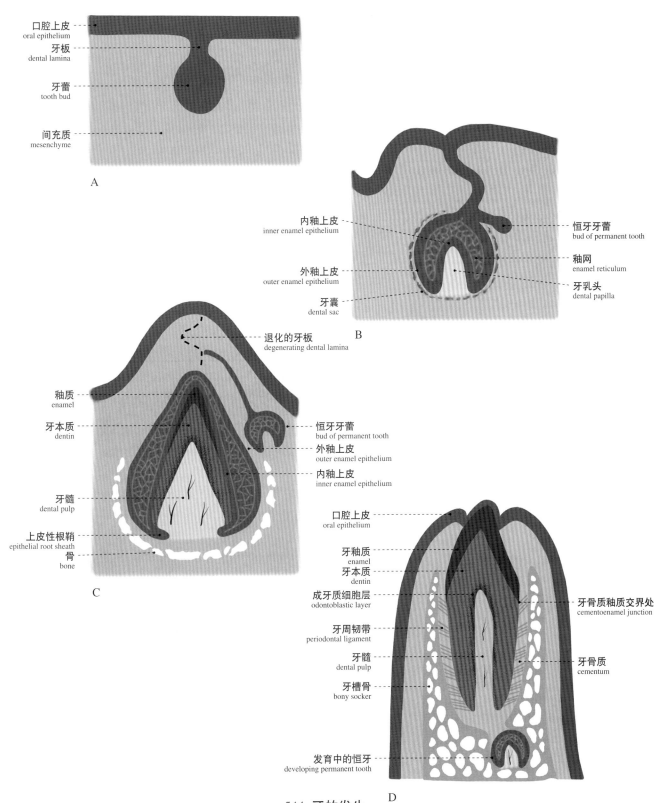

口腔上皮
oral epithelium

牙板
dental lamina

牙蕾
tooth bud

间充质
mesenchyme

A

内釉上皮
inner enamel epithelium

外釉上皮
outer enamel epithelium

牙囊
dental sac

恒牙牙蕾
bud of permanent tooth

釉网
enamel reticulum

牙乳头
dental papilla

B

退化的牙板
degenerating dental lamina

釉质
enamel

牙本质
dentin

牙髓
dental pulp

上皮性根鞘
epithelial root sheath

骨
bone

恒牙牙蕾
bud of permanent tooth

外釉上皮
outer enamel epithelium

内釉上皮
inner enamel epithelium

C

口腔上皮
oral epithelium

牙釉质
enamel

牙本质
dentin

成牙质细胞层
odontoblastic layer

牙周韧带
periodontal ligament

牙髓
dental pulp

牙槽骨
bony socker

发育中的恒牙
developing permanent tooth

牙骨质釉质交界处
cementoenamel junction

牙骨质
cementum

D

544. 牙的发生

Development of the teeth

A. 7 周；B. 10 周；C. 28 周；D. 出生后 6 个月

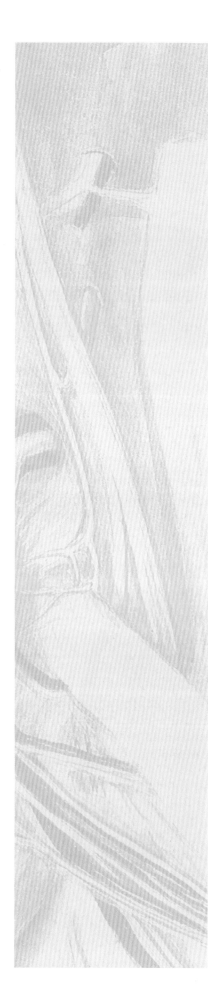

参考书目

[1] Schuenke M, Schulte E, Schumacher U. THIEME Atlas of Anatomy, Neck and Internal Organs. Thieme Stuttgart.

[2] Schuenke M, Schulte E, Schumacher U. THIEME Atlas of Anatomy, General Anatomy and Musculoskeletal System. Thieme Stuttgart.

[3] Schuenke M, Schulte E, Schumacher U. THIEME Atlas of Anatomy, Head and Neuroanatomy. Thieme Stuttgart.

[4] Putz R, Sobotta PR. Atlas der Anatomie des Menschen. Band 2, 21st edition. Elsevier, Pte Ltd.

[5] Standring S. GRAY'S Anatomy Susan Standring. Churchill Livingstone Elsevier.

[6] Netter FH. Atlas of Human Anatomy. SAUNDERS Elsevier.

[7] Bontrager KL, Lampignano JP. 王继琛译 . 放射技术与相关解剖 . 北京大学医学出版社 .

[8] Moore KL, Persaud TVN. The Developing Human. Saunders Elsevier.

[9] David W，Stoller MR. 廉宗澂译 . 关节镜和外科解剖图片集 . 天津科技翻译出版公司 .

[10] Agur AMR. Grant's Atlas of Anatomy. Lippincott Williams & Wilkins Inc.

[11] Stoller DW. MRI, Arthroscopy, and Surgical Anatomy of the Joints. Lippincott Williams & Wilkins Inc.

[12] 高士濂 . 实用解剖图谱，上肢分册 . 上海科学技术出版社 .

[13] 高士濂 . 实用解剖图谱，下肢分册 . 上海科学技术出版社 .

[14] 托尼·史密斯 . 左焕琛译 . 人体 . 上海科学技术出版社 .

[15] Agur AMR, Dalley AF. 左焕琛译 . Grant 解剖学图谱 . 上海科学技术出版社 .

[16] 金征宇 . 超高场 MR 全身应用图谱 . 中国协和医科大学出版社 .

[17] 张朝佑 . 人体解剖学 . 人民卫生出版社 .

[18] 郭光文，王序 . 人体解剖彩色图谱 . 人民卫生出版社 .

[19] 柏树令，段坤昌，陈金宝 . 人体解剖学彩色图谱 . 上海科学技术出版社 .

[20] 石玉秀，邓纯忠，孙桂媛，等 . 组织学与胚胎学彩色图谱 . 上海科学技术出版社 .

[21] 段坤昌，王振宇，李庆生 . 颅脑颈部应用解剖学彩色图谱 . 辽宁科学技术出版社 .

[22] 金连弘 . 人体断面解剖学彩色图谱 . 人民卫生出版社 .

[23] 姜树学，马述盛 . 断面解剖与 MRI、CT、ECT 对照图谱 . 辽宁科学技术出版社 .

[24] 梁长虹，赵振军 . 多层螺旋 CT 血管成像 . 人民军医出版社 .

[25] 徐达传 . 骨科临床解剖学图谱 . 山东科学技术出版社 .

[26] 姜宗来 . 胸心外科临床解剖学图谱 . 山东科学技术出版社 .

[27] 张正治 . 口腔颌面外科临床解剖学图谱 . 山东科学技术出版社 .

[28] 于春江，贾旺，张绍祥 . 神经外科临床解剖学图谱 . 山东科学技术出版社 .

[29] 孔祥玉，韩德民 . 眼耳鼻咽喉科临床解剖学图谱 . 山东科学技术出版社 .

[30] 刘树伟，柳澄，胡三元 . 腹部外科临床解剖学图谱 . 山东科学技术出版社 .

[31] 原林，王兴海 . 妇产外科临床解剖学图谱 . 山东科学技术出版社 .

[32] 丁自海，李忠华，苏泽轩 . 泌尿外科临床解剖学图谱 . 山东科学技术出版社 .

[33] 汪忠镐，舒畅 . 血管外科临床解剖学图谱 . 山东科学技术出版社 .

[34] 单鸿，姜在波，马壮 . 临床血管解剖学 . 世界图书出版公司 .

[35] 梁常虹，赵振军 . 多层螺旋 CT 血管成像 . 人民军医出版社 .

[36] 倪磊 . 膝关节镜彩色图谱 . 科学出版社 .

对提供参考书目的作者和出版社，在此一并表示衷心的感谢。